Lecture Notes in Computational Vision and Biomechanics

Editors

João Manuel R.S. Tavares
R.M. Natal Jorge

Address:
Departamento de Engenharia Mecânica
Faculdade de Engenharia
Universidade do Porto
Rua Dr. Roberto Frias s/n
4200-465 Porto
Portugal
{tavares, rnatal}@fe.up.pt

Editorial Advisory Board

For further volumes:
http://www.springer.com/series/8910

Lecture Notes in Computational Vision and Biomechanics
Volume 1

This book is the first to be published under the Book Series "Lecture Notes in Computational Vision and Biomechanics (LNCV&B)".

The research related to the analysis of living structures (Biomechanics) has been a source of recent research in several distinct areas of science, for example, Mathematics, Mechanical Engineering, Physics, Informatics, Medicine and Sport. However, for its successful achievement, numerous research topics should be considered, such as image processing and analysis, geometric and numerical modelling, biomechanics, experimental analysis, mechanobiology and enhanced visualization, and their application to real cases must be developed and more investigation is needed. Additionally, enhanced hardware solutions and less invasive devices are demanded.

On the other hand, Image Analysis (Computational Vision) is used for the extraction of high level information from static images or dynamic image sequences. Examples of applications involving image analysis can be the study of motion of structures from image sequences, shape reconstruction from images and medical diagnosis. As a multidisciplinary area, Computational Vision considers techniques and methods from other disciplines, such as Artificial Intelligence, Signal Processing, Mathematics, Physics and Informatics. Despite the many research projects in this area, more robust and efficient methods of Computational Imaging are still demanded in many application domains in Medicine, and their validation in real scenarios is matter of urgency.

These two important and predominant branches of Science are increasingly considered to be strongly connected and related. Hence, the main goal of the LNCV&B book series consists of the provision of a comprehensive forum for discussion on the current state-of-the-art in these fields by emphasizing their connection. The book series covers (but is not limited to):

- Applications of Computational Vision and Biomechanics
- Biometrics and Biomedical Pattern Analysis
- Cellular Imaging and Cellular Mechanics
- Clinical Biomechanics
- Computational Bioimaging and Visualization
- Computational Biology in Biomedical Imaging
- Development of Biomechanical Devices
- Device and Technique Development for Biomedical Imaging
- Digital Geometry Algorithms for Computational Vision and Visualization
- Experimental Biomechanics
- Gait & Posture Mechanics
- Grid and High Performance Computing for Computational Vision and Biomechanics
- Image-based Geometric Modeling and Mesh Generation
- Image Processing and Analysis
- Image Processing and Visualization in Biofluids
- Image Understanding
- Material Models
- Mechanobiology
- Medical Image Analysis
- Molecular Mechanics
- Multi-Modal Image Systems
- Multiscale Analysis in Biomechanics
- Multiscale Biosensors in Biomedical Imaging
- Multiscale Devices and Biomems for Biomedical Imaging
- Musculoskeletal Biomechanics
- Neuromuscular Biomechanics
- Numerical Methods for Living Tissues
- Numerical Simulation
- Software Development on Computational Vision and Biomechanics
- Sport Biomechanics
- Virtual Reality in Biomechanics
- Vision Systems

Renato M. Natal Jorge • João Manuel R.S. Tavares
Marcos Pinotti Barbosa • A.P. Slade
Editors

Technologies for Medical Sciences

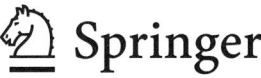 Springer

Editors
Renato M. Natal Jorge
Departamento de Engenharia Mecânica
Faculdade de Engenharia
Universidade do Porto
Rua Dr Roberto Frias s/n
4200-465 Porto
Portugal

João Manuel R.S. Tavares
Departamento de Engenharia Mecânica
Faculdade de Engenharia
Universidade do Porto
Rua Dr Roberto Frias s/n
4200-465 Porto
Portugal

Marcos Pinotti Barbosa
Departamento de Engenharia Mecanica
Laboratorio de Bioengenharia
Universidade Federal de Minas Gerais
Av. Antonio Carlos 6627
Belo Horizonte Minas Gerais
Brazil

A.P. Slade
College of Art, Science and Engineering
Medical Engineering Research Institute
University of Dundee
United Kingdom

ISSN 2212-9391   ISSN 2212-9413 (electronic)
ISBN 978-94-007-4067-9   ISBN 978-94-007-4068-6 (eBook)
DOI 10.1007/978-94-007-4068-6
Springer Dordrecht Heidelberg New York London

Library of Congress Control Number: 2012936068

Printed on acid-free paper

Springer is part of Springer Science+Business Media (www.springer.com)

Preface

This book presents novel and advanced Technologies for Medical Sciences in order to solidify knowledge in the related fields and define their key stakeholders.

The 15 chapters included in this book were written by invited experts of international recognition and address important Technologies for Medical Sciences, including: Computational Modeling and Simulation, Image Processing and Analysis, Medical Imaging, Human Motion and Posture, Tissue Engineering, Design and Development Medical Devices, and Mechanic Biology.

Different applications are addressed and described along the book, comprising: Biomechanical Studies, Prosthesis and Orthosis, Medical Diagnosis, Sport, and Virtual Reality.

Therefore, this book is of crucial effectiveness for Researchers, Students and Manufacturers from several multidisciplinary fields, as the ones related with Bioengineering, Biomechanics, Computational Mechanics, Computational Vision, Human Motion, Mathematics, Medical Devices, Medical Image, Medicine and Physics.

The Editors would like to take this opportunity to thank to all invited authors for sharing their works, experiences and knowledge, making possible their dissemination through this book.

Renato M. Natal Jorge
João Manuel R.S. Tavares
Marcos Pinotti Barbosa
A.P. Slade

Contents

**In-Silico Models as a Tool for the Design of Specific
Treatments: Applications in Bone Regeneration** 1
Esther Reina-Romo, María José Gómez-Benito,
Libardo Andrés González-Torres, Jaime Domínguez,
and José Manuel García-Aznar

Contact Finite Element with Surface Tension Adhesion 19
Rudolf A.P. Hellmuth and Raul G. Lima

**Biomechanical Characterization
and Modeling of Natural and Alloplastic Human
Temporomandibular Joint** 39
Michel Mesnard and Antonio Ramos

Blood Flow Simulation and Applications 67
Luisa Costa Sousa, Catarina F. Castro,
and Carlos Conceição António

**Measuring Biomechanics of the Vision Process, Sensory Fusion
and Image Observation Features** 87
Jaroslav Dušek and Tomáš Jindra

Motion Correction in Conventional Nuclear Medicine Imaging 113
Francisco J. Caramelo and Nuno C. Ferreira

OCT Noise Despeckling Using 3D Nonlinear Complex Diffusion Filter ... 141
C. Maduro, P. Serranho, T. Santos, P. Rodrigues, J. Cunha-Vaz,
and R. Bernardes

**Using an Infra-red Sensor to Measure the Dynamic Behaviour
of N$_2$O Gas Escaping Through Different Sized Holes**...................... 159
Alan Slade, Jan Vorstius, Daniel Gonçalves, and Gareth Thomson

**Plantar Pressure Assessment: A New Tool for Postural
Instability Diagnosis in Multiple Sclerosis** 179
João M.C.S. Abrantes and Luis F.F. Santos

Recent Progress in Studying the Human Foot 205
V.C. Pinto, M.A. Marques, and M.A.P. Vaz

**The Scapular Contribution to the Amplitude of Shoulder
External Rotation on Throwing Athletes** 227
Andrea Ribeiro, Augusto Gil Pascoal, and Nuno Morais

**Supercritical Solvent Impregnation of Natural Bioactive
Compounds in *N*-Carboxybutylchitosan and Agarose
Membranes for the Development of Topical Wound
Healing Applications**... 243
A.M.A. Dias, M.E.M. Braga, I.J. Seabra, and H.C. de Sousa

Improving Post-EVAR Surveillance with a Smart Stent-Graft 267
. Isa C.T. Santos, Alexandra T. Sepulveda, Júlio C. Viana,
António J. Pontes, Brian L. Wardle, S.M. Sampaio,
R. Roncon-Albuquerque, João Manuel R.S. Tavares,
and L.A. Rocha

**Synergic Multidisciplinary Interactions for Design
and Development of Medical Devices** 291
Ricardo Simoes

**A Process-Algebra Model of the Cell Mechanics of Autoreactive
Lymphocytes Recruitment** 311
Paola Lecca

Editors Biography

Renato M. Natal Jorge (rnatal@fe.up.pt)
IDMEC – Pole FEUP, Faculty
of Engineering, University of Porto
Rua Dr. Roberto Frias
4200–465 Porto
Portugal

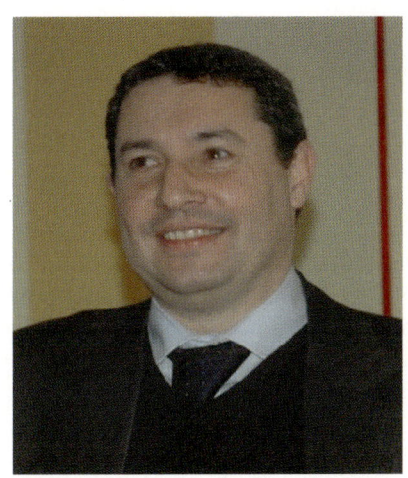

Associate Professor at the Faculty of Engineering, University of Porto (FEUP); Mechanical Engineer from the University of Porto, 1987; MSc from the University of Porto, 1991; Ph.D. from the University of Porto, 1999.

Present teaching and research interests: Computational methods in applied mechanics and engineering; New product development; Biomechanics and mechanobiology; Computational vision and medical image processing.

Between 2007 and 2011 was the Director of the "Structural Integrity Unit" research group of the Institute of Mechanical Engineering at FEUP (IDMEC – a R & D non-profit, private Research Institute). Member of the executive board of IDMEC-FEUP.

Responsible for the Supervision or Co-supervision of 12 Ph.D. students.

Co-chair of the following conferences: CompIMAGE; 14th International Product Development Management; VIPIMAGE; Fourteenth Annual Scientific Conference on WEB Technology, New Media, Communications and Telematics Theory, Methods, Tools and Applications; VIPIMAGE 2009; CompIMAGE 2010; Biodental;

iDEMi'09; Sixth International Conference on Technology and Medical Sciences, CIBEM 2011, among other mini-symposia within conferences.

Founder and Editor of the International Journal for Computational Vision and Biomechanics. Guest editor of several scientific journals.

Principal Investigator for several national and European scientific projects.

Co-author of more than 80 papers in international journals and more than 250 publications in international conferences.

João Manuel R.S. Tavares
Faculdade de Engenharia da Universidade
do Porto (FEUP)
Rua Dr. Roberto Frias, s/n
4200–465 Porto
Portugal
e-mail: tavares@fe.up.pt
url: www.fe.up.pt/tavares

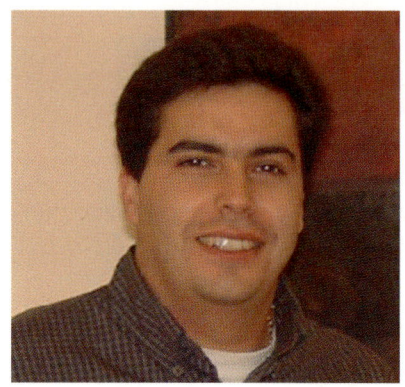

João Manuel R.S. Tavares graduated in Mechanical Engineering from the University of Porto – Portugal (1992); MSc in Electronic and Computer Engineering, in the field of Industrial Informatics, University of Porto (1995); Ph.D. in Electrical and Computer, University of Porto (2001). From 1995 to 2000 he was a researcher at the Institute of Biomedical Engineering (INEB).

Since 2001 he has been senior researcher and project coordinator at the Laboratory of Optical and Experimental Mechanics (LOME) at the Institute of Mechanical Engineering and Industrial Management (INEGI). Also, since 2001, he has been Assistant Professor at the Department of Mechanical Engineering (DEMec) of the Engineering Faculty of the University of Porto (FEUP).

He is co-author of more than 350 scientific papers in national and international journals and conferences and co-editor of 17 international books and guest-editor of several special issues of international journals. In addition, he is Co-Editor-in-Chief of the International Journal for Computational Vision and Biomechanics (IJCV&B) and of the International Journal of Imaging and Robotics (IJIR); Editor-in-Chief of the International Journal of Biometrics and Bioinformatics (IJBB); Associate Editor of the EURASIP Journal on Advances in Signal Processing (JASP), ISRN Machine Vision, and of the Journal of Computer Science (INFOCOMP) and reviewer of several international scientific journals.

Since 2001, he has been Supervisor and Co-Supervisor of several MSc and Ph.D. thesis and involved in several research projects, both as researcher and as scientific coordinator. Additionally, he is co-author of three international patents.

He has been Co-Chairman of various international conferences, such as: CompIMAGE 2006/2010/2012, VipIMAGE 2007/2009/2011, CIBEM 2011, BioDENTAL 2009/2012, TMSi 2010, IMAGAPP 2009 and EUROMEDIA 2008; and of numerous mini-symposia, workshops and thematic sessions. In addition, he has been a member of scientific and organizing committees of several national and international conferences.

His main research areas include Computational Vision, Computational Mechanics, Scientific Visualization, Human-Computer Interaction and New Product Development.

Marcos Pinotti Barbosa
Bioengineering Laboratory – Department
of Mechanical Engineering
Universidade Federal de Minas Gerais
Av. Antonio Carlos, 6627
Zip code: 31270–901
Belo Horizonte – MG
Brazil
e-mail: pinotti@ufmg.br
lapan.pinotti@gmail.com
url: www.demec.ufmg.br/grupos/labbio

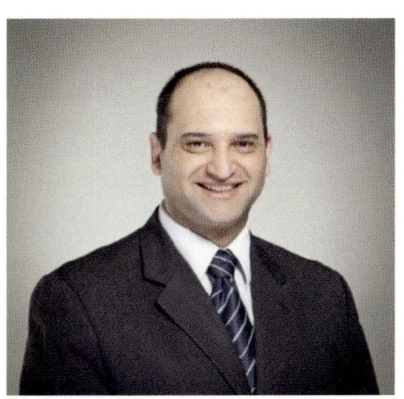

Marcos Pinotti Barbosa is graduated in Mechanical Engineering from State University of Campinas (1989), Masters in Mechanical Engineering from the University of Campinas (1992) and Ph.D. in Mechanical Engineering from the University of Campinas (1996). Since 1997 he has been Assistant Professor at the Department of Mechanical Engineering (DEMec) of the Universidade Federal de Minas Gerais. He is CNPq's Research Fellow (ranked 1B). In 2010, he participated, by invitation of the Eisenhower Fellowship (USA) 2010 Program Multinationals, enabling him closer relationships with agencies of the U.S. government and major university on the theme of Innovation. Also, he coordinates two research laboratories: LABBio and LAPAN. Laboratory of Bioengineering (LABBio) is dedicated to Cardiovascular Engineering, Biophotonics, Assistive Technology and Biomechanics. LABBio was recognized by FINEP (Federal Innovation Funding Agency) as "Innovative Laboratory" because of the expressive number of patents generated. Up to now, LABBio has launched three spin-offs companies: Aptivalux Bioengineering LTD. (established in 2005); Fanfarra Estúdio LTD. (established in 2008) and 3D Foot LTD. (established in 2009).

Neural Vision Applied Research Laboratory (LAPAN, in partnership with Eye Hospital – Dr. Ricardo Guimarães'clinic) is a multidisciplinary laboratory devoted to study and devise new technology on the field of neurosciences, specially related to the visual system. LAPAN is a unique experience of a public research laboratory located in a private hospital. This successful experience has catalyzed a new technological platform to perform screening tests for elementary school students – The Right Star Project. It aggregates a team of engineers, ophthalmologists, psychiatrists, speech therapists, psychologists, neuroscientists, computer scientists and physicists. Marcos Pinotti has been supervisor and co-supervisor of more than 30 MSc and 20 Ph.D. thesis. He is author of more than 30 scientific papers in national and international journals and conferences. Additionally, he is co-author of 38 patents. He has been invited and given seminars, or invited plenary talks, apart from Brazil, to scientific audiences in United States, China, Italy, Scotland and Argentina. Currently, he is second vice-chairman of the Latin American Society of Biomaterials, Artificial Organs and Tissue Engineering (SLABO); member of the Brazilian National Triennial Evaluation of the Mechanical Engineering Graduate Courses from Ministry of Education and chairman of the Technical Consultant Board of Assistive Technology – Brazilian Presidential's Office for Human Rights.

A.P. Slade (A.P.Slade@dundee.ac.uk)
Medical Engineering Research Institute
Division of Mechanical Engineering &
Mechatronics
Faculty of Engineering & Physical
Sciences
Room G6
Fulton Building
University of Dundee
Dundee,
Scotland
DD1 4HN

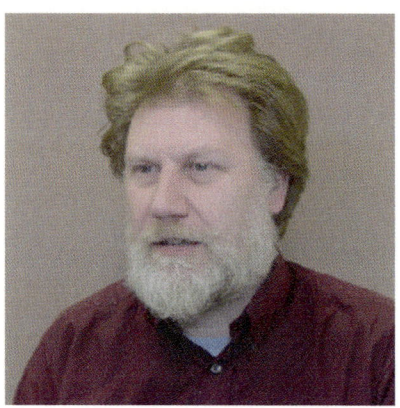

1982 – B.TEC. Electrical and Electronic Engineering, Higher Diploma. Loughborough Technical College.
1994 – M.Phil. Loughborough University of Technology.
2001 – Ph.D. University of Dundee.
1974–1994 – Loughborough University of Technology, Department of Mechanical Engineering.

Started in the I.C.E. Laboratory as general laboratory and workshop technician. Moved to Dynamics Laboratory in 1978 and was responsible for its rebuilding and supervision of student laboratory exercises. Started the Departments Mechatronic Research group with Professor J.R. Hewit in 1986.

During my time at Loughborough I was able to develop my skills in the machine shop and would now describe myself as a semi-skilled fitter with a knowledge of a wide range of machine tools and engineering principles. Since moving to the Dynamics, and latterly Mechatronics Group, I was able to pursue my interest in computers and robotics and was involved in a number of student projects which grew into full research projects over the years. The two which I consider to have been of the most importance to the department and myself are a robotic device for turning and sorting fabric garments and an FMS manufacturing/painting cell for the model industry. In both of these projects I was responsible for the design and building of the electronics and the basic computing elements, and also closely involved in the mechanical design and manufacture. From this last project a number of spin-off ideas have arisen and I am still involved with them with Professor Hewit. The area of medical mechatronic research is a relatively new field and I can see that there are many problems to be overcome. It is these areas which excite me and I believe that bringing an original mechatronic approach to them is the best way forward. Between 1984 and 1994 I was the First Aid Officer for the Department of Mecanical Engineering with responsibility for keeping the First Aid records up to date and dealing with accident reports.

1994 – University of Dundee Department of Applied Physics, Electronics and Mechanical Engineering.

Moved to the University of Dundee in October 1994 to undertake a Ph.D. in "Teleoperated manipulator for minimal access surgery".

1997 – Appointed as Teaching Associate to Deprtment of A.P.E.M.E. University of Dundee.

1999 – Appointed as lecturer in Robotics, Mechatronics and Contol in Department of A.P.E.M.E. University of Dundee.

2000 – Appointed as lecturer, Department of Mechanical Engineering, University of Dundee.

2001 – Appointed as lecturer, Division of Mechanical Engineering and Mechatronics, University of Dundee.

In-Silico Models as a Tool for the Design of Specific Treatments: Applications in Bone Regeneration

Esther Reina-Romo, María José Gómez-Benito, Libardo Andrés González-Torres, Jaime Domínguez, and José Manuel García-Aznar

Abstract Numerous pathologies related to bone regeneration such as bone healing or distraction osteogenesis are focus of intense research nowadays since there are many cues not well understood yet. Intense activity is performed in both experimental and computational fields. However, in silico models may play a relevant role since computer simulations allow considering and controlling factors that cannot be easily controlled or measured in experimental tests. In addition, experiments can be time-consuming, expensive and with a high difficulty to control all the parameters. This review addresses some of the main problems of in-silico models and focus on bone healing and distraction osteogenesis as mechanical based pathologies extensively investigated in the last decades.

1 Introduction

The design of new technologies in medicine and biology requires the development of in-vitro and in-vivo experiments needed to test different hypotheses that allow understanding observable phenomena. Identifying the molecular, cellular and macroscopic behavior of a specific pathology is essential to control the disease and significantly improve patient survival. However, these experiments can be time-consuming, expensive and with a high difficulty to control all the parameters.

In such cases, in-silico modeling can play a relevant role because computer simulations allow considering and controlling factors that cannot be easily controlled or

E. Reina-Romo (✉) • J. Domínguez
Department of Mechanical Engineering, University of Seville, Seville, 41092, Spain
e-mail: erreina@us.es; jaime@us.es

M.J. Gómez-Benito • L.A. González-Torres • J.M. García-Aznar
Aragon Institute of Engineering Research (I3A), University of Zaragoza, C/María de Luna 5,
"Agustín de Betancourt" Building, Zaragoza, 50018, Spain
e-mail: gomezmj@unizar.es; landresg@unizar.es; jmgaraz@unizar.es

R.M.N. Jorge et al. (eds.), *Technologies for Medical Sciences*, Lecture Notes
in Computational Vision and Biomechanics 1, DOI 10.1007/978-94-007-4068-6_1,
© Springer Science+Business Media B.V. 2012

measured in experimental tests. The fundamental role played by local mechanical factors on the biological processes involved in the bone regeneration phenomena make mechanical based pathologies suitable for a strong interest by the engineering community. Their research field includes experimental and analytical models that help to understand the skeletal response to mechanical factors. The purpose is to determine the quantitative rules that govern the effects of mechanical conditions on tissue differentiation, growth, adaptation and maintenance. However, the identification of the relevant mechanical parameters and their mechanisms of action are unresolved and continue to be investigated.

Currently, this trend of using in-silico models in different fields of biology and medicine is being highly extended. Indeed, a considerable progress has been made, for example, in the mathematical modeling of cancer growth [11]. Another field where the development of models has been very important is in orthopaedic biomechanics, where Finite-Element-Analysis (FEA) has been applied to the design of medical devices [43, 55]. In fact, FEA has also been widely used to simulate mechanobiological problems [65], where the main aim is to understand the way cells sense and respond to mechanical conditions, modifying and updating the extracellular matrix of the involved tissues. The potential of mechanobiology to contribute to clinical progress is very promising. Understanding the mechanobiology of mechanical based pathologies at the tissue level may reduce complications and enhance bone regeneration through the application of mechanical stimulation to guide differentiation of multipotent tissue.

In this review, a tissue differentiation theory is shown to be able to predict the effect of application of low magnitude high frequency (LMHF) mechanical stimulation in bone healing. However, to predict the outcome of the bone healing process, a complete in-silico model is needed. A differentiation theory is simulated together with other cell and matrix processes such as migration and proliferation. In addition, in order to simulate other features of bone and distraction osteogenesis processes such as reaction forces, different new variables and processes should be incorporated to the in-silico models. As an example, the model proposed by the authors is used to exemplify the extension of a bone healing model to distraction osteogenesis. In particular, the potential of this extended model was evaluated with the prediction of the most adequate distraction rate to achieve a successful outcome in a clinical process of long bone distraction and with its application to three-dimensions in a real clinical case of mandibular distraction osteogenesis.

2   Limitations of Computer Models: Process of Validation

As in many sciences, the integration of experimental and mathematical models within the orthopaedic field is critical to gain an understanding of the skeletal response to mechanical factors [65]. On the one hand, experimental modeling is needed to examine both tissue differentiation and adaptation to altered loading. On the other hand, in silico modeling proposes quantitative rules that govern the effects of mechanical loading on tissue differentiation, growth, adaptation and maintenance. In any case, it must be kept in mind that a computational model is a simplified and mathematical representation of a system to analyze its behavior under different conditions. Therefore, a model always requires experimental validation.

Model validation is an essential part in modeling. In order to validate a model it is necessary to compare predictions given by the model with results from in-vitro and in-vivo experiments. In fact, if a model is unable to reproduce some specific experiments, then the original hypotheses in which the model is based should be revised and updated. The experiments have to be designed in a way that the measured data contain information about the different parameters predicted by the model. Moreover, in-silico models can also improve experimental design by highlighting which measurements are needed to test a particular theory and whether additional information can be gained by collecting supplementary data.

3 Biological Background

During the last decades intense research has been performed in orthopaedic biomechanics. Bone healing and distraction osteogenesis in particular have been focus of numerous experimental studies [19, 32, 34, 35] since there are many cues not well understood yet. Next are described these processes briefly from a biological perspective.

3.1 Bone Healing

In the process of fracture healing, bone recovers its original shape and mass after fracture. It is a very complex process which involves intense cell migration, differentiation and proliferation within the fracture gap. A fracture callus is created and the bony union takes place by means of intramembranous and endochondral ossification. This is the most commonly way fractures heal and involve four overlapping phases (Fig. 1): inflammatory, soft callus, hard callus and remodeling to original bone contour [4]:

- *Inflammatory phase*. This phase starts immediately after the fracture occurs and as a result of vascular disruption an hematoma is formed and is converted into a clot. It lasts from 1 to 3 days at which the clot is replaced with granulation tissue [63].
- *Soft callus stage*: its starts once the pain has disappeared and ends with the bone fragments union by tissues with relative stability. It usually lasts approximately 2 weeks during which granulation tissue is converted to fibrous tissue by fibroblasts. Cartilage tissue also replaces the granulation tissue but in the periphery of the gap rather than in the central part [63].

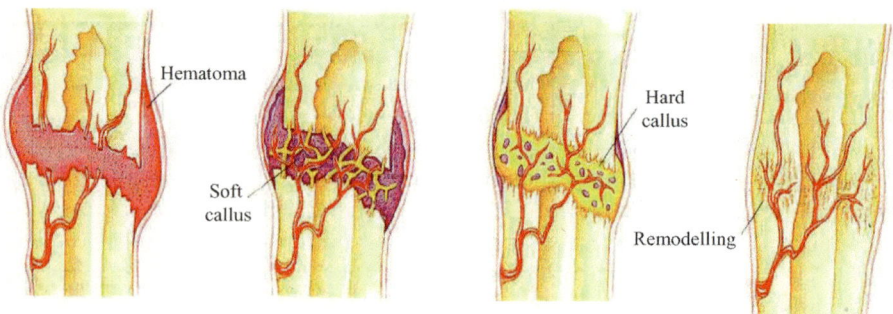

Fig. 1 Phases of bone healing [50]

- The *hard callus stage* lasts approximately 4 weeks [19] and ends with the bone fragments union by immature bone. Initially, the callus is formed by cartilage tissue predominately, with some areas of intramembranous ossification. In this phase, mineralization occurs although with a rhythm much slower than the preceding phases. The type of mineralization depends on the existing tissue within the soft callus, either intramembranous or endochondral ossification.
- The *remodeling phase* lasts approximately 1–4 years [19, 22] and consists of two phases. During the former, internal remodeling occurs and the immature bone is replaced by lamellar bone. During the latter, which is slower, external remodeling occurs, the size of the callus diminishes and the bone recovers its original shape.

3.2 Distraction Osteogenesis

Distraction osteogenesis is a unique biologic process of new bone formation between the surfaces of bone segments that are gradually separated. Under the influence of the tensional stress, the soft callus is maintained at the center of the distraction gap while routine fracture healing occurs at the periphery of the regenerate [63]. Many tissues besides bone have been observed to form under tension stress, including mucosa, skin, muscle, tendon, cartilage, blood vessels, and peripheral nerves [17, 34, 35]. Therefore, distraction osteogenesis as well as bone healing involve a process of continuum tissue formation.

In the distraction process, there are five fundamental sequential phases in which different biologic phenomena are produced (Fig. 2):

- *Osteotomy*. In this phase the bone is surgically divided into two segments, resulting in a loss of continuity and mechanical integrity. Bone fragments are then fixed by means of a distractor/external fixator to stabilize the new created gap [37].

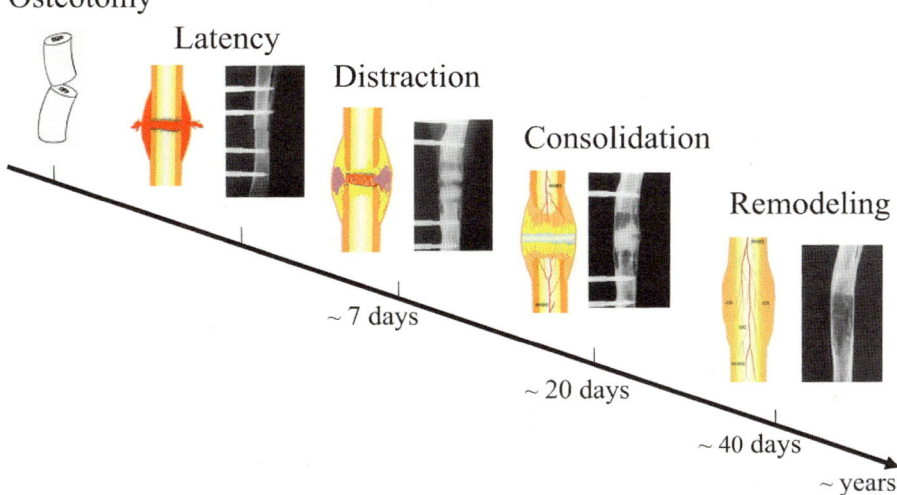

Fig. 2 Phases of distraction osteogenesis (Adapted from [63] and [45])

- *Latency phase*: it is the period between performance of osteotomy and start of the tension, during which the soft callus starts to be formed. This period coincides with the initial events in the normal process of bone healing.
- *Distraction*: it is the period in which the two ends of the osteotomized bone are gradually moved apart resulting in the formation of new bony tissues within the progressively increasing interfragmentary gap. Through the application of tensional stress, a dynamic microenvironment is created [18]. This environment stimulates changes at the cellular and subcellular level, including the prolongation of angiogenesis with increased tissue oxygenation and the increased fibroblast proliferation. The cells alter their phenotypic expression and become longitudinally oriented along the axis of distraction.
- *Consolidation*. The consolidation period is the time between the cessation of traction forces and removal of the distraction device. This period represents the time required for complete hard callus formation and mineralization of the regenerated tissue.
- *Remodeling*: it is the time from the removal of the distraction device (and thus application of full functional loading) to the complete remodeling of the newly formed bone. During this period, the initially formed bony scaffold is reinforced by parallel-fibered lamellar bone. Both the cortical bone and marrow cavity are restored.

4   In-Silico Models

In-silico models within the orthopaedic field can be roughly divided in two main groups: biomechanical and mechanobiological models. The former analyze the structure and function of biological systems applying laws of mechanics whilst the latter focus on how the mechanical environment regulates the cell behavior in different biological processes. Many of these models are based on different tissue differentiation theories [12, 16, 28, 53, 54] which try to provide quantitative or qualitative rules that relate a mechanical stimulus of an undifferentiated tissue with the tissue formed (see [27] for a complete review).

4.1   Tissue Differentiation Theories

Although existing tissue differentiation theories are different in details [12, 16, 53 28, 54], they share some characteristics. Firstly, they all propose that high mechanical stimulation favors the formation of fibrocartilage tissue, while non stimulated environments favor bone formation. Secondly, they all develop phenomenologic rules, with theories derived from empirical observations. Thirdly, they are not sufficiently validated despite being able to successfully reproduce the main patterns of fracture healing in specific mechanical environments. And finally, all these tissue differentiation theories are obviously related to mechanical stimuli, which is definitely executed by cells whose biological sensing and signaling activities are implicitly assumed but not directly considered. Two of these algorithms will be reviewed to analyze their ability to predict bone regeneration in fracture healing and distraction osteogenesis: the mechanoregulation theory developed by Prendergast et al. [54] and that proposed by Gómez-Benito et al. [28].

Prendergast et al. [54] developed a simple and different mechanoregulation concept as compared to the existing theories [12, 16, 53] assuming that tissues are biphasic with both fluid and solid phases. Existing models to date were static or linear elastic [12, 16, 53]. They proposed a mechanoregulation pathway regulated by two biophysical stimuli, the second invariant of the deviatoric strain of the solid, and the interstitial fluid velocity relative to the solid. Figure 3 shows how the tissue phenotype (granulation tissue, bone tissue, cartilage and fibrous tissue) is determined depending on its position in the mechano-regulation diagram. As far as the authors know, this differentiation law is the only which considers the frequency of stimulation, by means of the fluid flow. In contrast, Gómez-Benito et al. [28] and García-Aznar et al. [23] proposed a mathematical model driven exclusively by the second invariant of the deviatoric strain tensor, assuming that tissues are poroelastic.

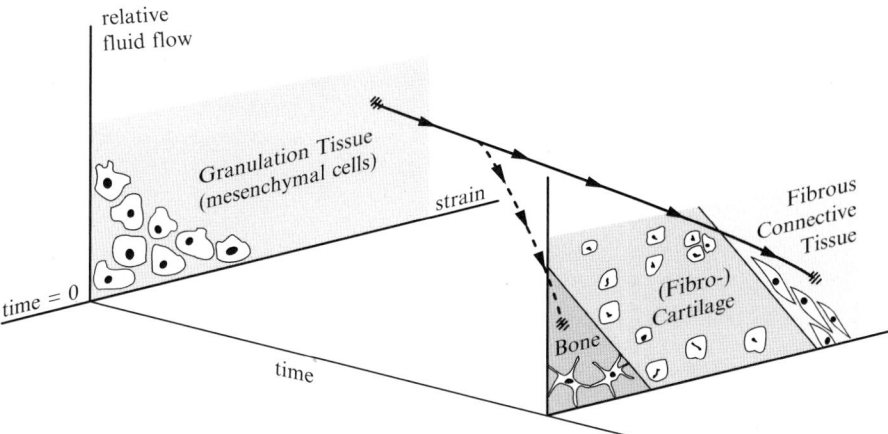

Fig. 3 Mechanoregulation diagram for bone formation and resorption based on mechanical strain and fluid flow [54]

4.1.1 Computational Simulations to Evaluate the Effect of External LMHF Cyclical Displacements

In this section it is shown that a differentiation theory alone is able to provide insight into the bone healing process. The differentiation theory proposed by Prendergast et al. [54] has been used to computationally determine the influence of an external mechanical stimulus based on a LMHF displacement of the fractured fragments on the bone healing process (see [30] for further details). In particular, it has been implemented to predict the most appropriate frequency of stimulation that optimizes the bone healing time [31]. An axisymmetric simplified model of the fracture callus in the metatarsus of a sheep was simulated [16] at two different time points, 1 and 4 weeks after fracture (see Fig. 4). A cyclical displacement of 0.02 mm was applied at the top of cortical bone with different frequencies of stimulation (1, 50 and 100 Hz) in order to evaluate their impact on tissue differentiation. Figure 4 shows the evolution of the magnitudes of some mechanical variables: octahedral strain, second invariant of the deviatoric strain tensor and fluid flow. It can be observed that the only mechanical stimulus affected by the frequency of stimulation is the fluid flow whilst the other mechanical variables (octahedral strain and second invariant of the deviatoric strain tensor) are just slightly modified. The major variations of the fluid flow occur for frequencies of stimulation higher than 50 Hz. According to the differentiation rule proposed by Prendergast et al. [54] an increase in the frequency of stimulation may promote chondrogenesis and endochondral ossification (Fig. 3).

This simulation provides the cues to perform experiments with the aim to improve the bone healing process. According to computational results, it was decided to stimulate the fracture site with a frequency higher than 50 Hz aiming

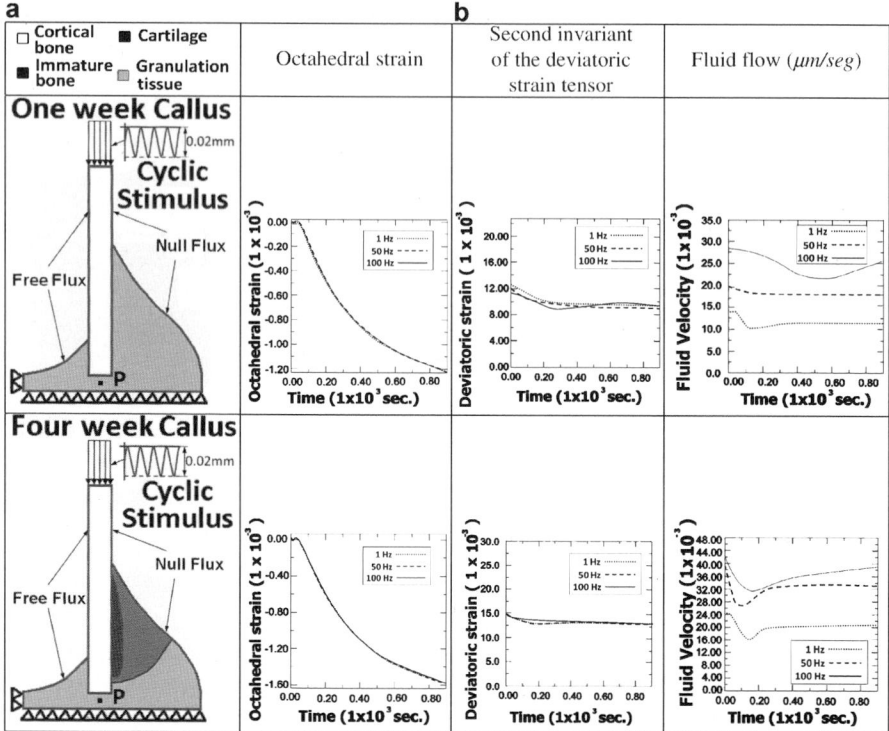

Fig. 4 (**a**) Tissue distribution and boundary conditions in the 1 and 4 week calluses (Adapted from [16]); and (**b**) evolution of the mean mechanical stimulus in one point of the gap (see (**a**)) when stimulating with different frequencies (1, 50 and 100 Hz) during 15 min [30]

to improve the endochondral ossification. As previous experimental works have used frequencies up to 90 Hz [40] to stimulate bone mass formation in osteoporotic conditions, this frequency was used experimentally in a long bone of a sheep animal model in order to evaluate its functionality [30, 33]. In fact, the findings of the mechanobiological model were corroborated with experiments: stimulation by LMHF mechanical stimulus with a frequency of 90 Hz improves the healing outcome. Thus, in this study, the mathematical model has been used in combination with experiments, showing the strong interaction needed within these research fields.

4.2 Continuum Evolutive Models

A further step in-silico models are the continuum evolutive models. Continuum evolutive models make use of the differentiation theories to predict from a computational perspective the evolution of the main patterns of different biological phenomena. For instance, Prendergast et al. [54] demonstrated the consistency of the model at implant to bone interfaces [54] and afterwards in a bone chamber [24–26] and osteochondral defects [41]. They also succeed in simulating the outcome of bone healing within the fracture callus for different gap sizes and loading magnitudes [46]. This model has then been taken up by Andreykiv et al. [2], Isaksson et al. [39], Byrne [10] and Boccaccio et al. [8]. In distraction osteogenesis, Isaksson et al. [38] have been able to predict the main tissue distributions for different frequencies of distraction and for moderate and low distraction rates in long bone distraction osteogenesis. Nevertheless, they were not able to reproduce the evolution of the reaction force during the distraction period. In mandibular distraction osteogenesis, Boccaccio et al. [6, 7] examined the influence of the rate of distraction and the latency period duration within the fracture callus of a human mandible submitted to symphyseal distraction osteogenesis.

Gómez-Benito et al. [28] and García-Aznar et al. [23] proposed a continuum evolutive model which considers as state variables the concentration of five cell phenotypes (mesenchymal stem cells, fibroblasts, cartilage cells, bone cells and dead cells). The evolution of the concentration of each skeletal cell type is considered to be function of the proliferation, migration and differentiation processes. In addition, they incorporated for the first time in their mechanoregulation model the mathematical formulation of callus growth. They succeeded in simulating the main processes that occur during fracture healing [23, 28]. In particular, this mechano-biological regulatory model predicted a geometry of the callus, tissue differentiation patterns and fracture stiffness similar to those reported in the literature with different gap sizes [28] and the influence of the interfragmentary movement on the callus growth, shape and tissue types [23]. Since fracture healing and distraction repair share similar biological processes and strain-related bone tissue reactions, this model could be applied to simulate distraction osteogenesis. In the model explained the differentiation process was function of the mechanical stimulus and time (the time that stem cells need to differentiate into specialized cells). However, with this differentiation concept, as there is a similar mechanical environment within the gap after the first days of distraction, a similar distraction osteogenesis outcome would be predicted with any mechanical factor analyzed (e.g. distraction rate). In fact, this model and others based on different mechanoregulatory differentiation rules [16, 28, 54] were used to simulate the influence of different distraction rates. They were able to successfully predict the distraction osteogenesis process for moderate and low distraction rates but not for high distraction rates (e.g. 2 mm/day). Therefore, the model needed to be extended further by introducing the effect of the load history on the process of cell differentiation. Cell differentiation was assumed to depend on the load history in such way that cells will differentiate only if they have been subjected to a specific mechanical environment during a period of time [62]. Thus, the maturation state of the cell type is included in the model as a state variable (see Reina-Romo et al. [56] for further details). The model incorporating the maturation state of the cells was just an extension of the previously proposed model. This extended model was also able to predict the regenerative process in different examples of fracture healing [23, 28, 29].

This extended model is applied to determine from a computational perspective the optimum rate of distraction in bone distraction prior to experimental performance [56] and to investigate its ability to predict the main tissue patterns during the course of the three dimensional lengthening procedure of the mandible ramus [60].

4.2.1 Long Bone Distraction Osteogenesis: Design of the Protocol of Distraction

Since distraction osteogenesis is a mechanical-based pathology, mechanical factors, such as axial alignment, stability and distraction rate affect both the quality and quantity of the regenerated bone [34,35]. For example, nonunions may occur when the bone ends move too much [21,34,64], the distraction rate is higher than a limit value [15,35,64,66], the frequency of distraction is not adequate [35], there is no latency phase [34,35,66] or due to damage of the bone marrow and periosteal soft tissues [34].

Therefore, in this section, the extended mechanobiological model of Gómez-Benito et al. [56] is applied to simulate different mechanical environments in order to determine the optimum rate of distraction from a computational perspective before experimental testing. Values of 0.3, 1 and 2 mm/day were applied to a sheep model [9]. These rates are commonly used in the experiments found in the literature [1, 3, 14, 20, 34–36, 42]. The distraction length was kept constant (20 mm) and therefore the distraction periods were modified accordingly for each distraction rate.

In order to test the reliability of the implemented model, the tissue distributions obtained were compared with experimental results. Results agree with the experimental ones: a moderate distraction rate is needed for successful bony bridging whist insufficient or excessive mechanical stimulation is adverse for distraction (Fig. 5).

With moderate distraction rates (1 mm/day), bone tissue appears in the peripherical zones, close to the cortical bone and periosteum (Fig. 5a). This is in agreement with the experimental findings, where bone forms from the host bones to the center of the gap (Fig. 5d) [45, 52, 61]. Similar computational results were presented by Isaksson et al. [38] simulating the same distraction protocol with a different evolutive model [54].

With insufficient mechanical stimulation (0.3 mm/day), there is a quick increase of the bone density during the first days of the distraction process (Fig. 5b, e). Computationally, this lower rate of distraction is accompanied by lower mechanical stimulation which promotes osteogenesis.

In contrast, excessive mechanical stimulation (2 mm/day) produces nonunion [48]. The mechanical stimulus (deviatoric strain) increases in the gap during the entire process of distraction osteogenesis, favoring the differentiation of MSCs to fibroblasts (Fig. 5c, f). Under this mechanical environment, the number of MSCs in the gap is limited and, consequently, they cannot contribute to the proliferation and differentiation processes producing a delay in bone tissue production. This is in agreement with most clinical results which consider that a rate of distraction of

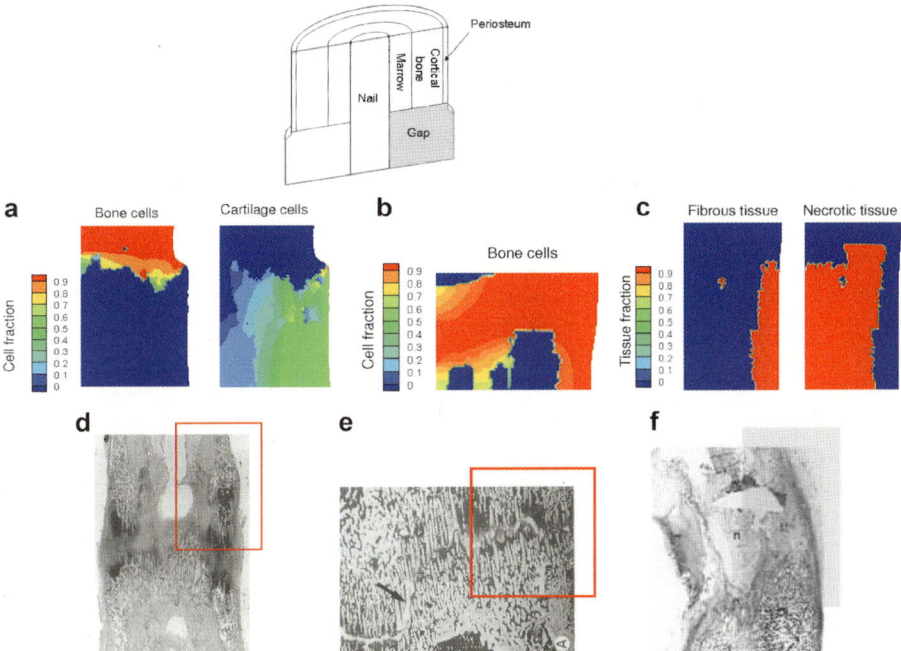

Fig. 5 Numerical results at a distraction rate of (**a**) 1 mm/day; (**b**) 0.3 mm/day and (**c**) 2 mm/day (From [56]). Experimental results showing (**d**) a successful bony bridging [52]; (**e**) a premature union [47]; (**f**) a nonunion [48]

around 1 mm/day produces the best effects on tissue regeneration [1, 34]. Nevertheless, higher distraction rates resulted in a predominantly fibrous interfragmentary gap [15].

Regarding the computed reaction force, the model is able to capture the gradual stiffening trend observed experimentally [9, 56]. However, the material properties are on the limit of the physiological range. With more realistic material properties, the model is not able to predict the stiffening behavior of the reaction forces. To solve this limitation and use a more realistic set of material properties, the pretraction stresses needed to be incorporated to the model (see Reina-Romo et al. [57] for further details). Reina-Romo et al. [58] showed that considering residual stresses is crucial for a correct reaction force prediction and material properties estimation. By contrast, tissue distributions were not affected significantly by these residual stresses [58].

4.2.2 Extension to Three Dimensions: Simulation of a Clinical Case

Distraction osteogenesis is an effective way to grow new bone and has been widely used in the last decades to correct bone deformities, either congenital or acquired, bone length discrepancies and bony defects. Its application to the craniofacial skeleton has gained wide acceptance, since its clinical introduction by McCarthy et al. [51], due to the huge possibilities this process offers. Previous studies of mandibular distraction osteogenesis have characterized the local bio-physical environment created within the osteotomy gap at different time points [5, 13, 44, 49, 59, 63] or during the whole process of distraction through mechanobiological models [6, 7, 60]. Reina-Romo et al. [60] studied the temporo-spatial evolution of the different tissues during distraction osteogenesis and the biomechanics in patients with severe deformities. The aim of this section is to review this work, in which the previously developed model of distraction osteogenesis [56] is used to investigate its ability to predict the main tissue patterns during the course of the three dimensional lengthening procedure of the mandible ramus.

This study was based on data from a 6-year-old male patient with unilateral mandibular hypoplasia of the right mandibular ramus, corresponding with a grade IIb according to Pruzanski criteria. This pathology is known as hemifacial microsomia (HFM) and consists of a congenital asymmetrical malformation of both the bony and soft-tissue structures of the cranium and face. The three-dimensional model of the mandible corresponded with the original morphology of the mandible before treatment. Four different regions were identified during the segmentation procedure of this model: gap, cancellous bone, cortical bone and teeth. The right ramus of the model was virtually cut simulating the osteotomy at the location indicated by the surgeon. With regard to the clinical distraction protocol, the full process includes a 7-day latency period and a phase of distraction of 20 days.

Figure 6 shows the evolution of the tissue distribution in the mandible through the process of distraction. It can be observed how this tissue distribution varies significantly. In the first days of the process the gap is mostly filled by damaged debris tissue, due to the high values of the mechanical stimulus. During the initial stage (1–10 days), tissue damage is gradually repaired due to the decreasing values of the strain magnitudes allowing granulation tissue to be deposited (Fig. 6). This granulation tissue is synthesized by MSCs that migrate from the marrow cavity, periosteum and surrounding soft tissues to the interfragmentary gap. By day 10, the first islands of cartilage tissue begin to appear within the distracted gap. As distraction proceeds, the low stimulated mechanical environment around the two bone fragments favor the formation of bone tissue. From day 15 until the end of the distraction process more amount of cartilage can be seen in the outer part of the callus. Immediately following completion of 20 mm, the distraction outcome shows a gap filled with cartilage tissue, which constitutes most of the regenerate surface. The area of new bone formation was located close to the host bones and the remaining gap was filled with cartilage tissue.

This model presents a preliminar three dimensional approach of distraction osteogenesis from a computational perspective. Although it should be further extended in the future, it shows the enormous potential it offers. It could be used to study different aspects of the distraction procedure such as the effect of the distraction rate, the best placement of the corticotomy or the time of the device removal amongst others once the model parameters have been adjusted.

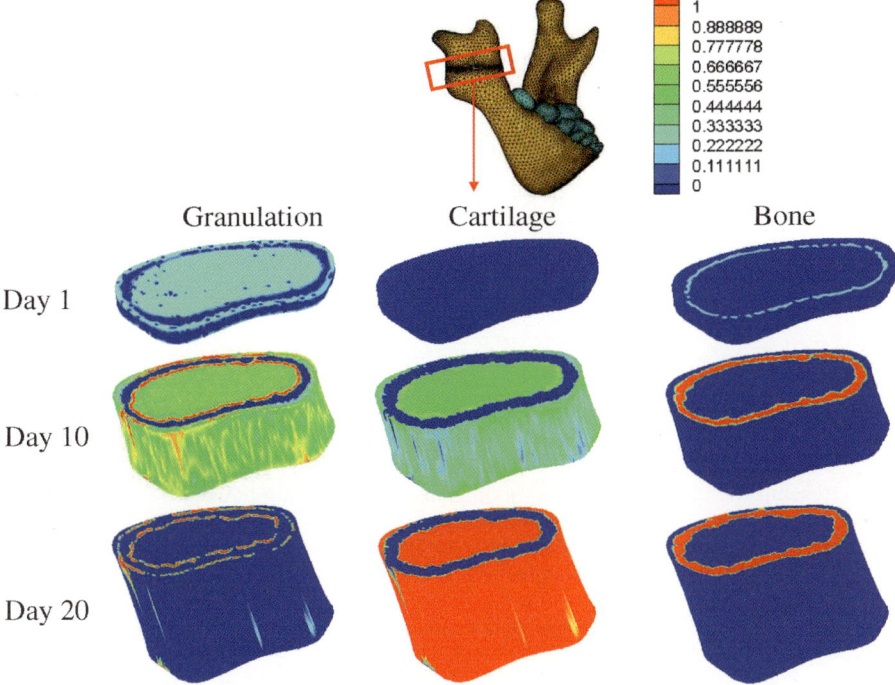

Fig. 6 Tissue distribution in within the distracted gap at days 1, 10 and 20 of the distraction procedure (Adapted from [60])

5   Discussion and Conclusions

In this review the computational results of three examples of application that involve intense bone regeneration have been presented: fracture healing, long bone distraction osteogenesis and mandibular distraction osteogenesis. The former provides a biomechanical approach based on the mechanoregulation theory proposed by Prendergast et al. [54] to design an external fixator able to stimulate mechanically the fracture at LMHF. The tissue differentiation theory of Prendergast et al. [54] is the only that considers the fluid flow and thus the effect of the frequency of stimulation on the tissue outcome. In contrast, the two remaining examples study from a mechanobiological perspective the process of distraction osteogenesis based on the model of fracture healing proposed by Gómez-Benito et al. [28]. This model was extended to simulate the process of distraction osteogenesis including the maturation cell level, thus considering cell plasticity [56, 62]. As far as the authors know, the extended tissue differentiation theory of Gómez-Benito et al. [28] is the only that includes the maturation state. In fact, when simulating highly stimulated mechanical environments in distraction osteogenesis (high distraction rates) existing models [16, 28, 54] are not able to predict the nonunion observed experimentally.

These results show the enormous potential in-silico tools have on treatments related to bone regeneration. The new developments in cellular, molecular and computational technologies will help to improve the treatment of pathologies related to bone formation. Therefore, engineers may play a crucial role in this emerging field since accurate simulations of the process and patient specific models can help the surgeon for a more precise performance. However, we have to be cautious since there are still many limitations that must be overcome.

Acknowledgements The authors gratefully acknowledge the research support of the project part financed by the European Union (European Regional Development Fund) through the grant DPI 2009-14115-C03-01.

References

1. Al Ruhaimi KA (2001) Comparison of different distraction rates in the mandible: an experimental investigation. Int J Oral Maxillofac Surg 30:220–227
2. Andreykiv A, van Keulen F, Prendergast PJ (2007) Simulation of fracture healing incorporating mechanoregulation of tissue differentiation and dispersal/proliferation of cells. Biomech Model Mechanobiol 7:443–461
3. Aronson J (1993) Temporal and spatial increases in blood flow during distraction osteogenesis. Clin Orthop Relat Res 301:124–131
4. Bailón-Plaza A, van der Meulen MC (2001) A mathematical framework to study the effects of growth factor influences on fracture healing. J Theor Biol 212:191–209
5. Boccaccio A, Lamberti L, Pappalettere C, Carano A, Cozzani M (2006) Mechanical behavior of an osteotomized mandible with distraction orthodontic devices. J Biomech 39:2907–2918
6. Boccaccio A, Pappalettere C, Kelly DJ (2007) The influence of expansion rates on mandibular distraction osteogenesis: a computational analysis. Ann Biomed Eng 35:1940–1960
7. Boccaccio A, Prendergast PJ, Pappalettere C, Kelly DJ (2008) Tissue differentiation and bone regeneration in an osteotomized mandible: a computational analysis of the latency period. Med Biol Eng Comput 46:283–298
8. Boccaccio A, Kelly DJ, Pappalettere C (2011) A mechano-regulation model of fracture repair in vertebral bodies. J Orthop Res 29:433–443
9. Brunner UH, Cordey J, Schweiberer L, Perren SM (1994) Force required for bone segment transport in the treatment of large bone defects using medullary nail fixation. Clin Orthop Relat Res 301:147–155
10. Byrne DP (2008) Computational modelling of bone regeneration using a three-dimensional lattice approach. PhD thesis, Trinity College Dublin, (Ireland)
11. Byrne H (2010) Dissecting cancer through mathematics: from the cell to the animal model. Nat Rev Cancer 10:221–230
12. Carter DR (1987) Mechanical loading history and skeletal biology. J Biomech 20:1095–1109
13. Cattaneo PM, Kofod T, Dalstra M, Melsen B (2005) Using the Finite Element Method to model the biomechanics of the asymmetric mandible before, during and after skeletal correction by distraction osteogenesis. Comput Method Biomech Biomed Eng 8:157–165
14. Choi IH, Shim JS, Seong SC, Lee MC, Song KY, Park SC, Chung CY, Cho TJ, Lee DY (1997) Effect of the distraction rate on the activity of the osteoblast lineage in distraction osteogenesis of rat's tibia. Immunostaining study of the proliferating cell nuclear antigen, osteocalcin, and transglutaminase C. Bull Hosp Jt Dis 56:34–40
15. Choi P, Ogilvie C, Thompson T, Miclau T, Helms JH (2004) Cellular and molecular characterization of a murine non-union model. J Orthop Res 22:1100–1107

16. Claes LE, Heigele CA (1999) Magnitudes of local stress and strain along bony surfaces predict the course and type of fracture healing. J Biomech 32:255–266
17. Cope JB, Samchukov ML, Cherkashin AM (1999) Mandibular distraction osteogenesis: a historic perspective and future directions. Am J Orthod Dentofac Orthop 115:448–460
18. Delloye C, Delefortrie G, Coutelier L, Vincent A (1990) Bone regenerate formation in cortical bone during distraction lengthening: an experimental study. Clin Orthop 250:34–42
19. Einhorn TA (1998) The cell and molecular biology of fracture healing. Clin Orthop Rel Res 355:S7–S21
20. Farhadieh RH, Gianoutsos MP, Dickinson R, Walsh WR (2000) Effect of distraction rate on biomechanical, mineralization, and histologic properties of an ovine mandible model. Plast Reconstr Surg 105:889–895
21. Fischgrund J, Paley D, Suter C (1994) Variables affecting time to bone healing during limb lengthening. Clin Orthop Relat Res 301:31–37
22. Frost HM (1989) The biology of fracture healing an overview for clinicicians. part i and ii. Clin Orthop 289:283–309
23. García-Aznar JM, Kuiper JH, Gómez-Benito MJ, Doblaré M, Richardson JB (2007) Computational simulation of fracture healing: influence of interfragmentary movement on the callus growth. J Biomech 40:1467–1476
24. Geris L, Van Oosterwyck H, Vander Sloten J, Duyck J, Naert I (2003) Assessment of mechanobiological models for the numerical simulation of tissue differentiation around immediately loaded implants. Comput Method Biomech Biomed Eng 6:277–88
25. Geris L, Andreykiv A, Van Oosterwyck H, Vander Sloten J, van Keulen F, Duyck J, Naert I (2004) Numerical simulation of tissue differentiation around loaded titanium implants in a bone chamber. J Biomech 37:763–769
26. Geris L, Vandamme K, Naert I, Vander Sloten J, Duyck J, Van Oosterwyck H (2009) Numerical simulation of bone regeneration in a bone chamber. J Dent Res 88:158–163
27. Geris L, Schugart R, Van Oosterwyck H (2010) In silico design of treatment strategies in wound healing and bone fracture healing. Philos Trans A Math Phys Eng Sci 368:2683–2706
28. Gómez-Benito MJ, García-Aznar JM, Kuiper JH, Doblaré M (2005) Influence of fracture gap size on the pattern of long bone healing: a computational study. J Theor Biol 235:105–119
29. Gómez-Benito MJ, García-Aznar JM, Kuiper JH, Doblaré M (2006) A 3D computational simulation of fracture callus formation: influence of the stiffness of the external fixator. J Biomech Eng 128:290–299
30. Gómez-Benito MJ, González-Torres LA, Reina-Romo E, Grasa J, Seral B, García-Aznar JM (2011) Influence of high frequency cyclical stimulation on bone fracture healing process: mathematical and experimental models. Philos Transact A Math Phys Eng Sci 369:4278–4294.
31. González-Torres LA, Gómez-Benito MJ, Doblaré M, García-Aznar JM (2010) Influence of the frequency of the external mechanical stimulus on bone healing: a computational study. Med Eng Phys 32:363–371
32. Goodship AE, Kenwright J (1985) The influence of induced micromovement upon the healing of experimental tibial fractures. J Bone Jt Surg Br 67:650–655
33. Grasa J, Gómez-Benito MJ, González-Torres LA, Asiaín D, Quero F, García-Aznar JM (2010) Monitoring in vivo load transmission through an external fixator. Ann Biomed Eng 38:605–612
34. Ilizarov GA (1989) The tension-stress effect on the genesis and growth of tissues. Part I: the influence of stability of fixation and soft-tissue preservation. Clin Orthop 238:249–281
35. Ilizarov GA (1989) The tension-stress effect on the genesis and growth of tissues. Part II: the influence of the rate and frequency of distraction. Clin Orthop 239:263–285
36. Ilizarov GA (1990) Clinical application of the tension–stress effect for limb lengthening. Clin Orthop Relat Res 250:8–26
37. Ilizarov GA, Ledyaev VI (1992) The replacement of long tubular bone defects by lengthening distraction osteotomy of one of the fragments. 1969. Clin Orthop Relat Res 280:7–10
38. Isaksson H, Comas O, Van Donkelaar CC, Mediavilla J, Wilson W, Huiskes R, Ito K (2007) Bone regeneration during distraction osteogenesis: mechano-regulation by shear strain and fluid velocity. J Biomech 40:2002–2011

39. Isaksson H, van Donkelaar CC, Huiskes R, Ito K (2008) A mechanoregulatory bone-healing model incorporating cell-phenotype specific activity. J Theor Biol 252:230–246
40. Judex S, Lei X, Han D, Rubin C (2007) Low-magnitude mechanical signals that stimulate bone formation in the ovariectomized rat are dependent on the applied frequency but not on the strain magnitude. J Biomech 40:1333–1339
41. Kelly DJ, Prendergast PJ (2005) Mechano-regulation of stem cell differentiation and tissue regeneration in osteochondral defects. J Biomech 38:1413–1422
42. King NS, Liu ZJ, Wang LL, Chiu IY, Whelan MF, Huang GJ (2003) Effect of distraction rate and consolidation period on bone density following mandibular osteodistraction in rats. Arch Oral Biol 48:299–308
43. Kluess D, Mittelmeier W, Bader R (2010) From theory to practice: transfer of fea results into clinical applications. J Biomech 43S1:S3–S14
44. Kofod T, Cattaneo PM, Melsen B (2005) Three-dimensional finite element analysis of the mandible and temporomandibular joint on simulated occlusal forces before and after vertical ramus elongation by distraction osteogenesis. J Craniofac Surg 16:421–429
45. Kojimoto H, Yasui N, Goto T, Matsuda S, Shimomura Y (1988) Bone lengthening in rabbits by callus distraction. J Bone Jt Surg Br 70-B:543–549
46. Lacroix D, Prendergast PJ (2002) A mechano-regulation model for tissue differentiation during fracture healing: analysis of gap size and loading. J Biomech 35:1163–1171
47. Li G, Simpson HRW, Kenwright J, Triffitt JT (1997) Assessment of cell proliferation in regenerating bone during distraction osteogenesis at different distraction rates. J Orthop Res 15:765–772
48. Li G, Simpson HRW, Kenwright J, Triffitt JT (2000) Tissues formed during distraction osteogenesis in the rabbit are determined by the distraction rate: localization of the cells that express the mRNAs and the distribution of types I and II collagens. Cell Biol Int 24:25–33
49. Loboa EG, Fang TD, Parker DW, Warren SM, Fong KD, Longaker MT, Carter DR (2005) Mechanobiology of mandibular distraction osteogenesis: finite element analyses with a rat model. J Orthop Res 23:663–670
50. Marieb EN (2004) Bone and skeletal tissues part A. Human anatomy and physiology. Power point lecture slide presentation by Vicen Austin, University of Kentchucky, 6th edn. Pearson education, New York, publishing as Benjamin Cummings
51. McCarthy JG, Schreiber J, Karp N, Thorne CH, Grayson BH (1992) Lengthening the human mandible by gradual distraction. Plast Reconstr Surg 89:1–8
52. Ohyama M, Miyasaka Y, Sakurai M, Yokobori AJ, Sasaki S (1994) The mechanical behavior and morphological structure of callus in experimental callotasis. Biomed Mater Eng 4:273–281
53. Perren SM (1979) Physical and biological aspects of fracture healing with special reference to internal fixation. Clin Orthop 138:175–195
54. Prendergast PJ, Huiskes R, Soballe K (1997) Biophysical stimuli on cells during tissue differentiation at implant interfaces. ESB Research Award 1996. J Biomech 30:539–548
55. Prendergast PJ, Lally C, Lennon AB (2009) Finite element modelling of medical devices. Med Eng Phys 31:419
56. Reina-Romo E, Gómez-Benito MJ, García-Aznar JM, Domínguez J, Doblaré M (2009) Modeling distraction osteogenesis: analysis of the distraction rate. Biomech Model Mechanobiol 8:323–335
57. Reina-Romo E, Gómez-Benito MJ, García-Aznar JM, Domínguez J, Doblaré M (2010) Growth mixture model of distraction osteogenesis: effect of pre-traction stresses. Biomech Model Mechanobiol 9:103–115
58. Reina-Romo E, Gómez-Benito MJ, García-Aznar JM, Domínguez J, Doblaré M (2010) An interspecies computational study on limb lengthening. Proc Inst Mech Eng H 224:245–1256
59. Reina-Romo E, Sampietro-Fuentes A, Gómez-Benito MJ, Domínguez J, Doblaré M, García-Aznar JM (2010) Biomechanical response of a mandible in a patient affected with hemifacial microsomia before and after distraction osteogenesis. Med Eng Phys 32:860–866
60. Reina-Romo E, Gómez-Benito MJ, Sampietro-Fuentes A, Domínguez J, García-Aznar JM (2011) Three-dimensional simulation of mandibular distraction osteogenesis: mechanobiological analysis. Ann Biomed Eng 39:35–43

61. Richards M, Goulet JA, Weiss JA, Waanders NA, Schaffler MB, Goldstein SA (1998) Bone regeneration and fracture healing: experience with distraction osteogenesis model. Clin Orthop Relat Res 355S:S191–S204
62. Roder I (2003) Dynamical modeling of hematopoietic stem cell organization. PhD thesis, University of Leipzig, Leipzig
63. Samchukov ML, Cope JB, Cherkashin AM (2001) Craniofacial distraction osteogenesis. Springer, Heidelberg, pp 22–23. Mosby, Inc. St. Louis
64. Tajana GF, Morandi M, Zembo M (1989). The structure and development of osteogenic repair tissue according to Ilizarov technique in man. Characterization of extracellular matrix. Orthop 12:515–523
65. van der Meulen MC, Huiskes R (2002) Why mechanobiology? A survey article. J Biomech 35:401–414
66. White SH, Kenwright J (1990) The timing of distraction of an osteotomy. J Bone Jt Surg Br 72:356–361

Contact Finite Element with Surface Tension Adhesion

Rudolf A.P. Hellmuth and Raul G. Lima

Abstract This work is a contribution on the development of a computational model of lung parenchyma capable to simulate mechanical ventilation manoeuvres. This computational model should be able to represent adhesion caused by surface tension and be able suffer collapse and alveolar recruitment. Therefore, a contact finite element was developed and then simulated in a structure with structural properties of the same order of magnitude of a real alveolus. The simulation was performed with the non-linear finite element method. The implementation of the arc-length method was also necessary in order to prevent divergence at limit points. The numerical results of the simulation of a single alveolus, including the surface tension and adhesion, are qualitatively similar to experimental data obtained from whole excised lungs. Both present hysteresis and transmural pressures of the same order of magnitude.

1 Introduction

Many patients in intensive care units (ICU) are unable to breathe spontaneously and therefore they can only survive by means of mechanical ventilation. In many clinical cases the patient's condition is so weak that the physician must choose between a ventilation manoeuvre or other procedures that would perhaps help in the recovery of the patient. However, there is a lack of information about the lung's current condition and the efficacy of such therapeutic procedure can't be well predicted. So, any improvement in knowledge about the physical and biological phenomena involved in lung dynamics would be very useful both for critical decisions at the bedside and for the development of new pulmonary therapy manoeuvres.

R.A.P. Hellmuth (✉) • R.G. Lima
Escola Politécnica da Universidade de São Paulo, Av. Prof. Mello Moraes,
2231 – 05508-970, São Paulo, SP, Brazil
e-mail: rudolf.hellmuth@gmail.com; lima.raul@gmail.com

R.M.N. Jorge et al. (eds.), *Technologies for Medical Sciences*, Lecture Notes
in Computational Vision and Biomechanics 1, DOI 10.1007/978-94-007-4068-6_2,
© Springer Science+Business Media B.V. 2012

In order to exchange gases the lung depends on a harmonious relationship between ventilation and perfusion. The air and blood are guided by a complex branching system [1], where they are exposed to variations of transmural and transpulmonary pressures [2]. Thus, the ability of this organ to perform its essential function is intimately related to both its mechanical behaviour and its geometry. Moreover, there is a strong dependence of function and structure [3]. Therefore, many pulmonary diseases either are caused by failures on the structure or directly affect the structure (e.g. asthma, emphysema, atelectasis etc.).

A major challenge for the next generations of physiologists is to integrate the large amount of biological information (in rapid growth) in consistent quantitative models [4]. The models summarize briefly the information, and interacting with experiments, show properties and remove contradictions, which are not evident by simple description of its parts.

1.1 Mechanical Properties of Lung Parenchyma

The lung parenchyma is the tissue where the exchange of gases occurs. It is composed of alveoli and alveolar ducts. Tensile testings of the lung parenchyma show stress–strain curves with all characteristics of a soft tissue [5–7]. The extracellular matrix of soft tissues is rich in collagen and elastin fibres. The concentration and spatial organization of collagen and elastin fibres are the main factors which defines the mechanical properties of each type of soft tissue [8]. At small deformations elastin provides stiffness and stores most of the strain energy. The collagen fibres are comparatively inextensible and usually wavy at rest. With increasing deformation the collagen bundles are gradually stretched at the direction of deformation, what strongly increases the tissue's stiffness. This composite behaviour is analogous to the fibrous tissue of a nylon stocking, where elastin does the role of the rubber band and collagen the nylon's.

1.2 Idealized Geometry of the Pulmonary Alveolus

Recent descriptions based on histological analysis have shown that the the alveolar walls are shared between neighbour alveoli and form a structure similar to a honeycomb [9, 10]. Therefore, the airways in the lung parenchyma are series of branching corridors with polygonal walls and their dead ends are called alveoli. There are no "inner" and "outer" parts of the alveoli, instead there are septa which divide either an alveolus from another or an alveolus from an alveolar duct.

Dale [11] proposed a geometric model in which the parenchyma takes the form of a tessellation of second order regular polyhedra with 14 faces, see Fig. 1. This kind of polyhedron is also know as tetrakaidecahedran, truncated octahedron or simply 14-hedron. It has the advantages of being regular, being convex, filling the

Fig. 1 14-hedra tessellation filling the space

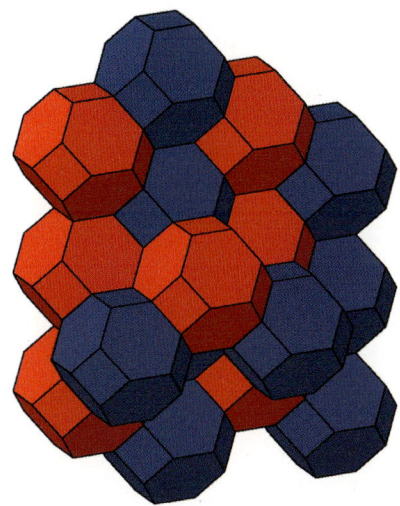

space when tessellated and having the smallest ratio of surface to volume among the space filling polyhedra [12]. The airways are then formed by removing some walls from the tessellated 14-hedra. The estimated difference for the surface-volume ratio between the parenchyma modelled this way and the values found in literature for real parenchyma is very small, around 2.7% [13], which corroborates this geometrical approximation.

1.3   Surface Tension in Alveoli

Because the lungs are very efficient mass exchangers with very thin wall between air and blood, some water diffuses from the blood vessels to alveolar cavity. The surface tension of the water film on the septa affects significantly the alveolar mechanics. To reduce surface tension of the air–water interface, some epithelial cells produce a very efficient surfactant mixture. Surfactant molecules have a water affinity polar side and an air affinity apolar side [14].

1.4   Structural Effect and Hysteresis

The surface tension magnitude depends on the concentration of the surfactant molecules at the air–liquid interface. During the respiratory cycle changes in the total area of the lung alter the air–liquid interface area. Consequently the surfactant concentration at the interface vary together with the surface tension magnitude. That is, surface tension increases during inspiration and decreases during expiration.

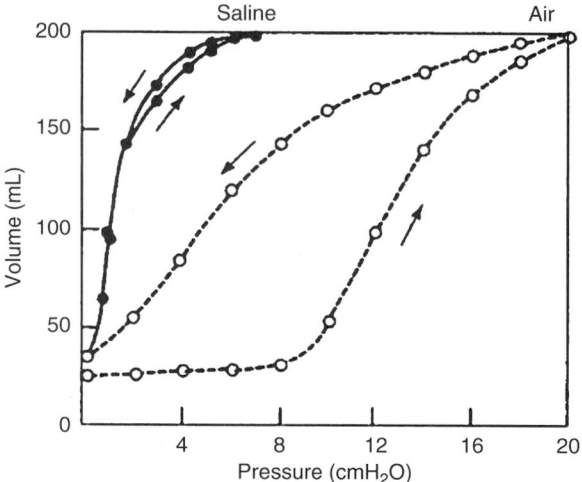

Fig. 2 Pressure–volume graphs of cat excised lungs. Lungs inflated with saline (*solid line*) and air (*dashed line*)

During inspiration, an excess surfactant molecules are recruited to the interface when the concentration there drops below the saturation level, and at expiration the decrease in interface area causes the expulsion of surplus molecules [15]. The dynamics of interface area, concentration of surfactant at the interface and surface tension causes part of the lung hysteresis, see Fig. 2, although much of the hysteresis is caused by successive collapses and recruitments of pieces of lung parenchyma.

The surface tension also has structural function, because it increases the stiffness of the lung parenchyma and supports part of the load. Fortunately, this increased stiffness is much higher in lung volumes near total lung capacity, since the increased surface area of parenchyma reduces the concentration of surfactant at the interface [16].

1.5   Atelectasis

Atelectasis is a lung condition in which part of the lung collapses preventing air flow there. Atelectasis can be acute or chronic and can affect the entire lung or part of it. From the physical point of view atelectasis occurs when moist membranes of the parenchyma touch themselves, leading to the fusion of the liquid layers, what consequently reduces the surface energy. The collapsed region can only be recruited if subjected to a higher contrary pressure to the adhesion pressure. The surfactant is very important to detach the adhered membranes because it makes easier to increase the area of the interface liquid–air with lower surface tension.

Despite the biomedical literature addressing the surface tension as the cause of atelectasis, no tribological studies of the septa surfaces were found. The mechanism of adhesion of the septa and the forces involved in it are still not well understood [17].

2 Objective

A fundamental building block for developing a structural model capable of simulating pulmonary alveolar recruitment manoeuvres is an element of contact with adhesion caused by the surface tension. A constitutive equation for this element is proposed and evaluated numerically in a simple structure using the non-linear finite element method.

3 Methodology

A constitutive equation for the contact with adhesion finite element is formulated. In order to validate this model a simulation of the contact between a simplified membrane and a undeformable surface is conducted. This simulation is performed with the finite element method (FEM). Because problems involving large deformations, rotations, and particularly contact are not linear, an algorithm for finding equilibrium configurations had to be used. Since the contact element's constitutive equation introduce critical points to the system, the arc-length method was implemented to avoid numerical instabilities.

3.1 Constitutive Equation

The adhesive contact model developed here is simplified. The surface tension is considered constant and the geometry of the meniscus is approximated. The formulation is based on a number of assumptions announced below, which are illustrated in the Fig. 3.

h1. The liquid film is continuous on both membrane surfaces. At height h from the surface, molecular attraction forces start to be significant (see Fig. 3g). At greater distances, $d > 2h$, the attraction forces are negligible.

h2. At a distance $d \approx 2h \doteq d_2$ the liquid films begin to attract each other (see Fig. 3b) and a meniscus is formed between both surfaces (see Fig. 3c).

h3. The pressure inside the meniscus (or on the contact region) is stated by the Young–Laplace Law [18],

$$p_{YL} = \gamma \left(\frac{1}{r_1} + \frac{1}{r_2} \right). \tag{1}$$

h4. The surface of the meniscus has two curvature radii, but only the one proportional to distance is considered $r = r_1 = d/2$ (see Fig. 3d).

(continued)

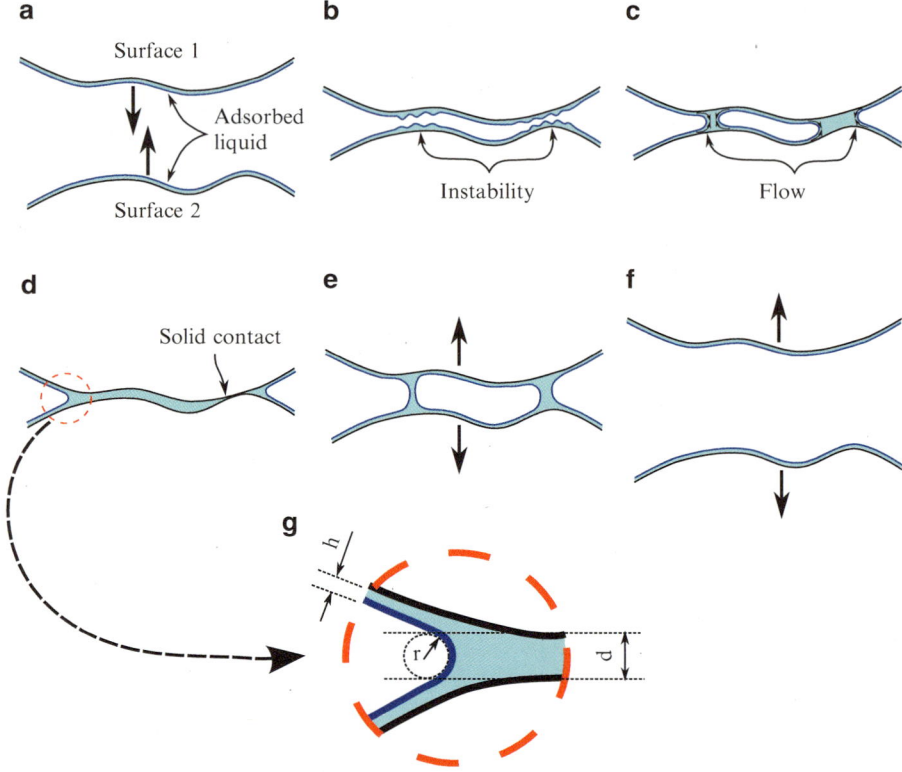

Fig. 3 Outline of the adhesive contact between two surfaces. (**a**) Approaching. (**b**) The force of molecular attraction draws the liquid into the region where the surfaces are closer. (**c**) When liquid films fuse and the meniscus is formed, more liquid is attracted to the region. (**d**) The approach ends when the roughness of the surfaces touch themselves. (**e**) Withdrawing. (**f**) Detached surfaces. (**g**) Detail of the contact showing the geometric variables

(continued)

The second radius is neglected in (1), because it is much higher than the first ($r_2 \gg r_1$). The adhesion pressure becomes

$$\tilde{p}_{YL}(d) = -\frac{2\gamma}{d}. \tag{2}$$

h5. At a distance d_1 when the roughness of the surfaces touch each other a reaction force arises, for the contact between solids (see Fig. 3d). At this distance the adhesion pressure is maximal, i.e. $\max\left(p_{YL}(d)\right) = p_{YL}(d_1)$. For preventing the interpenetration of the solid surfaces, the reaction forces must increase with greater intensity than the adhesion forces as the distance approaches zero.

h6. The adhesion work is reversible. That is, the work to detach the surfaces is equal to the work to join them.

3.2 Formulation

Since $d \in \mathbb{R}_+$, (2) is a negative hyperbole. In order to include the hypotheses h1 and h5, the adhesion pressure must act only within the range of $d_1 < d < d_2$ and the solid contact reaction in $d < d_1$. To satisfy all hypotheses the constitutive equation $p_\gamma(d)$ should be formulated with the following characteristics: $p_\gamma(0) < 0$, $p_\gamma(d) \approx \tilde{p}_{YL}(d) < 0$ within $d_1 < d < d_2$, $p_\gamma(d) \approx 0$ for $d < d_2$. Finally, to allow the application of the Newton-Raphson algorithm for finding equilibrium configurations, the constitutive equation's first derivative $p_\gamma'(d)$ have to be smooth.

There are some possibilities for $p_\gamma(d)$ function, which can be split in a portion of contact reaction $p_c(d)$ and another of adhesion $p_{ad}(d)$,

$$p_\gamma(d) = p_c(d) + p_{ad}(d), \tag{3}$$

whose derivative is

$$p_\gamma'(d) = p_c'(d) + p_{ad}'(d). \tag{4}$$

The contact reaction was defined as

$$p_c(d) = p_{c_0} e^{-\alpha d}, \tag{5}$$

where $p_{c_0} = p_c(0)$. It is defined such that at the distance d_1 the contact pressure is one percent of that at $d = 0$, therefore α is a constant obtained by

$$p_c(d_1) = 0,01 p_c(0) \qquad \Leftrightarrow \qquad \alpha = \ln \frac{100}{d_1}. \tag{6}$$

The derivative of the contact pressure is

$$p_c'(d) = -\alpha p_{c_0} e^{-\alpha d}. \tag{7}$$

The class of sigmoid functions have interesting properties to approximate (2) in $d_1 < d < d_2$. They form a smooth step function ("S" shaped curve in Fig. 4) inside the range and are asymptotically constant outside it. Some examples of sigmoid functions are the logistic function, arctangent, hyperbolic tangent and *erf* error function. For convenience, the logistic function will be used:

$$p_{lg}(t) = \frac{1}{1 + e^{-t}}, \tag{8}$$

Fig. 4 Graph of the logistic
function, (8)

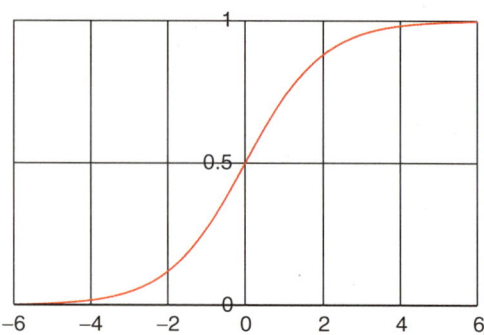

whose derivative is

$$p'_{lg}(t) = \frac{e^{-t}}{(1 + e^{-t})^2} = p_{lg}(1 - p_{lg}), \qquad (9)$$

whose graphic can be seen in Fig. 4.

For (8) to approximate (2) some adjustments must be made. Transforming the range $d : [d_1, d_2]$ to $t : [-5, 5]$ of (8) leads to

$$t(d) = \frac{10}{d_2 - d_1} \left[d - \left(\frac{d_1 + d_2}{2} \right) \right] \qquad (10)$$

and

$$t'(d) = \frac{10}{d_2 - d_1}. \qquad (11)$$

To $p_{ad}(d_1) \approx \tilde{p}_{YL}(d_1)$ and $p_{ad}(d_2) \approx 0$, (8) and (9) are transformed into

$$p_{ad}(d) = \frac{2\gamma}{d_1} \left[1 - p_{lg}(t(d)) \right] \qquad (12)$$

and

$$p'_{ad}(d) = \frac{2\gamma}{d_1} t'(d) p'_{lg}(t(d)). \qquad (13)$$

Finally, a value for p_{c_0} in (5) is chosen, such that $p_\gamma(0) = \tilde{p}_{c_0}$. By stressing (5) and (12) inside (3) at $d = 0$,

$$p_\gamma(0) = p_{c_0} - \frac{2\gamma}{d_1} = \tilde{p}_{c_0} \quad \Leftrightarrow \quad p_{c_0} = \tilde{p}_{c_0} + \frac{2\gamma}{d_1}. \qquad (14)$$

With p_{c_0} of (14) in (5) and (12), (3) can be fully rewritten,

$$p_{ad}(d) = \left(p_{c_0} + \frac{2\gamma}{d_1} \right) e^{-\ln\left(\frac{100}{d_1}\right)d} + \frac{2\gamma}{d_1} \left\{ 1 - \frac{1}{1 + e^{-\frac{10}{d_2 - d_1}\left[d - \left(\frac{d_1 + d_2}{2}\right)\right]}} \right\}. \qquad (15)$$

Equations 3 and 4 are illustrated in Figs. 5 and 6, respectively.

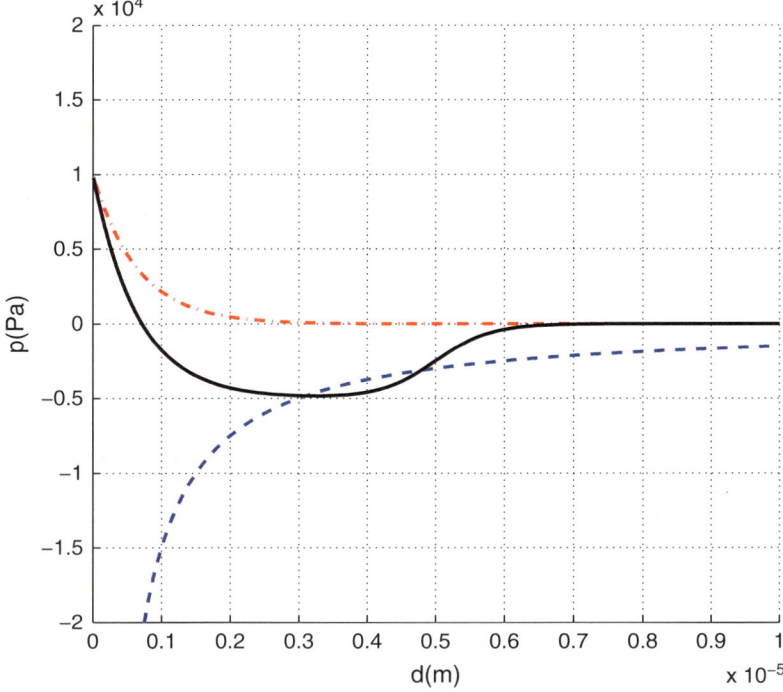

Fig. 5 Graphs showing the pressure of Young–Laplace's Law in *dashed line* ($\tilde{p}_{YL}$ of (2)), dry contact in *dashed-dot line* (p_c, (5)) and the constitutive equation of surface tension adhesive contact in *continuous line* (p_y, (3)). The parameters of the equations are: $\gamma = 7.5 \cdot 10^{-3}$ N/m, $d_1 = 3 \cdot 10^{-6}$ m, $d_2 = 7 \cdot 10^{-6}$ m, $p_{c_0} = 2 \cdot 10^4$ Pa

3.3 Viability Test

Because the significance of capilarity effects relies on the length scale, the proposed constitutive equation have to be evaluated on a structure with the length scale of an alveolus. In order to reduce the test's numerical complexity, a simple approximate geometry was used. The human alveoli have an average diameter of $D \approx 0.3$ mm [19]. Simplifying to 2D, a central section of a sphere of this diameter is a circle with perimeter $P = \pi D \approx 0.9$ mm. A rectangle with the same perimeter can then be taken $P = 2(l_1 + l_2) \approx 2(0.30 + 0.15)$ mm, as shows Fig. 7. This is a fairly reasonable approximation since some portions of the lung tend to deform in a non-uniform way.

The membrane of the inter-alveolar septum is simulated with non-linear first-order isoparametric truss elements [20], with the Kirchhoff material model [21] as constitutive equation. The value of Young's modulus for collagen, $E = 10^9$ Pa [8], was chosen as material constant. Despite the Young's modulus (E) and Kirchhoff material's constant (C^{SE}) relate different strain measures, they differ very little for small uniaxial strains. That is, at small strains the first Piola–Kirchhoff stress

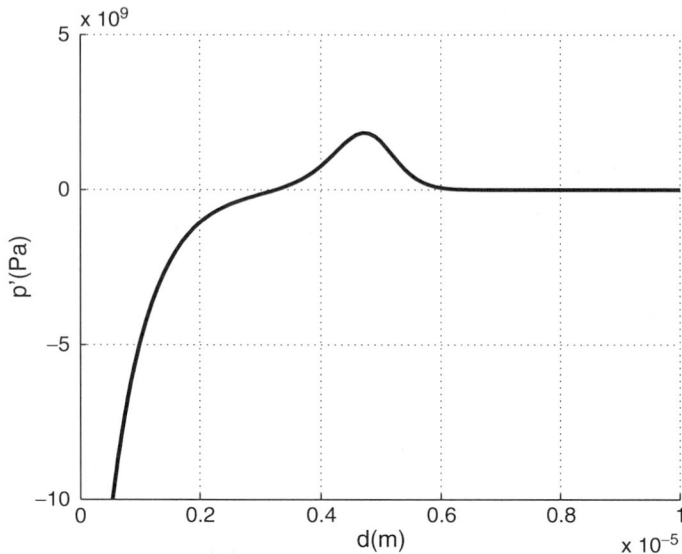

Fig. 6 Graphs of the constitutive equation of surface tension adhesive contact derivative (p'_γ of (4)). Same parameters of Fig. 5

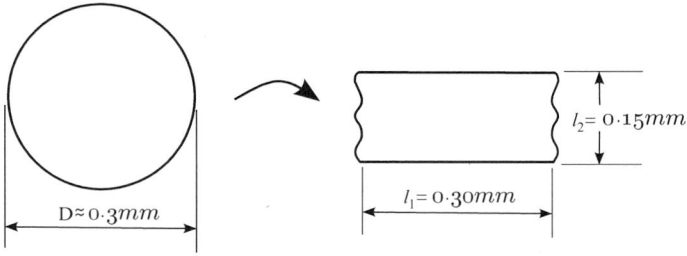

Fig. 7 Geometric approximation of a circle to a rectangle with the same perimeter

tensor is approximately equal to the second Piola–Kirchhoff: $P \approx S$, and the engineering strain is approximately equal to the Green–Lagrange's ($\epsilon \approx E$). As the collagen maximum strain level is low, $\epsilon_{max} = 2\%$ [8, 22], the approximation error of E to C^{SE} is 1%, which makes this approach acceptable. Using the collagen Young's module is reasonable since this is the fibre that resists large soft tissues' deformations.

The thickness of the collagen structural section is difficult to estimate, since at this scale the collagen is presented as fibre bundles and not as continuum. However the collagen bundles usually have an average diameter between 0.2 and 12 μm [8]. Considering the section of the membrane geometry as seen in Fig. 7, which by one side has the length of the alveolus (l_1) and by the other the height (h) equivalent to the fibre thickness, a reasonable area for the bar section could be $A_{bar} = l_1 \cdot h = 3 \cdot 10^{-4} \cdot 1.3 \cdot 10^{-6} \approx 4 \cdot 10^{-10}$ mm.

The height of the liquid film was arbitrarily defined as $3.5\,\mu m$, which means by the hypothesis h2 that the adhesion starts at a distance between membranes of $d_2 = 7 \cdot 10^{-6}$ m. The distance of the roughness interference (hypothesis h5) was also chosen arbitrarily as $d_1 = 3 \cdot 10^{-6}$ m. The value of surface tension was chosen as $7.5 \cdot 10^{-3}$ N/m, which is a physiological value [15].

3.4 Numerical Stability

The algorithm used to search the non-linear solution was the Newton–Raphson method [23]. Because the system has limit points, it was necessary to employ a continuation method to prevent divergence close to these points. The continuation method here applied was the arc-length method [24] linearised by Schweizerhof and Wriggers [25].

4 Results

From Figs. 8–16 a sequence of configurations related to different transmural pressures p_{tm} is shown. The thick lines represent the truss elements current position, the dash lines their initial positions and the circles represent the nodes. The fixed thin line indicate the opposed surface and the dash-dot line the distance d_2 from the opposed surface, or the position where the adhesion forces start and cease to affect the above membrane. The application of the arc-length algorithm makes it possible to find states of unstable equilibrium. Otherwise, an unstable degree of freedom could present big variations between iterations, which would induce numerical diversion.

It is interesting to observe the free nodes vertical trajectory, following the numerical steps. In Fig. 17 the trajectory of half-symmetric structure is shown. Figure 18 shows the adhesion of the central nodes in detail.

Figure 19 is a graph of pressure to cross-sectional area of the alveolus (analogous to the volume in excised lungs), which clearly shows the hysteresis caused by the adhesion. The magnitude of the cross-sectional area was calculated by the trapezoid integration method. Each point in evidence in Fig. 19 is a configuration of a pre-set transmural pressure. Most of these configurations are shown in Figs. 8–16.

Figure 20 shows the equilibrium trajectory got by the arc-length method. The arc-length method prevent numerical snap-through and snap-back, which would destabilize the simulation.

5 Discussion

The sequel from Figs. 8–16 rebuilds the intuitively expected mechanics. The curve in Fig. 19 has the same pattern of hysteresis observed experimentally for whole lung, see Fig. 2. The difference of inclination level between the recruitment paths

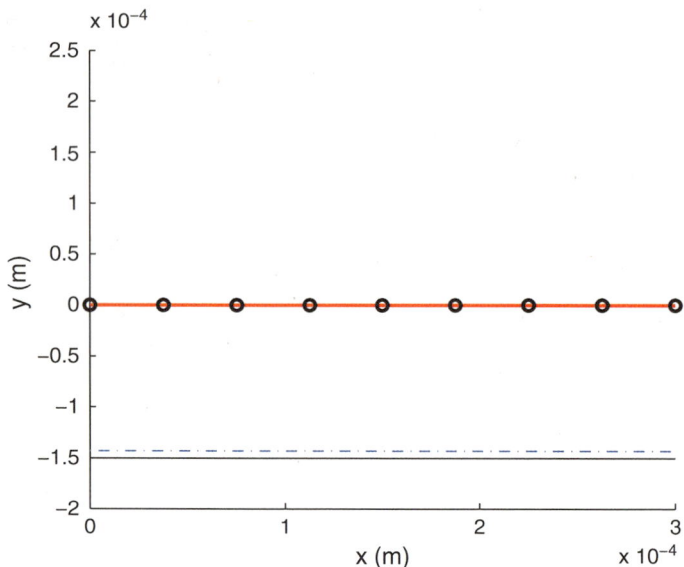

Fig. 8 Initial configuration at $p_{tm} = 0.0$ cmH$_2$O

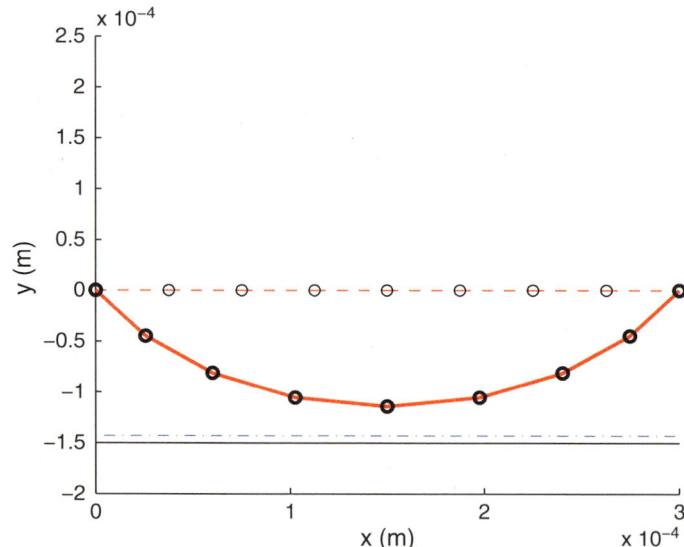

Fig. 9 Configuration at $p_{tm} = -4.0$ cmH$_2$O

of Figs. 19 and 2 results from the fact that the whole lung has many collapsed alveoli being recruited with different pressure levels. The variation of surfactant's concentration on the interface also affects the curve loop in Fig. 19, but this effect was neglected in Fig. 2.

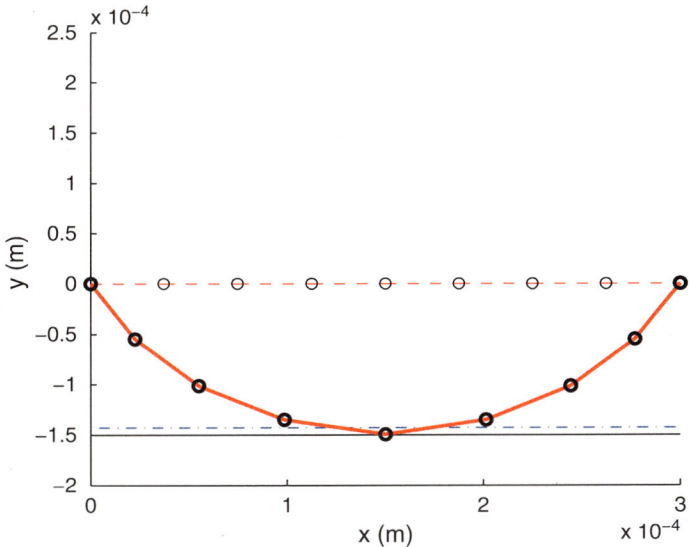

Fig. 10 Configuration at $p_{tm} = -8.0$ cmH$_2$O

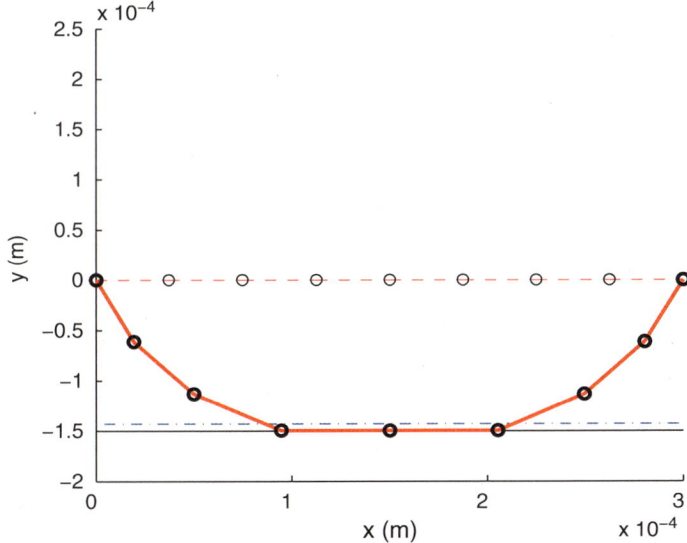

Fig. 11 Configuration at $p_{tm} = -12.0$ cmH$_2$O

Figure 17 shows the element nodes vertical trajectory as a function of transmural pressure. Two peaks of pressure can be seen, which correspond to attachment and detachment of the central node (node 5) and the nodes next to it (node 4 and its symmetric pair, node 6). The lowest transmural pressure level ($p_{tm} \approx 14$ cmH$_2$O)

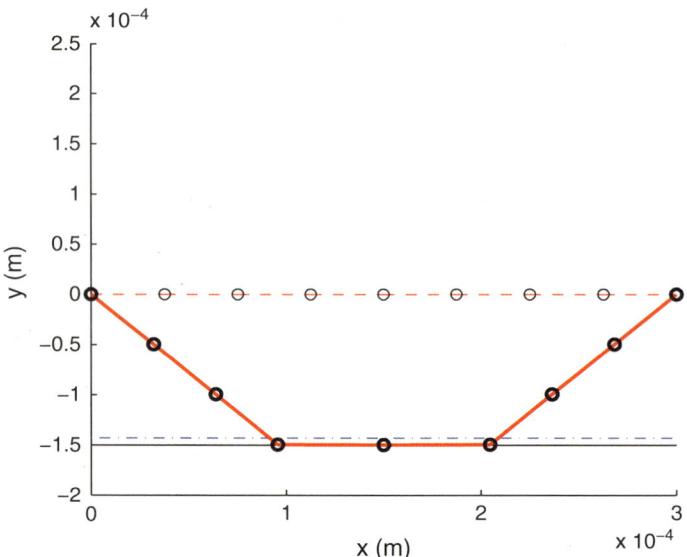

Fig. 12 Configuration at $p_{tm} = 0.0$ cmH$_2$O

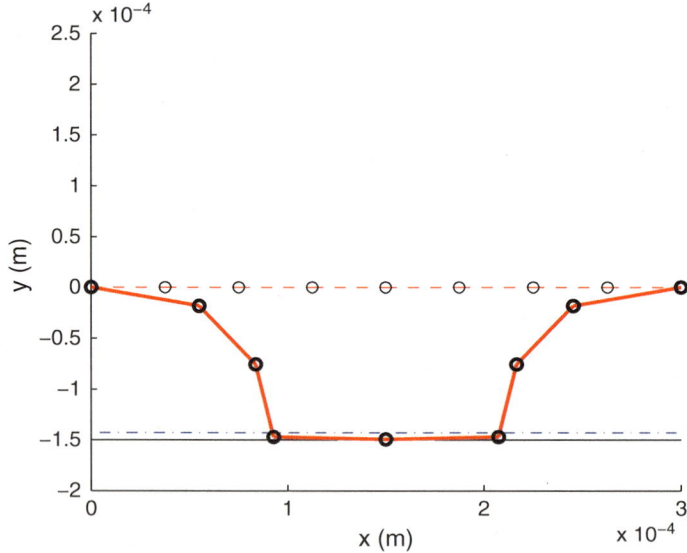

Fig. 13 Configuration at $p_{tm} = 30.0$ cmH$_2$O

corresponds to the adhesion pressure of the central node and the highest ($p_{tm} \approx$ 30 cmH$_2$O) to the nodes next to the central one. Figure 18 highlights the movement of the central nodes, the ones which undergo adhesion. It is important to remember hypothesis h6, which means that the work needed either to attach or detach are conservative.

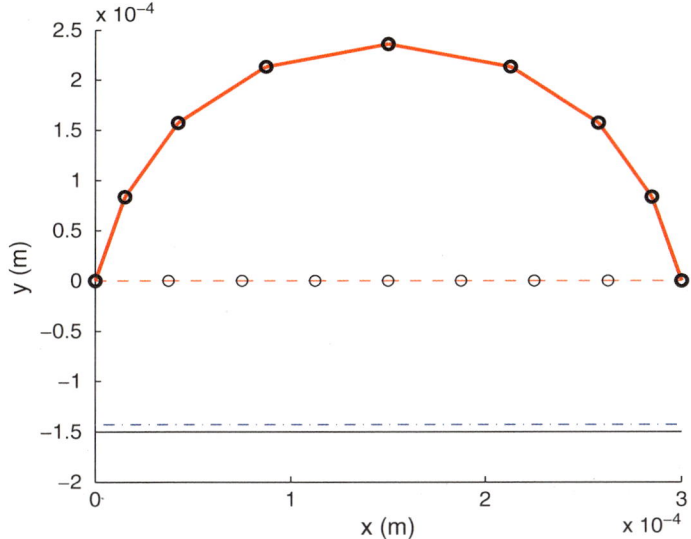

Fig. 14 Configuration at $p_{tm} = 30.5$ cmH$_2$O

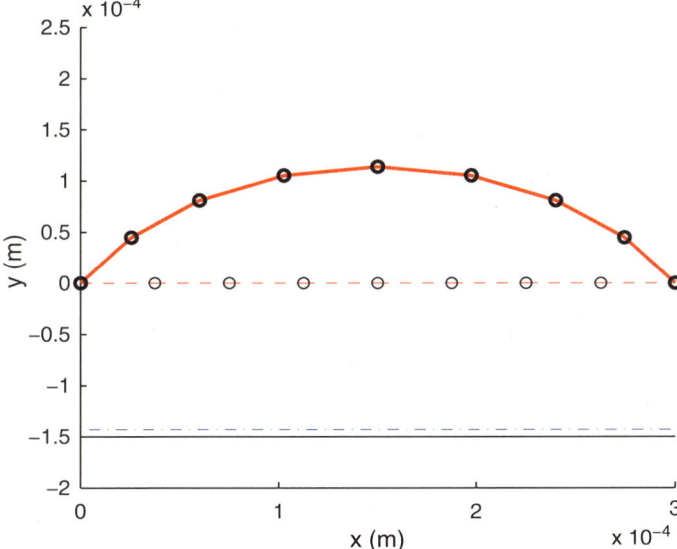

Fig. 15 Configuration at $p_{tm} = 4.0$ cmH$_2$O

From the standpoint of structural stability, there are limit points at the adhesion zone border, and therefore it was necessary to apply the arc-length method. Without the arc-length method each node entering or quitting the adhesion configuration would snap-through, which leads to numerical instabilities. The degrees of freedom near limit points present almost horizontal derivatives. Then big displacements

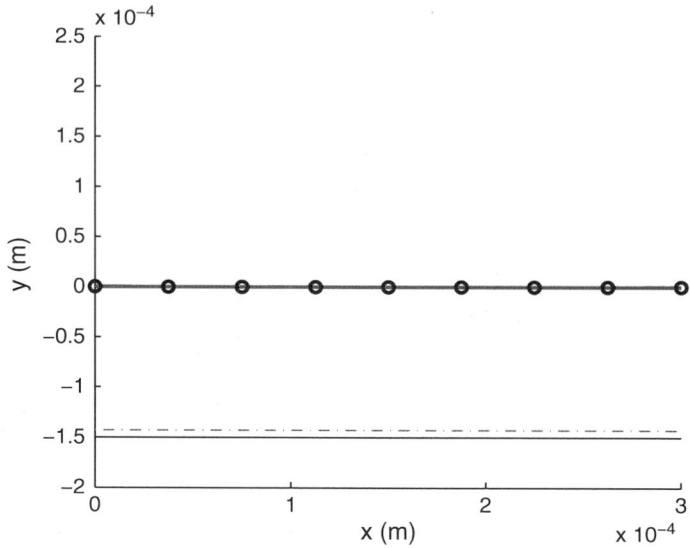

Fig. 16 Final configuration at $p_{tm} = 0.0$ cmH$_2$O

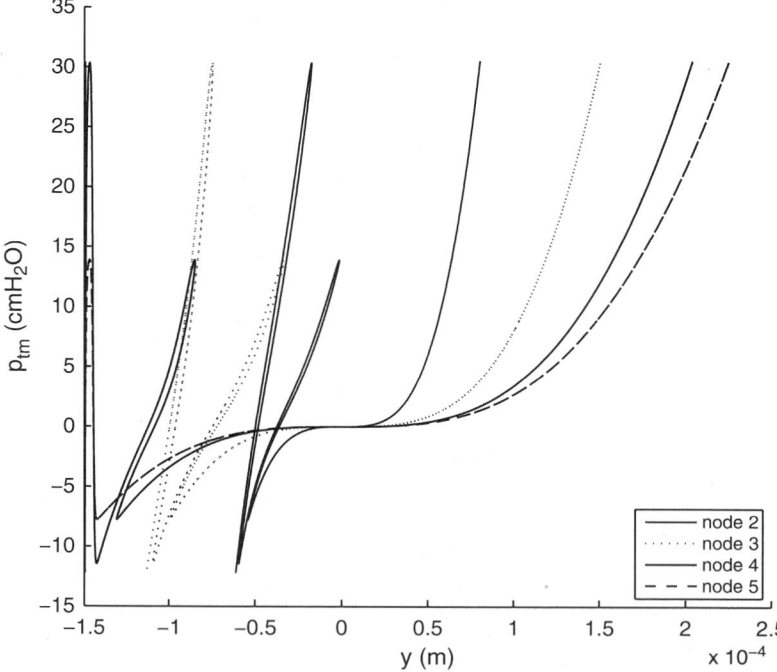

Fig. 17 Graphs of pressure to vertical displacement of the nodes of the membrane half-symmetric part

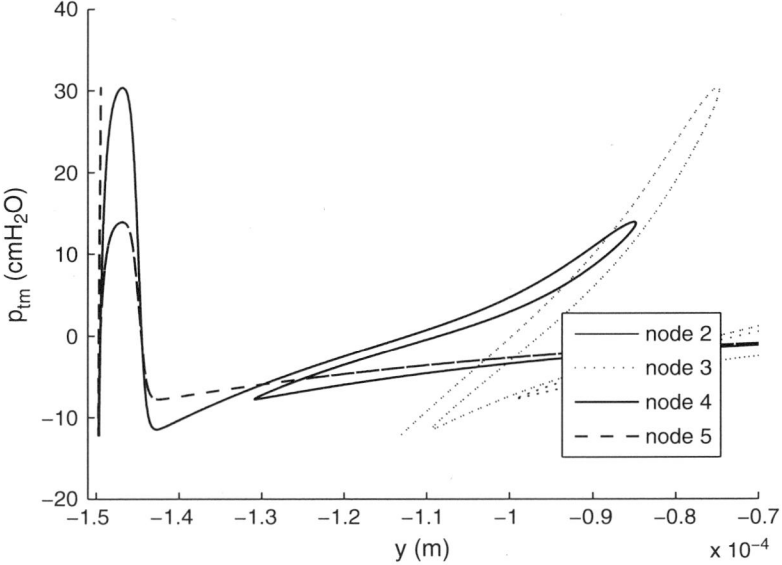

Fig. 18 The same curves of Fig. 17, highlighting the central nodes 4 and 5

are inevitably produced by the Newton–Raphson method in these soft stiffness configurations. A big displacement of one degree of freedom may unduly drag other degrees of freedom to either inside or outside the adhesion zones. Abrupt variations of derivative magnitudes usually lead to either numerical instability or wrong results.

Controlling step evolution allows to find intermediate equilibrium positions to snap-through and snap-backs. These results are almost impossible to be observed experimentally. To reconcile the numerical results with ones experimentally observed, Fig. 19 shows only some stable equilibrium configurations found for desired transmural pressure levels (points in evidence) and disregards the equilibrium path that might show unstable configurations. If the whole arc-length trajectories were regarded, path morphology would be like in Fig. 20. It would not be a closed curve and the energy barriers of the adhesive contact would be visible.

The open curve in Fig. 20 indicates that the adhesion work with continuous surface tension is conservative, which is consistent with the hypothesis of h6. Hysteresis is a characteristic of non-conservative systems and it just appears in the results when snap-through is considered. The snap-through occurs when the equilibrium of the whole system is not quasi-statically controlled. Since it is impracticable to completely control a continuum medium, a theoretical conservative system end up becoming non-conservative. Both the attached and detached conditions are conditions of minimum potential energy, with an energy barrier between them. In Fig. 20 it is possible to see the nodes 4 and 5 getting up and down not through an energy barrier but through a transmural pressure barrier, with peaks near $y = -1.43 \cdot 10^{-4}$ m.

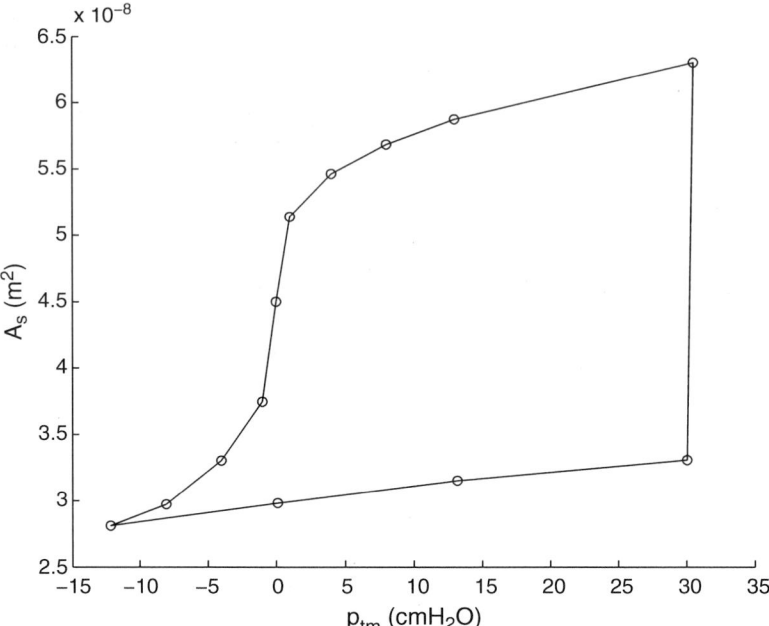

Fig. 19 Graph of pressure vs. cross-sectional area of the alveolus, showing hysteresis

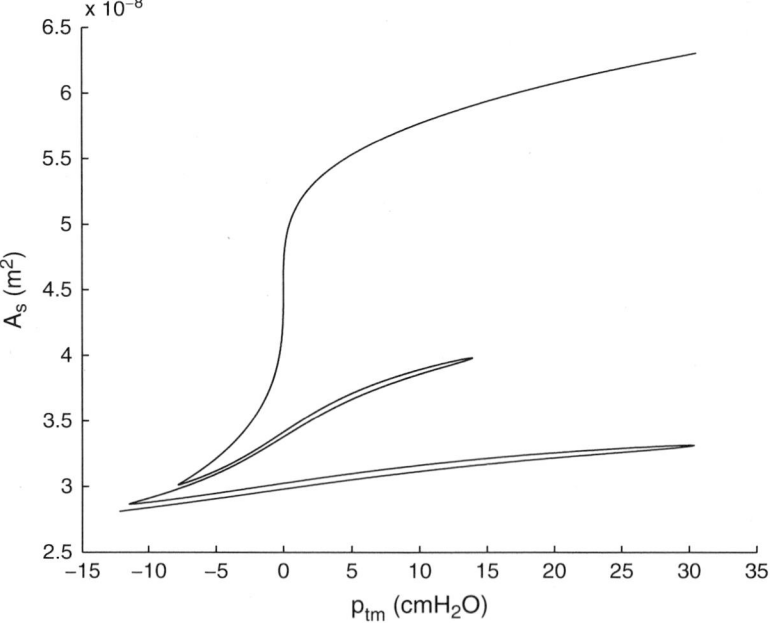

Fig. 20 Graph of pressure vs. cross-sectional area of the alveolus, showing the equilibrium path

6 Conclusions

The adhesive contact element proposed here can reproduce the hysteresis loop observed in the collapse and recruitment of a group of alveoli, in agreement with the order of magnitude of the involved physical measures. Recruitment is triggered at higher pressures than the collapse, which is the same asymmetry observed experimentally. However it does not reproduce the viscous dissipative aspects of lung dynamics, such as liquid flow, variation of surfactant concentration and tissue viscoelasticity.

This finite element simulations can be applied to large populations of alveoli, which would allow a more realistic structural analysis. Another big advantage of this element is that its parameters can be adjusted with experimental measurements. However the adhesion magnitude on the surface of the alveoli still has to be measured by tribological experiments. The relationship between the surfactant, the liquid film and the surface of the epithelial cell membrane also needs to be better understood.

Even without reliable parameters for a more accurate assessment for the estimation of the intensity of the adhesion forces, this contact element can already simulate aspects not found in the literature.

Acknowledgements This work was supported by the National Counsel of Technological and Scientific Development ("Conselho Nacional de Desenvolvimento Cientfico e Tecnolgico" – CNPq) 135262/2007-0.

References

1. Moore KL, Dalley AF (2001) Anatomia orientada para a clínica, 4th edn. Guanabara Koogan, Rio de Janeiro
2. Fung YC (1975b) Dose the surface tension make the lung inherenthly unstable? Circ Res 37:497
3. Fung YC (1975a) Stress, deformation, and atelectasis of the lung. Circ Res 37:481
4. Bassingthwaighte JB (2000) Strategies for the physiome project. Ann Biomed Eng 28:1043
5. Hoppin FG, Lee GC, Dawson SV (1975) Properties of lung parenchyma in distortion. J Appl Physiol 39(5):742
6. Vawter DL, Fung YC, West JB (1978) Elasticity of excised dog lung parenchyma. J Appl Physiol 45(2):261
7. Zeng YJ, Yager D, Fung YC (1987) Measurement of mechanical properties of the human lung parenchyma. J Biomech Eng 109:169
8. Fung YC (1993) Biomechanics: mechanical properties of living tissues, 2nd edn. Springer, New York
9. Hansen JE, Ampaya EP, Bryant GH, Navin JJ (1975) The branching pattern of airways and air spaces of a single human terminal bronchiole. J Appl Physiol 38(6):983
10. Hansen JE, Ampaya EP (1975) Human air space shapes, sizes, areas, and volumes. J Appl Physiol 38(6):990
11. Dale PJ, Matthews FL, Schroter RC (1980) Finite element analysis of lung alveolus. J Biomech 13:865

12. Fung YC (1988) A Model of the lung structure and its validation. J Appl Physiol 64:2132
13. Tawhai MH, Burrowes KS (2003) Developing integrative computational models of pulmonary structure. Anat Rec B New Anat 275B:207
14. Veldhuizen R, Nag K, Orgeig S, Possmayer F (1998) The role of lipids in pulmonary surfactant. Biochim Biophys Acta 1408:90
15. Schürch S, Lee M, Gehr P (1992) Pulmonary surfactant: surface properties and function of alveolar and airway surfactant. Pure Appl Chem 64:1745
16. Schürch S, Bachofen H, Goerke J, Possmayer F (2001) Surface activity in situ, in vivo, and in the captive bubble surfactometer. Comp Biochem Physiol A 129:195
17. Hills BA (1999) An alternative view of the role(s) of surfactant and the alveolar model. J Appl Physiol 87:1567
18. Butt HJ, Kappl M (2010) Surface and interfacial forces. Wiley-VCH Verlag GmbH & Co. KGaA, Weinheim, Alemanha
19. McArdle WD, Katch FI, Katch VL (2006) Exercise physiology: energy, nutrition, and human performance, 6th edn. Lippincott Williams & Wilkins, Baltimore, EUA
20. Felippa C (2001) Nonlinear finite element method. Department of Aerospace Engineering Sciences and Center for Space Structures and Controls: University of Colorado, Boulder. http://www.colorado.edu/engineering/CAS/courses.d/NFEM.d/Home.html
21. Reddy JN (2008) An introduction to continuum mechanics. Cambridge University Press, Cambridge/Reino Unido
22. Maksym GN, Bates JHT (1997) A distributed nonlinear model of lung tissue elasticity. J Appl Physiol 82(1):32
23. Wriggers P (2008) Nonlinear finite element methods. Springer, Berlin
24. Crisfield MA (1981) A fast incremental/iterative solution procedure that handles "snap-through". Comput Struct 13:55
25. Schweizerhof KH, Wriggers P (1986) Consistent linearization for path following methods in nonlinear FE analysis. Comput Method Appl Mech Eng 59:261

Biomechanical Characterization and Modeling of Natural and Alloplastic Human Temporomandibular Joint

Michel Mesnard and Antonio Ramos

Abstract To improve reduced functions of the temporomandibular joint, total replacement involves removing the non-functional joint and replacing it with an artificial one. Recent prostheses may lead to different cases of failure that require additional surgical procedures. Some solutions are available to improve the artificial joint survival rate. Materials and geometry play important key roles in enhancing the long-term life of the joint, but the biomechanics of the human masticatory system must also be well characterized. Forces applied to the mandible by muscles, articular joints and teeth need to be determined to assess the strain and stress patterns of the whole mandible and particularly of the condyle area to control the effects of stress shielding. While the femur, for example, is a well-documented bone structure, this is not the case for the mandible bone; there seems to be little investigation in the literature into the biomechanics of the mandible.

The first part of the study describes the characterization of the muscular actions, i.e. the forces exerted by the elevator muscles that were considered: deep and superficial masseters, pterygoid and temporal. In vivo electromyography and MRI contributed to quantifying force intensities when the mandible was loaded. This load between the teeth was recorded using a sensor which also adjusted the mouth aperture. The description of the articular surfaces and the calculations of the muscular insertion co-ordinates were obtained from four cadaver dissections.

In the second part of the study, the synthetic mandible was digitized with a laser scanner device to build the finite element model. The solid model of the mandible was created with a modeling package after digitizing the surfaces. The study proved that the finite element model of the mandible can reproduce experimental strains

M. Mesnard (✉)
Université de Bordeaux, Institut de Mécanique et d'Ingénierie,
CNRS UMR 5295, Bordeaux, France
e-mail: michel.mesnard@u-bordeaux1.fr

A. Ramos
Department of Mechanical Engineering, University of Aveiro, Aveiro, Portugal

R.M.N. Jorge et al. (eds.), *Technologies for Medical Sciences*, Lecture Notes
in Computational Vision and Biomechanics 1, DOI 10.1007/978-94-007-4068-6_3,
© Springer Science+Business Media B.V. 2012

within an overall agreement level of 10%. The model correctly reproduced bone strains under different load configurations. For this reason, it adequately reproduces the mechanical behavior of the mandible and has therefore become an essential tool for predicting biomechanical changes in the mandible and long-term failure.

First, we describe mandible strains under natural loads. Using simulations we were able to define the worst boundary conditions for the condyle and the associated mandible behavior. Next, a plate implant was screwed onto one of the mandible ramus. The results were then used to determine the strains at the end of the plates and around the screws; the modified mandible strain patterns and mandible displacements are compared to demonstrate the influence of the implant on mandible behavior.

1   Introduction

The most common reason for replacing the temporomandibular joint (TMJ) is to relieve pain and to improve reduced function caused by arthritis [1].

Total replacement of the TMJ involves removing the non-functional joint and replacing it with an artificial one [2]. Due to the nature of the bone structures involved in this joint, prosthesis design is somewhat complex, and materials and geometry play an important key role in enhancing the long-term life of the artificial joint [1]. The most commonly applied TMJ implants are plates that are flat and rigid and surgeons can spend some hours bending a plate to fit it to the contours of the patient's bones [3].

Total TMJ replacement has seen several different stages of development from 1945 until now [4]. In the 1990s a negative experience with the Vitek-Kent prosthesis brought some discredit to TMJ replacements [1] and some were abandoned [5, 6]. The new prosthesis introduced in the last decade has increased its application in Europe [7].

1.1   Prosthesis Design

TMJ prosthesis design can be categorized into prostheses providing replacements for the fossa only (Fig. 1a), reconstruction plates to replace the condyle, and combined prostheses for fossa and condyle (Fig. 1b, c).

The evolution of TMJ joints in the UK resulted in a reevaluation of the principal models applied, the Christensen and Vitek-Kent prostheses. The TMJ-concept is the most popular, with a current estimated annual total of between 60 and 65 patients in the UK. The most common problem in TMJ revision is infection in 2% of cases, with problems occurring overall in around 9% or 170 cases (1999–2006) [1]. Surgeons are currently reported to charge from £15,000 to £19,000 for a TMJ prosthesis procedure.

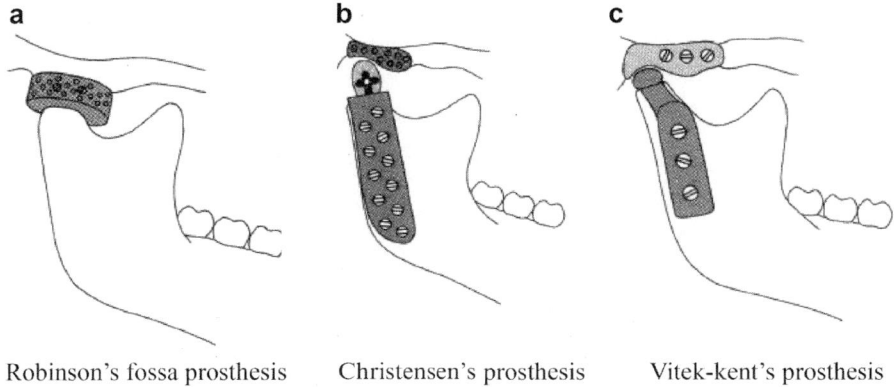

a	b	c
Robinson's fossa prosthesis	Christensen's prosthesis	Vitek-kent's prosthesis

Fig. 1 TMJ prostheses [8]

The first type of prosthesis, characterized by introducing an alloplastic material between the fossa and condyle, was used before the 1950s before 50th years. The applied materials were Tantalum, Cr-Co alloy, UHMWPE by different commercial prosthesis. The prosthesis used to replace the condyle was made of Titanium and Cr-Co alloy, and normally consisted of a plate with a flat geometry and fixed by screws.

Reconstruction with metallic materials modifies the physiological behavior of the mandible (stress and strain patterns and condyle displacements). As a result of the changing bone strains the TMJ and articular contacts must be adapted. Replacing a single condyle is preferable as a temporary TMJ replacement, maintaining the glenoïd fossa. Another type of TMJ implant is the custom-made variety; this may have some advantages related to its being a perfect fit [9], but they have to be evaluated in a long term-study to justify the extra costs.

Comparative studies of recent prostheses [3, 10] point out that the inter-incisor opening is almost 20 mm. Occlusion corrections clearly give the patient both psychological and physical comfort. On the other hand, these studies and Karray [11] point out different cases of failures that sometimes require additional surgical procedures:

– *Inflammation* can occur due to the choice of material, with persistence of pain revealing imperfect osteointegration (bone screws) consequently accompanied by implant micro-displacements with respect to the bone [12],
– *Prosthesis fracture* (rare) happens near a screw or in a sharp variation of the implant section where stresses tend to concentrate,
– *Bone connection fracture* is the result of an insufficient number of screws and/or a too high intensity of loads on the mandible condyle [13, 14].

There are several solutions available to improve the TMJ survival rate, but the most frequent consists of a plate and fixation screws [13, 14].

The analogical and empirical approach to prosthesis design relies on practices, tools, choices, etc. specific to the medical and industrial sectors concerned.

Before a reconstruction of the natural joint can be produced, it first has to be characterized and then the model is gradually built up. From observing the physical phenomena involved (geometry and behavior on contact, etc.) perspectives for experimental analysis can be decided on [15, 16]. This characterization provides a set of results and input data on which a preliminary model can be based. By exploiting the possibilities of this model and assessing its robustness it can be further strengthened and validated.

Simulation can often lead to more creative proposals for solutions, using new technologies (material, treatments, production, etc.) or innovative functional diagrams.

1.2   Protocol to Characterize TMJ Biomechanics

First, using a "mechanism theory" approach, the temporomandibular joint is likened to a mechanical joint between two undeformable solid bodies. The term joint here refers to the "contact" between the two elements. By its nature (localized, applied linearly or across a surface) and its geometry (surface area), this contact partially enables the six possible relative movements to take place and ensures that articular forces are transmitted.

The relationship between degrees of freedom (mobility) of the natural joint and forces that can be transmitted was characterized using results from three types of experimental reading:

- Cadaver dissections[1] to study functional anatomy and the geometry of the articular surfaces,
- Electromyography[2] and MRI[3] to study muscle actions,
- 3-D video analysis to study kinematics and observe articular displacements.

1.2.1   Cadaver Dissection

In the protocol, fresh cadavers were dissected so that the contact zones (nature of the contact) and the muscle anchor points could be observed. The directions of the muscle forces were determined experimentally by photographic readings and calculations.

---

[1] Dissections carried out with JC. Coutant in the Medical-Surgical Anatomy Department, University of Bordeaux.

[2] Electromyography readings taken at the University of Perm as part of the International Project on Scientific Cooperation CNRS-RFBR n°4280.

[3] MRI images produced at the University Teaching Hospital, Bordeaux.

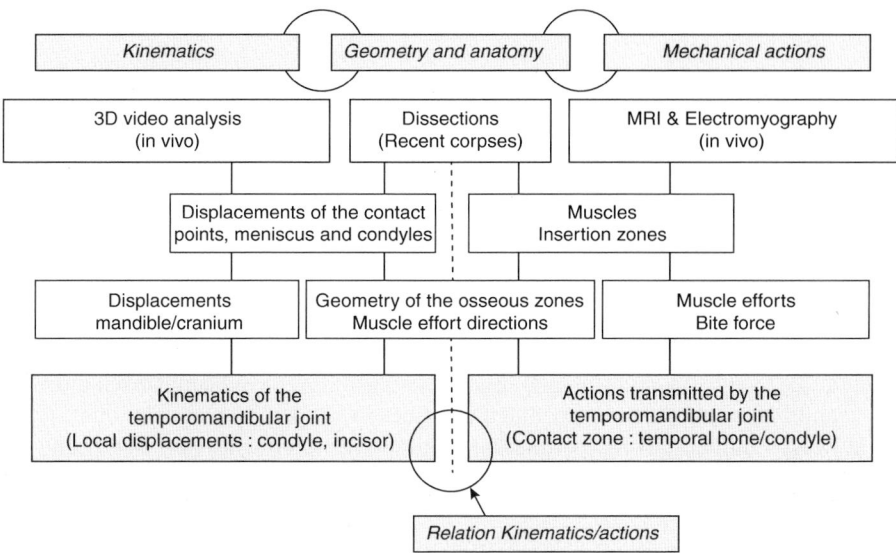

Fig. 2 Experimental protocol to characterize the TMJ

1.2.2 Electromyography and MRI

The protocol used electromyography and IRM data to evaluate the intensity of the action of the elevator muscles under loading. This load was measured by a sensor which also regulated the distance between the incisors. Articular contact forces could be determined by calculation.

1.2.3 3D Video Analysis

The protocol used 3D video analysis techniques to describe the overall kinematics of the mandible without loading. Displacements from a point on the mandible or from the centre of the joint were then obtained by calculation. From a population of 32 volunteers, the study established a correlation between the kinematic characteristics of the joint and the disk-condyle trajectories. The geometrical characteristics of the articular tubercle slope and inter-individual variations were quantified, which will be useful in TMJ prosthesis design [15–17].

1.2.4 Experimental Protocol

The organizational chart below shows the relationships between three types of experimental readings. The study of articular geometry and muscle forces are described in Sect. 2 (Fig. 2).

1.3   Finite Element Modeling of the Mandible

Numerical pre-clinical testing using Finite Element Models (FEM), for example, is becoming more important as an alternative to animal testing. This numerical technique has no ethical requirement or patient involvement in clinical trials [1, 18]. In this respect, computational modeling will be one of the most important tools for detecting implant performance in the short and long term. The design of TMJ prostheses presupposes the use of numerical tools like finite element analysis (FEA) [19, 20]. The finite element simulation has been criticized because of the lack of validation; however, it is the only way forward to explore 'possible' solutions. These FE models must be applied carefully and it is sensible that they should be "calibrated" using an experimental model. Some studies have been carried out with the mandible, applying experimental techniques to validate numerical models [21].

However, numerical or experimental simulation can influence and undermine the results of biomechanical analyses, by introducing configurations into the problem and associated variables. There are many issues in Finite Element Analysis [19, 22–27] that one must be aware of as well as data resulting from commercial FEA applications. FEM results must be examined with care, because this model presents some variables associated with the solution.

The FEM model results depend on simulation parameters like geometry replication, bone properties, boundary conditions and type of elements. The geometry of bone is irregular and finite element modeling is increasingly carried out using digitized images generated from computer tomography scanning [28–30] or micro-computer tomography for better resolution with small problems [30].

Another variable in FEM is bone materials, which are normally assumed to be isotropic and homogeneous, whereas it is known that they are highly anisotropic and inhomogeneous. This variable is a limitation when using FE models, because it is very complex to simulate the biological process and bone evolution.

Boundary conditions are relevant input conditions that can considerably alter and undermine the reliability of results. Loads applied to finite element models have been very much simplified and many published papers have analyzed all sorts of loading configurations. The model in [22, 31–34] presents 10 muscles, but other models present more [35]. Thus, there is a degree of uncertainty in determining which muscles are important, and their relevance to mechanical testing.

The biomechanics of the mandible and the TMJ is an extremely complex problem and the correct knowledge of the functioning of muscles and ligaments is unknown. Predicting muscle forces should be treated with caution since many assumptions are made when calculating them.

The finite element mesh is a key factor for an efficient analysis and much research has been done on meshing and element performance. Finite element models must be sufficiently refined to accurately represent the geometry [36, 37]. The results of these models are meshing sensitive and ideally a convergence test should be performed to test the model's accuracy [38].

Another difficulty in FEM simulation is related to the biomechanical boundary conditions applied to the mandible and how important they are in replicating physiological loading and kinematics.

Modeling the mandible using the finite element technique is described in Sect. 3.

2 Characterization of the Temporomandibular Joint

Three localized dissections, carried out on recently deceased patients, provided the qualitative and quantitative information needed for the geometrical analysis of the articulation. The protocol required information on morphological anatomy, the articular surfaces and the main masticatory muscles.

Three dissection planes (superficial, medial and deep) were observed to describe the articular surfaces and to determine the directions of the muscle actions. A geometric scale was used to for the subsequent exploitation of photographic data.

2.1 Geometry and Contacts of the Articular Surfaces

The parts of the temporal and mandibular surfaces involved and also their contacts evolve according to the interincisal opening. The contact model is not continuous and as a result, several loading configurations or examples must be considered.

2.1.1 Centric Occlusion and Occlusion from the Rest Position

Centric or maximum intercuspation occlusion, with a null opening and dental contact (occlusal faces of the dental crowns), corresponds to the swallowing position or also to those moments when mastication begins and ends. The mandibular condyle is situated at the base of the temporal glenoid. The contact, or more exactly the glenoid-condyle relationship, is established via the meniscus which does not support much weight.

The rest position (comfort occlusion), with lips closed, and with a slight dental opening (no dental contact), corresponds to reduced muscle tone, strong enough only to overcome gravity. The mandibular condyle is placed in the upper area of the temporal condyle without exerting any significant pressure on the disc. The space between the first two antagonistic premolars is then about 1–2 mm.

The obstacle of the incisor influences the positioning of the mandible. To overcome this obstacle, all propulsion movement starts by an opening movement needed to pass from the centric position to a null interincisor distance.

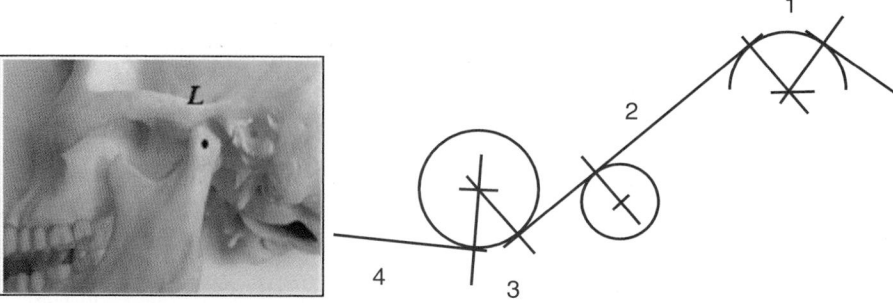

Fig. 3 Geometry of the temporal and mandibular surfaces (Bones *left* and model *right*)

2.1.2 Geometry of Articular Surfaces, Nature of Contacts

Geometric readings were taken of the bony areas at the end of dissection. The results established at this time were later confirmed in the 27-case statistical study [17].

The functional temporal articular surface consists essentially of the temporal slope (Fig. 3). Tension in the external lateral ligament limits the extent of the contact zone around the condyle eminence. Accidental anterior luxation and the blocking of the mandibular fossa in the mandibular condyle in the zygomatic fossa result from ligament distension or even rupture.

The temporal condyle, the root of the zygomatic arch, forms a double convex eminence, transversally and from front to back (frontal and sagittal planes). It extends forwards along an almost plane surface and backwards towards the glenoid fossa, which is doubly concave.

The glenoid fossa is about *7 mm* deep and the walls are *1 mm* thick at the bottom of the fossa. Around the condylar eminence, cortical thickness can be *10 mm*.

Only the anterior zone of the mandibular condyle is involved during contact. The condyle head, which is doubly convex, very often seems to be almost ellipsoid. The horizontal view of the semi-mandible shows an angle of about *90°* between the transverse axis of the condyle and the lateral axis of the mandible. When viewed from behind, the angle formed by the transverse axis and the rising branch is also about *90°*.

Except in pathological situations (perforation of the meniscus), the mandibular condyle and the temporal area do not come into direct contact. The meniscus, which is deformable, is interposed and takes on the shape of the two articular surfaces to modify the distribution of pressure on contact.

2.1.3 Elementary Contacts, First Models

When plane opening and protrusion movements are extremely wide they displace the centre of the mandibular condyle by about 22 mm. The relative position of the

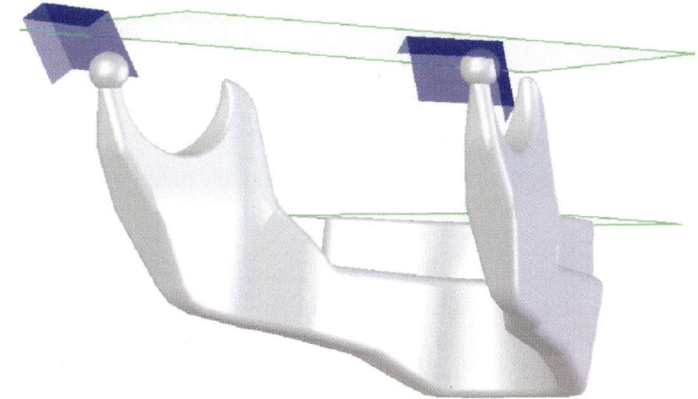

Fig. 4 Geometrical model of the TMJs under asymmetrical loading

two bony areas, and hence the location of the contact, changes with the displacement and/or the mandible loading.

The model associated with the elementary joint is for the most part the result of the local geometry of the articular surfaces. As this geometry of the temporal surface evolves, the area is divided into four simple geometric sectors (Fig. 3).

Under plane loading on the mandible (symmetrical tightening), the elementary joint can thus be modeled by an isolated contact which, depending on the opening, is located in sector 2 or sector 3 (Fig. 3). The perpendicular to the tangent plane, which is common to the two surfaces, is not contained in a horizontal or parasagittal plane.

When loading is asymmetrical (unilateral tightening), the median plane of the mandible is not combined with the sagittal plane. This displacement of the jaw results in different configurations for the two elementary joints. For the "open" or "working" profile, the mandibular condyle comes into contact occasionally with the temporal slope mainly as a result of the action of the masseters (sectors 2 or 3). The opposite condyle tends to move back simultaneously into the glenoid towards its highest point (sector 1). The geometries of the local surfaces that are in contact tend to be directed towards modeling a linear annular type of joint. The ligaments (mainly the external lateral) restrict the amplitude of transversal displacement to 1 or 2 mm when movements are almost plane (excluding lateral excursion). In this configuration, the hinge joint then takes on the same behavior as a kneecap.

The model (Fig. 4) corresponding to asymmetrical loading (with the sensor in position 34 or 36) presents one point of contact for the left mandible condyle or a "ball-and-plane pair" (1BPP) and a "spherical pair" (1SP, joint with two links allowing spherical motion of one link relative to the other) for the right condyle. This model is described further in Sect. 3 when defining the limiting conditions for modeling the mandible.

2.2　Actions of the Jaw-Closing Muscles

This section presents a 3D method analyzing and quantifying the muscle forces exerted on the mandible under loadings. The experimental protocol is described and data from four volunteers are presented.

A sensor had been designed to simulate and register the bite force between two teeth, when placed successively between two incisors, two premolars and then two molars.

We were able to describe contacts between the mandible condyles and the temporal bone and also the insertions of the jaw closing-muscles after carrying out dissections. The directions of the muscular forces were thus determined in a morphological coordinate system. Using in vivo MRI and electromyography data, we were able to evaluate the magnitudes of six muscle forces on each side of the face.

2.2.1　Biomechanical Model and Volunteers

The morphological symmetry of the face was admitted with respect to the sagittal plane.

Reference Coordinate System

Most papers analyzing actions exerted on the mandible exploit an undefined or exotic coordinate system to express the results. This study used a functional and anatomical reference coordinate system attached to the Camper's plane (Fig. 5). This coordinate system (noted S_c), like the one used to study the jaw motion, was associated to the three morphological points defining the plane: point N, the sub nasal point, points L and R, the centers of the left and right condyles in the intercuspidation position. Using the 3D video analysis to determine the co-ordinates of these three points, the coordinate system S_c was the following:

- The origin C was the middle of the segment defined by the two condyle centers,
- The x-axis passed through the two TMJ centers (positive x-axis towards the left),
- The z-axis was defined by points C and N (positive z-axis from C towards N),
- The y-axis completed the system (perpendicular to the Camper's plane, positive y-axis upward). The basis associated to these three axes was noted b.

Jaw-Closing Muscles

Three pairs of muscles on the left and right sides of the face mainly rise up from the mandible and contribute to transmitting the forces that are used for speaking or for chewing: the masseter muscles, the medial pterygoid muscle and the temporal

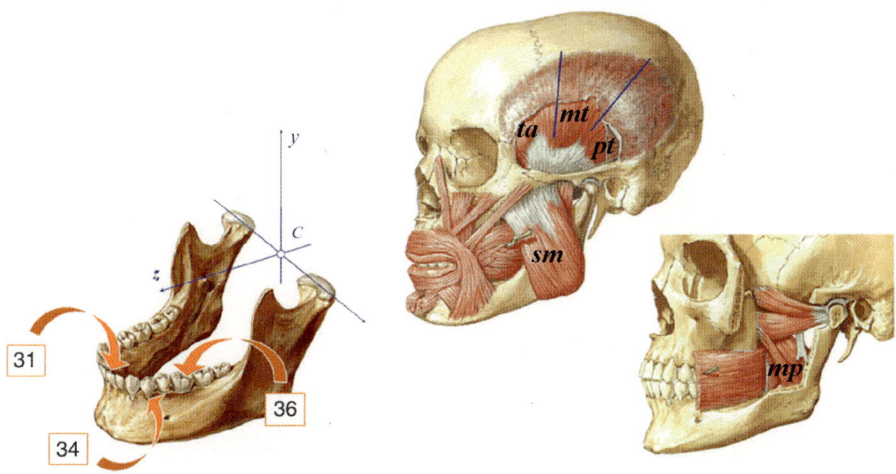

Fig. 5 Biomechanical model, mandible and jaw-closing muscles

muscles (Fig. 5). These three pairs of muscles were taken into account to build a mathematical model of the TMJ forces in order to increase the precision of the results [39].

The masseter muscle, which is short and wide, presents two parts. The thick surface masseter (noted *sm*) arises from the anterior part of the zygomatic arch. Its fibers are inserted into the mandible angle and constitute a powerful elevator. Its direction contributes to mandible propulsion. The deep masseter (noted *dm*), which is smaller, arises from the posterior part of the zygomatic arch. Its fibers are inserted into the lateral surface of the mandible coronoid process and remain almost normal to the occlusion plane.

The medial pterygoid muscle (noted *mp*) remains parallel to the inner side of the mandible. It is inserted just above the medial surface of the lateral pterygoid plate and into the lower and back part of the medial surface of the mandible ramus. It is a powerful elevator that also helps in propelling and side to side movement of the jaw.

The temporal muscle arises from the temporal fossa, passes through the zygomatic arch and is inserted onto the mandible coronoid process. Broad and flat, it can be subdivided into three bundles to model its action by three forces (Fig. 5). The anterior bundle (noted *ta*) simultaneously propels and lifts the mandible. The medial bundle (noted *mt*) whose fibers are virtually orthogonal to the occlusion plane primarily lifts the jawbone. Finally, the fibers of the posterior bundle (noted *pt*), which also present some insertions on the TMJ meniscus contribute to the retro-propelling movement.

2.2.2 Location of the Insertion Points, Directions of the Muscle Forces

Four dissections were carried out to investigate the contacts between the mandibular condyles and the temporal bone, and the insertions of the six jaw-closing muscles

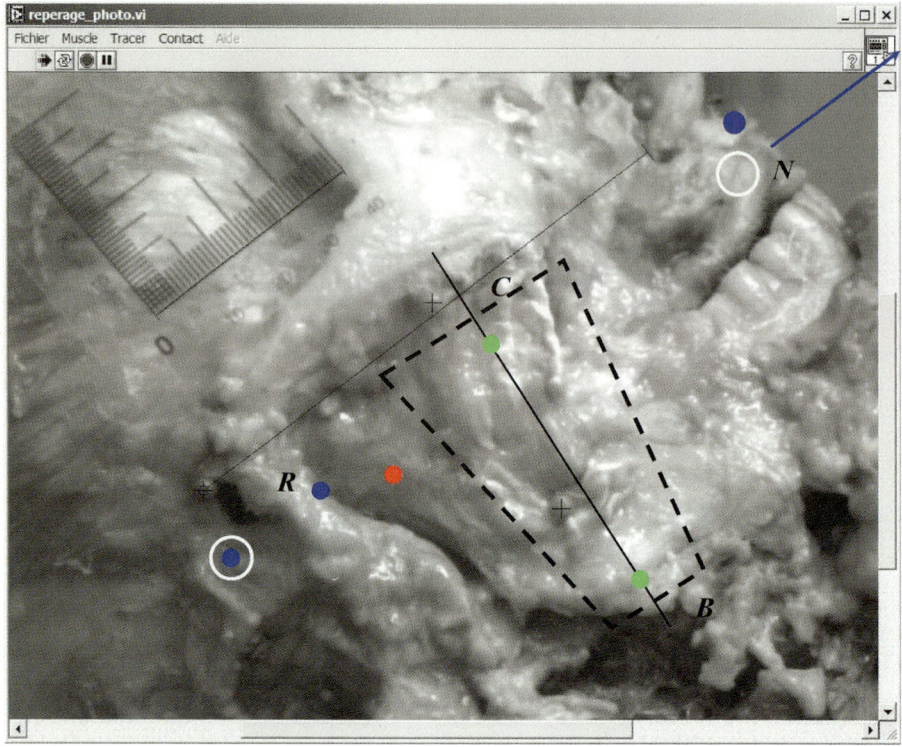

Fig. 6 Determination of the directions of the muscle forces (deep masseter)

being considered. Photographs and image processing software developed in the laboratory (using Labview) were used to determine experimentally the points of contact (left point L, right point R) and the muscle insertion centers in the Camper's morphological coordinate system (Fig. 6). Calculation of the directions of the muscular forces was computer-assisted. The mouth openings corresponded to the two thicknesses (5 and 15 mm) successively adjusted with the sensor. The co-ordinates used to calculate the directions of the articular forces corresponded to the averages from the four dissections.

2.2.3 Magnitudes of the Jaw-Closing Muscle Forces

In vivo electromyography and MRI data were used to measure the six jaw-closing muscle forces [40].

Electromyographic Activities of the Muscles

In significant voluntary contractions, the global EMG provides information about muscle fiber activity and the magnitudes of the muscle forces. The maximum magnitude for these forces can be reached only when almost all the fibers are involved in the contraction process. The electrical activity was here intercepted in an intramuscular bipolar mode. As the two muscle extremities did not present any relative displacement, muscle length remained constant and contraction was isometric.

Locating the surface masseter and the temporal muscle was straightforward. The deep masseter, on the other hand, is located in a dense anatomical zone and the pterygoid muscle can only be reached from the oral cavity. Intramuscular thread electrodes were used for the six closing muscles. Two wires (platino-iridium, diameter 20–30 μm), isolated by a nylon sheath, were introduced into a hypodermic needle. The extremities were then burned to remove the insulator. The two electrodes thus obtained were bent in order to improve anchoring when the needle was withdrawn.

Because of the techniques being used, a strict legal framework was necessary. The room had been approved by the DRASS (Direction Régionale des Affaires Sanitaires et Sociales) after advice from the CCPPRB (Comité Consultatif pour la Protection des Personnes de Bordeaux). The electrode implantations were carried out by a medical Doctor.

Under the isometric conditions described, there is a linear relation between the EMG signal and the muscular force. This relation is frequently used in the literature [41, 42]. If the force developed by the muscle is written as F, the maximum value can be then noted $F\ max$. In the same way, $EMGr$ and $EMGr\ max$ indicate the current and the maximum root mean square values (RMS) of the EMG signal. Then, linearity makes it possible to write the following equation:

$$F\,muscle = (F\,muscle\,max / EMGr\,max) \times EMGr, \text{where}$$

$$EMG_{RMS} = \left(1/T \int_{t-T/2}^{t+T/2} (EMG)^2\ dt \right)^{1/2} \quad (mV)$$

During the voluntary contraction, when almost all the muscle fibers are involved (maximum bite force exerted by the volunteer), an equally linear relation exists between the maximum muscle force and its main physiological section at rest. If the area of this section is written as $S\ max$ and if K indicates a constant coefficient that characterizes the muscular group, the equation can be written:

$$F\,muscle\,max = S\,max \times K$$

The values suggested for the coefficient $K\ (N/m^2)$ vary with the muscle morphology. They were taken from the literature [41–45] and the current muscular force was expressed by:

$$F\,muscle = (S\,max \times K / EMGr\,max) \times EMGr$$

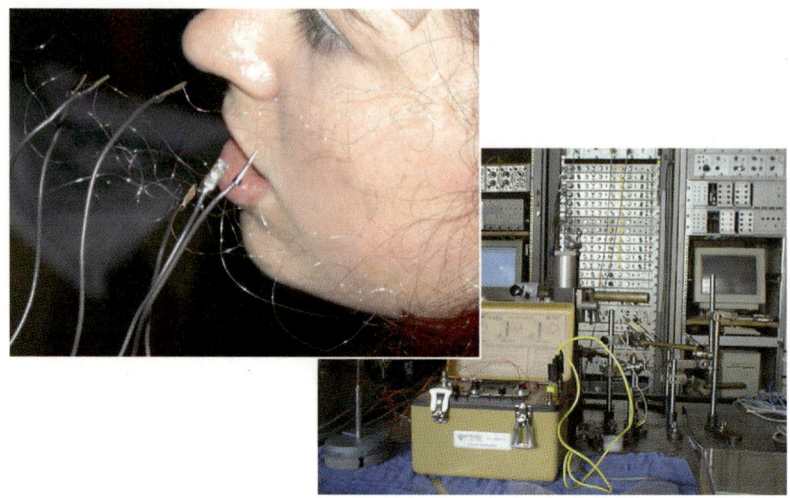

Fig. 7 Determining the muscle EMG signals

To exploit this relation, for each jaw-closing muscle, it was thus necessary to determine:

– *EMGr max*, repeating isometric voluntary maximum contractions and,
– *S max*, starting from an MRI examination.

In recording the EMG signals (Fig. 7), the device provided several successive functions:

– Signal capture using thread electrodes, amplification and filtering,
– Data recording and computer-assisted processing.

To reduce the strong discomfort imposed on the volunteer, the morphological symmetry of the face was admitted. Consequently, the areas of the muscle sections were read only on the left profile. The electrodes were distributed evenly on the left profile and the sensor was positioned successively between the incisors (31/21), the first premolars (34/24) and the first molars (36/26).

Admitting the perfect geometrical symmetry of the face, the situation (31/21), corresponded to a case of plane loading. On the other hand, for an asymmetrical loading, between premolars for example, the sensor was first positioned on tooth 34. The electrodes and the sensor were then located on the same profile and the sensor was moved to tooth 44. The electrodes and the sensor were thus located on different profiles. Using this technique, EMG signals of the two profiles (ipsi and contro) could be quantified while avoiding bilateral electrode implantation.

Physiological Muscle Sections

MRI provides images with a high degree of accuracy. To determine the main muscle section, the principal direction (or the positions of the insertion centers) needed to

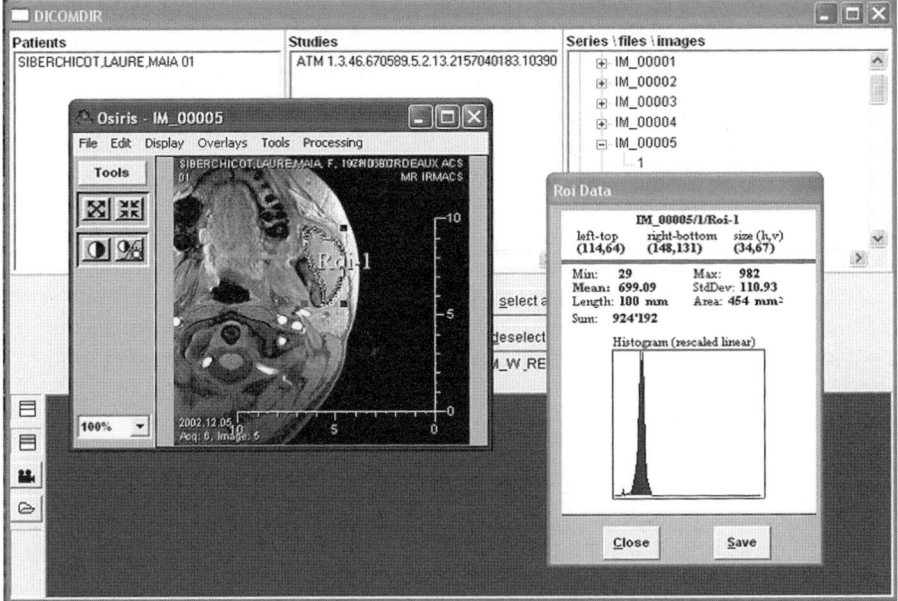

Fig. 8 Determining the muscle sections

be known. Several parallel and close recordings, orthogonal with this longitudinal muscle axis, were then made.

The digitized images were analyzed using image processing software (Osiris, Hopitaux Universitaires de Genève, Switzerland). A module makes it possible to select one area of the image and characterize it. Thus this area of interest can, for example, delimit the two masseters (Fig. 8). The software revealed here a total area of the section of nearly *454 mm²*.

2.2.4 Evolutions of the Protocol and Accuracy of the First Results

The contribution of the posterior temporal muscle remained weak compared to that of the other two muscle bundles (medial, and anterior): dividing the temporal muscle into two bundles therefore seemed sufficient. The objective was first to improve the precision of the results and to circumvent the difficulty of vectorizing this fan-like muscle. Because of the volunteers' hair, surface electrodes could be used only for the anterior bundle of the temporal muscle. This suppression of four thread electrodes was interesting, however, because it simplified the experimental procedure and reduced the pain experienced by the volunteers. Reducing volunteer pain will also probably improve the accuracy of results.

Table 1 presents the magnitudes of the forces for the six pairs of jaw-closing muscles. In each position, three tests were carried out for each of the four volunteers. Averages were calculated on the basis of 12 values.

Table 1 Jaw-closing muscle forces (N)

Muscles	Ref.	Loads (N)		
		x	y	z
Deep masseter (dm)	M1,2	7.8	127.2	22.7
Superficial masseter (sm)	M3,4	12.9	183.5	12.1
Medial pterygoid (mp)	M5,6	140.4	237.8	−77.3
Temporal anterior (ta)	M7,8	0.06	0.37	−0.13
Medial temporal (mt)	M9,10	0.97	5.7	−7.4

The directions of the forces exerted by the masseter and the medial pterygoid muscles remained almost parallel and it is thus possible to consider substituting the pterygoid electrode in the oral cavity by assigning a corrected section to the masseter.

Six jaw-closing muscles have been selected here, while the jaw-opening muscles have not been taken into account. Since a muscle does not act in isolation but in synergy with several other muscles, the protocol described in this paper is not limitative and does offer equally the possibility of taking jaw-opening muscles into account. The next step will be to quantify the relative contribution of the opening and closing muscles and test the hypothesis formulated by Caix [46]. We will also improve numerical results by using a larger population sample [47].

3   Finite Element Model

The mandible bone presents a complex geometry and boundary conditions need to be correctly specified, otherwise these can undermine the reality of results. In this sense, it is essential that numerical models are tested and validated experimentally [27, 48, 49]. Finite element and experimental models have been used to determine stresses and strains on the surface of bone structures with relevant conclusions [35, 50, 51]. These models can be used for different biomechanical analyses and to predict the performance of implants. Defining numerical models needs to be broken down into stages; the first stage involves the geometric model or a CAD model.

3.1   CAD Model

The geometry of the mandible is the first step in constructing the FE model, and geometry acquisition was normally by CT scan. In this work the model of the mandible was based on a polymeric replica of a human mandible from Sawbones® (model 1337 was selected). This model has adequate geometric accuracy for the experiments [52]. The geometry of the model was obtained using a 3D laser scanning device (Roland LPX 250 machine). The complexity of the geometry required ten scans with different orientations. The scan resolution was 0.2 x 0.2 mm and the final geometry is shown in Fig. 2.

Fig. 9 Mandible CAD
Model with a TMJ implant in
left condyle

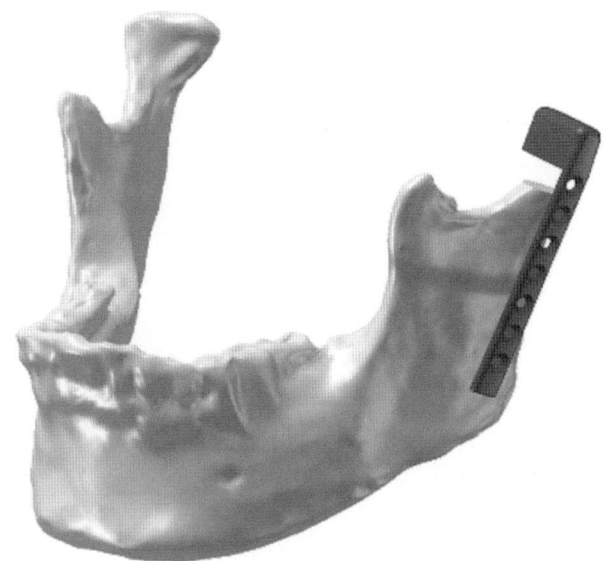

The final model of the mandible was obtained with dedicated CAD software (Solidworks, Dassault Systems). A solid homogeneous polymeric model was considered which, due to the nature of the study, does not compromise the results and discussion. Ichim et al. [35] and Liu et al. [53] concluded that the thickness of the mandible cortical bone and cancellous bone does not have significant influence on the strain distribution in the external surface. The polymeric model enabled us to obtain the geometric model. However, we considered real cortical bone properties for the FE simulations applied by other studies [20, 27, 35].

The CAD model of the implants was obtained based on an experimental implant designed at the University of Bordeaux and is depicted in Fig. 9. This implant has a straight geometry and seven holes aligned for the screws. The diameter of the holes is 2.1 mm.

3.2   FE Model

The next step is to discretize the CAD model into Finite elements; the FEM is composed of 71,280 tetrahedral linear elements with four nodes and 51,245 degrees of freedom (DOF) (Fig. 10). The model we analyzed had teeth but other authors conclude that these in fact have marginal influence on the biomechanics of the mandible and particularly on the behavior of the condyles [54]. This hypothesis was validated through experimental studies by Mesnard et al. [27] which also defined the boundary conditions applied in FE simulations. For the convergence tests, the maximal displacements and the maximal equivalent strains were assessed in the

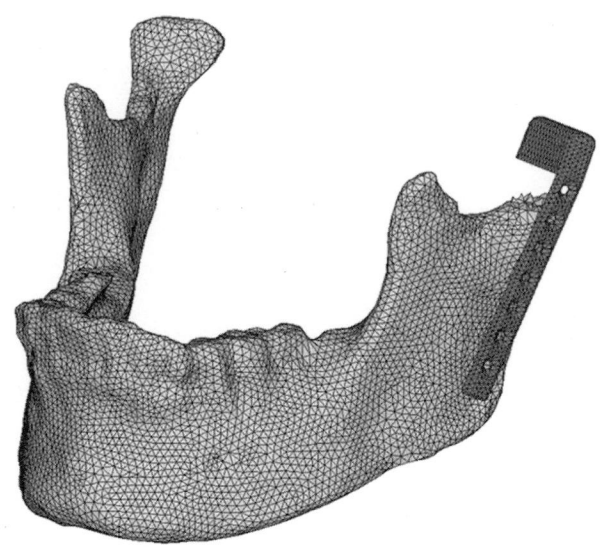

Fig. 10 Mandible FE model with a TMJ implant in *left* condyle

regions where the rosettes were placed on the mandible. The convergence rate for the displacements and the equivalent strains was reached for a mesh of more or less 40,000 DOF. Other authors, e.g. Hart et al. [51], considered convergence for 25,000 DOF and Lovald et al. [50] used a model with 47,525 elements with a model convergence.

The simulations took into account the mechanical properties of the mandible, where cortical bone was considered to have a Young's modulus of 14,700 MPa and a Poisson coefficient of 0.3, similar to models used by other authors [24, 35] for experimental validation. The implants were fixed with four screws and, as is often the case, there was no screw in the proximal position, which was also suggested by a surgeon. The Young's modulus (titanium alloy) and Poisson coefficient of the implant and screws were 110 GPa and 0.3 respectively.

The implant was applied to the left side of the mandible. The implant position with respect to the mandible was defined by the surgeon. In this study we used the same upper part of implant in the same position because the main goal was to analyze the behavior of the condyle region where the implant was placed.

The screw positions were also chosen by the surgeon. As in a real clinical situation, four screws were used to fix the implant to the mandible. Screws of 2 mm diameter were used and these have been considered as the minimum diameter that can provide sufficient stability [55, 56]. To simulate the screws they were considered completely bound to cortical bone. For the screw-implant contact we considered a touching contact situation. We also considered the contact between implant and bone with a 0.3 coefficient of friction.

Fig. 11 Boundary condition
applied in FE model

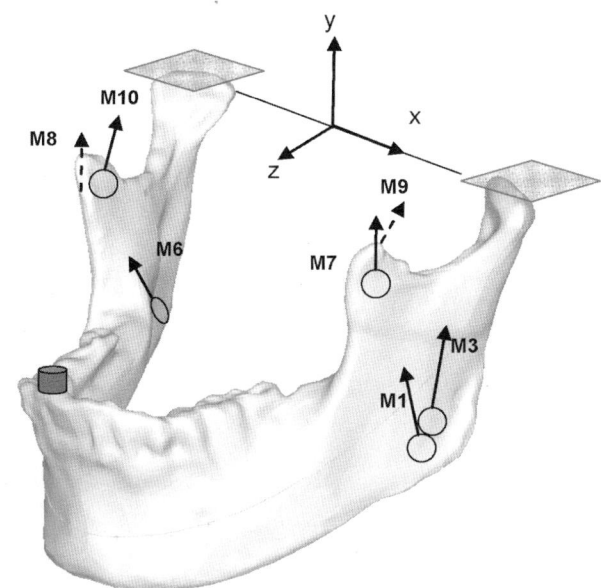

3.3 *Boundary Conditions, Validation and Sensibility*

The boundary condition presents an important role in the results. For the boundary conditions the incisor was fixed in three directions but could rotate, and the condyle could slide on the plane surface of a support as shown in Fig. 11. The variation in aspects like mandible size, mandible shape, bone properties, bite forces do not allow to determine the stress and strain data in a real situation. These variations can be differentiated by some aspects like gender, age and size.

The loads are included in Table 1 for a mouth opening of 5 mm on the incisor, which is the condition that causes the most critical situation on the condyle [27, 57], and which presents most tension and displacement in the condyle compared with the other two support positions (canine and molar teeth) and different mouth apertures (5, 10, 15, 20, 25, 30 mm) [27].

The muscular actions applied were the ones presented [32] and five principal muscles were included in the loading configuration: deep and superficial masseter, medial pterygoid, temporalis and medial temporal. The muscle forces were considered in the same insertion zones and with symmetrical x direction.

These insertions have been observed through MRI images by Mesnard et al. [27] based on dissections made to investigate contact between the condyles and the temporal bone and the insertion centers of the muscles [57]. Calculation of the muscular force directions was thus computer-assisted for three different sensor thicknesses (5, 10 and 15 mm). The co-ordinate values used to calculate the articular forces corresponded to the averages of the values obtained from the four dissections, and was used in the FE models.

Fig. 12 Synthetic mandible
with locations of rosette
strain gauges. Bone strains
were measured with four
gauges glued onto the
external mandible surface

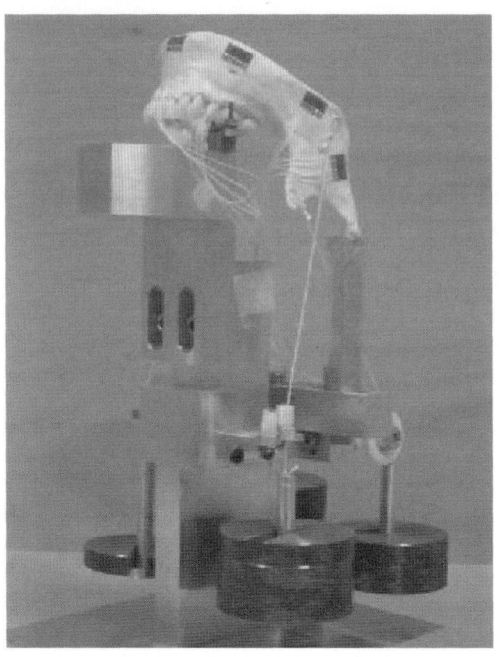

The FEM used in the present study has been validated [58]. The model was experimentally validated with tri-axial strain gauges (CEA-06-062UR-350, Vishay Electronic GmbH, Germany) and the fiber brag sensors technique. To validate the accuracy of the FE model, simplified boundary conditions were used, as shown in the apparatus Fig. 12. In the model, validation strain was only applied to two muscles in each side, with a lower magnitude 5 and 10 N. Four nylon wires were glued at the anatomical insertions of the masseter and temporal muscles and used to load the mandible by placing weights at the end of them. In this validation the material properties of the mandible in FEM was the Sawbones with 460 MPa Young's modulus.

In this experiment, three different mandible support situations were considered, incisor, canine and molar teeth. Four load situations were analyzed, Load_1 applied masseter muscle with 5 N, Load_2 the same muscle with 10 N, Load_3 configuration includes the master muscles with a force of 10 N and the temporal muscle force of 5 N. Load_4 configuration included forces of 12 N, 6 N, 2 N respectively for the right masseter, right temporal and left masseter muscles. No force was considered for the left temporal (Tleft) muscle. The experimental and numerical results are presented in Fig. 13 for canine teeth support.

The results revealed a good correlation between FEM and experimental results and considering all FE and measured strains, the correlation value R^2 and slope of the regression line are 0.98 and 0.93 for the maximum and minimum principal strains presented in Fig. 14.

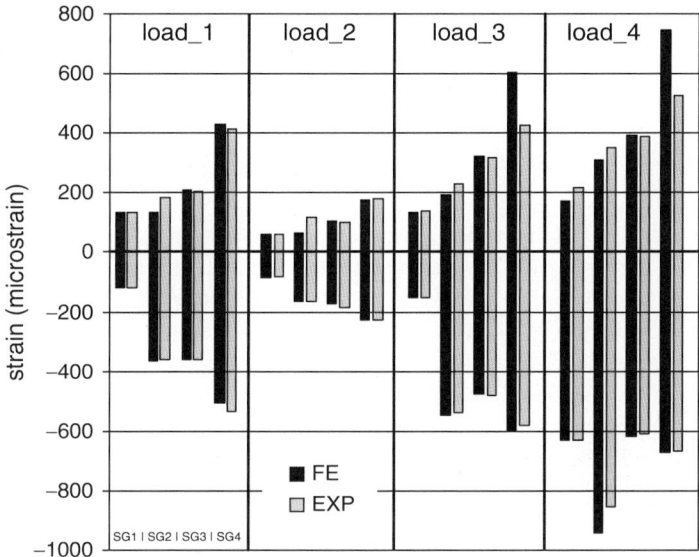

Fig. 13 Comparison of the FE and mean measured principal strains for each gauge location and for all load configurations with support in incisor teeth

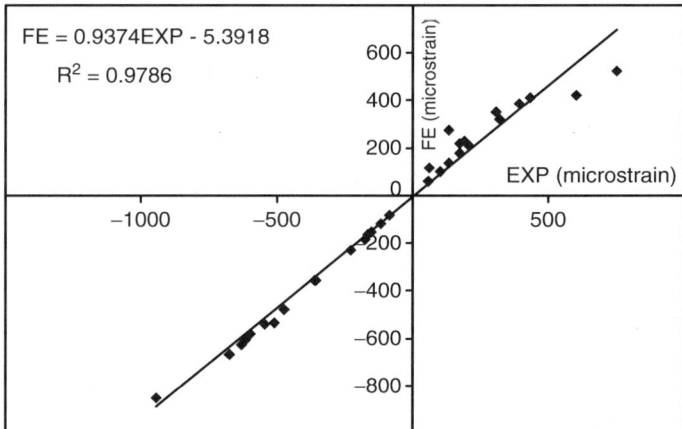

Fig. 14 Linear regression analyses were performed to determine the overall correspondence between FE and mean measured strains in all supports

The intercept value is small (6 $\mu\varepsilon$) and the RMSE value of the measured strains is 1%. By separating the minimal strains from the maximal strain, relevant differences can be observed. The other load configurations present similar results [58].

This study proved that FE models of the mandible can reproduce experimental strains within an overall agreement level of 10%. The FE models correctly reproduced bone strains under different load configurations. For this reason, the FE model adequately reproduces the mechanical behavior of the mandible and is essential for predicting biomechanical changes in the mandible and long-term failure.

4   Results and Discussion: Stiffness and Screw Distributions

Within this study we compared the behavior of an intact mandible and one implanted with a TMJ, assessing the displacements and strain distributions on the external mandible surface. We also analyzed the influence of screws. Strain distribution is important because the implant fixation is a critical factor for its success [13, 59]. Figure 15 represents displacement in the z direction for the intact mandible and the one with a TMJ implant. Overall, the results evidence a non-symmetrical mechanical behavior for both the intact and implanted mandibles. However, the implanted mandible provoked a more pronounced symmetrical behavior in the z direction. The TMJ implanted on the left condyle influences the behavior of the right condyle. A 10% difference in maximum displacement was observed in the opposite condyle.

On the left condyle, where the implant was placed, maximum displacement was observed for the TMJ implant (3.20 mm) compared with the intact situation which was (3.16 mm). The difference on this condyle was around 5%, due to the rigidity of the implant. Implant stiffness is an important factor for condyle mobility.

It was observed that the x displacements were not significantly affected by the implant. Displacements in the x direction were similar for TMJ implant and the intact mandible. The displacement distributions were symmetrical for all simulated cases.

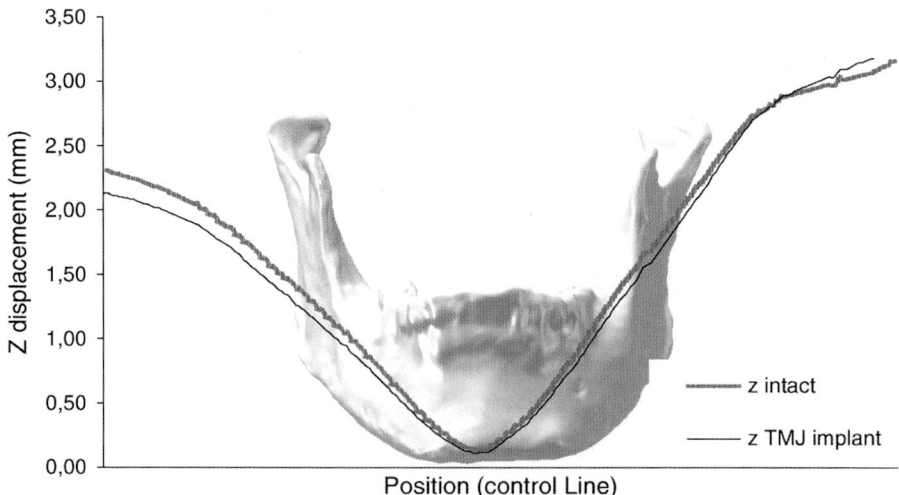

Fig. 15 Comparative displacement on intact and implanted mandible in z direction

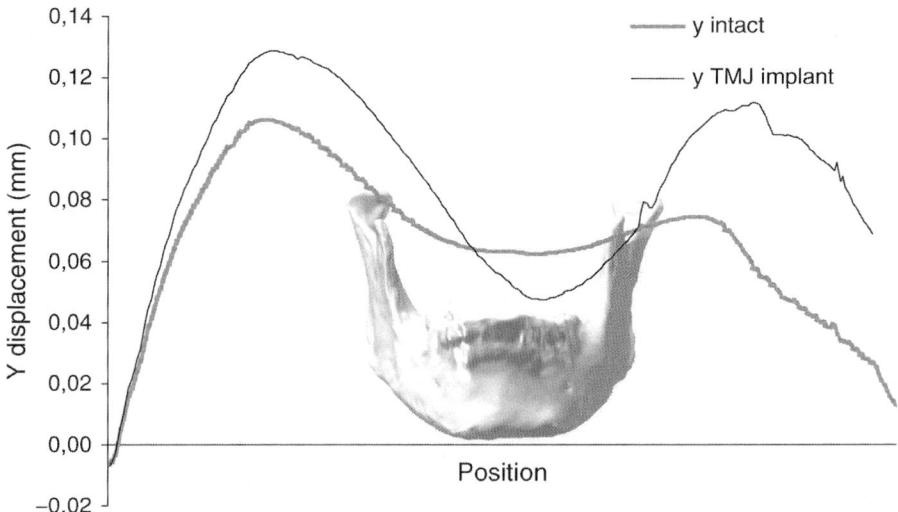

Fig. 16 Comparative displacement on intact and implanted mandible in the y-direction

The magnitudes of the displacements in the y direction in Fig. 16 are small when compared with those in the z direction. Differences can be seen between the intact mandible and the TMJ implant mandible. The TMJ implant not only affects the left region of the mandible. On the left side displacement increased (50% more) and also the relative displacement between implant and bone.

We observed that the minimum principal stress is the most important design factor, but the distribution was almost the same as the equivalent stress. On the right condyle the influence of the TMJ implant increases the stresses on the mandible. Identical influence was also verified in the frontal mandible region.

The straight implant also generated a high level of tensile stresses near the first screw, and this was highest compared with the other implants. The highest magnitude stress was seen on the right condyle, 20.7 MPa, 14% more than on the intact mandible.

The minimal principal strain on the external mandible surface is in Fig. 17. The TMJ implant increases the strain level in the condyle region, similar to the intact mandible, and affects the right side of the mandible. In the frontal region of the mandible the TMJ increases the strain on the TMJ side, and increases the bone formation.

The screw positions are an important factor in the success of mandible kinematics. The four screws were considered and the minimal principal strains are presented in Fig. 18. These results reveal two different points. First, when we analyze the influence of screws we observe that the first and last screws are in the most critical positions. The geometry of the implant and its stiffness lead to critical strain distribution around these screws.

The principal strain distributions near the screws are shown in Fig. 19. The first and last screws present a μstrain of 5,330 and 5,610, respectively. To cause

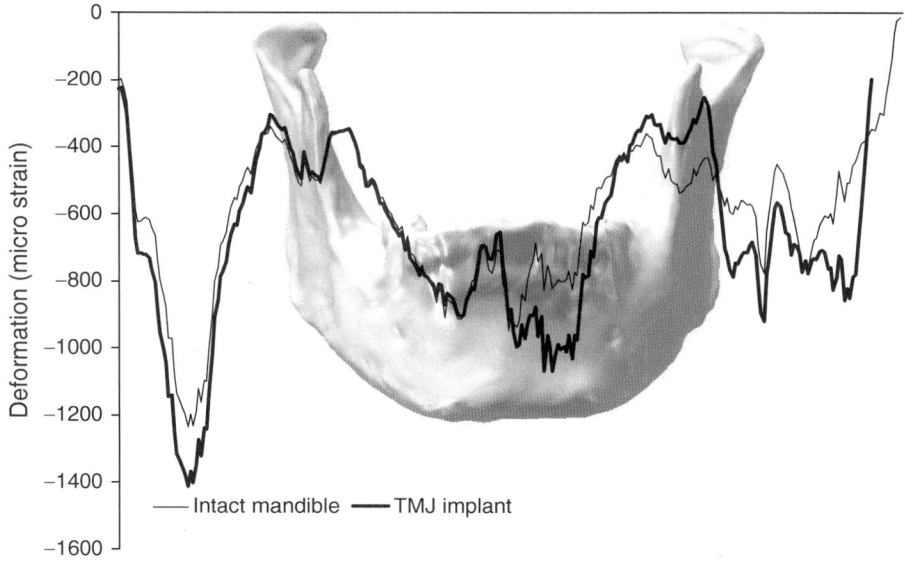

Fig. 17 Distribution of minimum principal strain

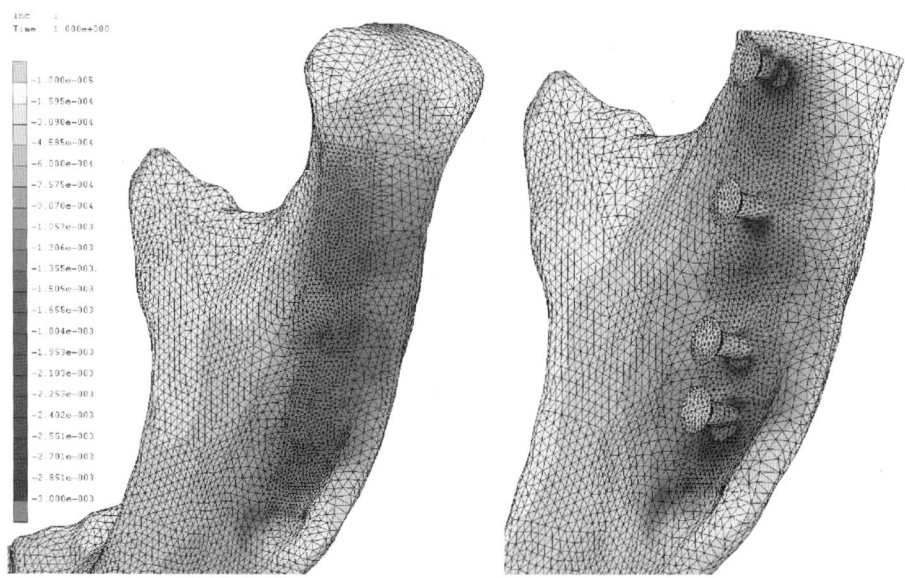

Fig. 18 Minimum principal strain distribution near the TMJ fixation

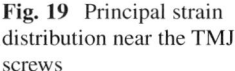

Fig. 19 Principal strain distribution near the TMJ screws

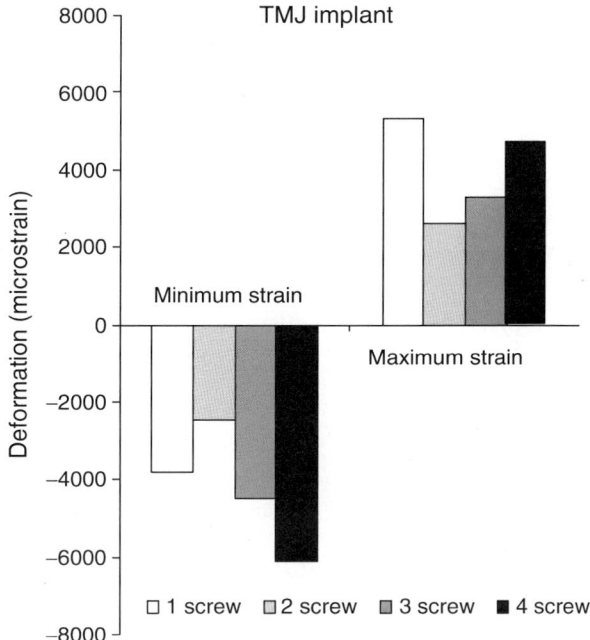

hypotrophy to the bone, a strain higher than 4,000 µstrain is required according to Roberts et al. [60], therefore it is expected that there will be bone growth or hypotrophy on the first and last screws. To reduce the strains near these screws more screws will need to be applied in the first part of TMJ implant (for example parallel to the first screws). With this process, it will be possible to reduce strain and promote the bone maintenance process. For the second and third screws, the strains are below the hypotrophy limit presented by Roberts et al. [60] and then the bone may grow.

This study proved that FE models can reproduce important information for TMJ implant design. The knowledge obtained within this study provides a good basis for other studies that can be performed with real bones for further development of standardized FE pre-clinical tests for TMJ implants. Rigidity and structural integrity of the implant are key issues to be observed.

5   Conclusions

This study proved that FE models can produce important information for TMJ implant design. The knowledge obtained within this study provides a good basis for further analyses that have to be performed with real bone characteristics to develop standardized FE pre-clinical tests for TMJ implants. Rigidity and structural integrity of the implant are key issues that can be observed.

The methodology adopted presents good correlation between experimental and numerical models. The results show the influence of strain distribution around TMJ replacement.

The screw position and implant geometry and stiffness will be determining factors in the fixation and stabilization of TMJ implants.

References

1. Speculand B (2009) Current status of replacement of the temporomandibular joint in the United Kingdom. Br J Oral Maxillofac Surg 47(1):37–41
2. Guarda-Nardini L, Manfredini D, Ferronato G (2008) Temporomandibular joint total replacement prosthesis: current knowledge and considerations for the future. Int J Oral Maxillofac Surg 37(2):103–110
3. Speculand B, Hensher R, Powell D (2000) Total prosthetic replacement of the TMJ: experience with two systems 1988–1997. Br J Oral Maxillofac Surg 38(4):360–369
4. Driemel O et al (2009) Historical development of alloplastic temporoman-dibular joint replacement after 1945 and state of the art. Int J Oral Maxillofac Surg 38(9):909–920
5. Dimitroulis G (2005) The role of surgery in the management of disorders of the temporomandibular joint: a critical review of the literature Part 2. Int J Oral Maxillofac Surg 34(3):231–237
6. Dimitroulis G (2005) The role of surgery in the management of disorders of the temporomandibular joint: a critical review of the literature – part 1. Int J Oral Maxillofac Surg 34(2):107–113
7. van Loon JP et al (2002) Groningen temporomandibular joint prosthesis. Development and first clinical application. Int J Oral Maxillofac Surg 31(1):44–52
8. van Loon J-P, de Bont LGM, Boering G (1995) Evaluation of temporomandibular joint prostheses: review of the literature from 1946 to 1994 and implications for future prosthesis designs. J Oral Maxillofac Surg 53(9):984–996
9. Mercuri LG et al (1995) Custom Cad-Cam total temporomandibular-joint reconstruction system – preliminary multicenter report. J Oral Maxillofac Surg 53(2):106–115
10. Wolford LM et al (2003) Comparison of 2 temporomandibular joint total joint prosthesis systems. J Oral Maxillofac Surg 61(6):685–690
11. Karray F et al (1999) The interface of living tissue and inert material. Can J Phys 77(9): 745–750
12. Mercuri LG (1999) Considering total temporomandibular joint replacement. Cranio 17(1): 44–48
13. Mercuri LG, Giobbie-Hurder A (2004) Long-term outcomes after total alloplastic temporomandibular joint reconstruction following exposure to failed materials. J Oral Maxillofac Surg 62(9):1088–1096
14. Mercuri LG, Ali FA, Woolson R (2008) Outcomes of total alloplastic replacement with periarticular autogenous fat grafting for management of reankylosis of the temporomandibular joint. J Oral Maxillofac Surg 66(9):1794–1803
15. Coutant JC et al (2008) Discrimination of objective kinematic characters in temporomandibular joint displacements. Arch Oral Biol 53(5):453–461
16. Mesnard M et al (2006) Métrologie articulaire tridimensionnelle, déplacements et morphologie temporo-mandibulaires. Morphologie 90(289):86–86
17. Modschiedler T (1989) La place de la prothèse dans la chirurgie reconstructive de l'articulation temporo-mandibulaire. In: Sciences Médicales. Université Bordeaux 2, Bordeaux
18. Ramos A, Fonseca F, Simoes JA (2003) The effect of cemented femoral stem cross-section geometry in total hip replacement. Simulat Biomed V 7:323–331

19. Casas EBL et al (2008) Comparative 3D finite element stress analysis of straight and angled wedge-shaped implant designs. Int J Oral Maxillofac Implants 23(2):215–225
20. Tanaka E, Tanne K, Sakuda M (1994) A 3-dimensional finite-element model of the mandible including the Tmj and its application to stress-analysis in the Tmj during clenching. Med Eng Phys 16(4):316–322
21. Silva JCC et al (2005) Fibre Bragg grating sensing and finite element analysis of the biomechanics of the mandible. In: 17th international conference on optical fibre sensors, pts 1 and 2, vol 5855, p 102–105
22. Ramos A et al (2009) The strain patterns of the mandible for different loadings and mouth apertures. In: Jorge RMN, Santos SM, Tavares JMRS, Campos R, Vaz MAP (eds) Biodental engineering, CRC Press, pp 133–137
23. Li T et al (2011) Optimum selection of the dental implant diameter and length in the posterior mandible with poor bone quality – A 3D finite element analysis. Appl Math Model 35(1): 446–456
24. Motoyoshi M et al (2009) Bone stress for a mini-implant close to the roots of adjacent teeth-3D finite element analysis. Int J Oral Maxillofac Surg 38(4):363–368
25. Knets I et al (2001) Stress analysis in the human mandible during simulated tooth clenching. Comput Methods Biomech Biomed Engin 3:661–666
26. Bujtar P et al (2010) Finite element analysis of the human mandible at 3 different stages of life. Oral Surg Oral Med O 110(3):301–309
27. Mesnard M et al (2006) Numerical-experimental models to study the temporo-mandibular joint (TMJ). J Biomech 39(Supplement 1):S458–S458
28. Gao JX, Xu W, Ding ZQ (2006) 3D finite element mesh generation of complicated tooth model based on CT slices. Comput Methods Programs Biomed 82(2):97–105
29. Zhao LP et al (2001) Medical imaging genesis for finite element-based mandibular surgical planning in the pediatric subject. In: Proceedings of the 23rd annual international conference of the ieee engineering in medicine and biology society, vols 1–4, 23, pp 2509–2512
30. Limbert G et al (2010) Trabecular bone strains around a dental implant and associated micromotions-A micro-CT-based three-dimensional finite element study. J Biomech 43(7):1251–1261
31. de Zee M et al (2007) Validation of a musculo-skeletal model of the mandible and its application to mandibular distraction osteogenesis. J Biomech 40(6):1192–1201
32. Iwasaki LR et al (2003) Muscle and temporomandibular joint forces associated with chincup loading predicted by numerical modeling. Am J Orthod Dentofacial Orthop 124(5):530–540
33. Natali AN, Carniel EL, Pavan PG (2010) Modelling of mandible bone properties in the numerical analysis of oral implant biomechanics. Comput Methods Programs Biomed 100(2):158–165
34. Iwasaki LR et al (2004) Individual variations in numerically modeled human muscle and temporomandibular joint forces during static biting. J Orofac Pain 18(3):235–245
35. Ichim I, Kieser JA, Swain MV (2007) Functional significance of strain distribution in the human mandible under masticatory load: numerical predictions. Arch Oral Biol 52(5): 465–473
36. Ramos A, Simoes JA (2006) Tetrahedral versus hexahedral finite elements in numerical modelling of the proximal femur. Med Eng Phys 28(9):916–924
37. Gröning F et al (2009) Validating a voxel-based finite element model of a human mandible using digital speckle pattern interferometry. J Biomech 42(9):1224–1229
38. Relvas C et al (2010) The influence of data shape acquisition process and geometric accuracy of the mandible for numerical simulation. Comput Methods Biomech Biomed Engin 3:1–8
39. Throckmorton GS, Rasmussen J, Caloss R (2009) Calibration of T-Scan((R)) sensors for recording bite forces in denture patients. J Oral Rehabil 36(9):636–643
40. Bouisset S, Zattara M (1988) Is joint fixation during an intentional movement in man due to tonic activation of antagonistic muscles. J Physiol-London 406:P30–P30
41. El-Bilay T, Abdelhameed M (2004) Quantitative calculations of temporomandibular joint reaction forces as a function of mandibular lengthening. TMJ 3(7):1–11

42. Pruim GJ, de Jongh HJ, ten Bosch JJ (1980) Forces acting on the mandible during bilateral static bite at different bite force levels. J Biomech 13(9):755–763
43. Moller E (1996) The chewing apparatus. Acta Physiologica Scandinavia, Copenhagen
44. Pruim G, Ten Bosch JJ, De Jongh HJ (1978) Jaw muscle EMG-activity and static loading of the mandible. J Biomech 11:389–395
45. Nahmias I (2000) Contribution à l'étude de la cinématique mandibulaire. In: Orthodontie. Université Paris 5, Paris
46. Caix PaJC (2000) Anatomie fonctionnelle. In: L.d.A.M.-F.e.(ed) Chirurgicale, Université Bordeaux 2, Bordeaux
47. Mesnard M, Coutant JC, Aoun M, Morlier J, Cid M, Caix Ph (2012) Correlation between geometry and kinematic characteristics in the temporomandibular joint. Comput Meth Biomech Biomed Eng 15(4):393–400
48. DeVocht JW et al (2001) Experimental validation of a finite element model of the temporomandibular joint. J Oral Maxillofac Surg 59(7):775–778
49. Vollmer D et al (2000) Experimental and finite element study of a human mandible. J Cranio-Maxillofac Surg 28(2):91–96
50. Lovald S et al (2010) Biomechanical optimization of bone plates used in rigid fixation of mandibular symphysis fractures. J Oral Maxillofac Surg 68(8):1833–1841
51. Hart RT et al (1992) Modeling the biomechanics of the mandible – a 3-dimensional finite-element study. J Biomech 25(3):261–286
52. De Santis R et al (2004) Continuous fibre reinforced polymers as connective tissue replacement. Compos Sci Technol 64(6):861–871
53. Liu Z, Fan YB, Qian YL (2007) Biomechanical simulation of the interaction in the temporomandibular joint within dentate mandible: a finite element analysis. In: 2007 Ieee/Icme international conference on complex medical engineering, vols 1–4, pp 1842–1846
54. Korioth TWP, Romilly DP, Hannam AG (1992) 3-dimensional finite-element stress-analysis of the dentate human mandible. Am J Phys Anthropol 88(1):69–96
55. Maurer P, Holweg S, Schubert J (1999) Finite-element-analysis of different screw-diameters in the sagittal split osteotomy of the mandible. J Cranio-Maxillofac Surg 27(6):365–372
56. Scaf de Molon R et al (2011) In vitro comparison of 1.5 mm vs. 2.0 mm screws for fixation in the sagittal split osteotomy. J Cranio-Maxill Surg 39(8):574–577
57. Mesnard M et al (2011) Biomechanical analysis comparing natural and alloplastic temporomandibular joint replacement using a finite element model. J Oral Maxil Surg 69(4):1008–1017
58. Ramos A et al (2011) Numerical and experimental models of the mandible. Exp Mech 51(7):1053–1059
59. Mercuri LG, Edibam NR, Giobbie-Hurder A (2007) Fourteen-year follow-up of a patient-fitted total temporomandibular joint reconstruction system. J Oral Maxillofac Surg 65(6):1140–1148
60. Roberts WE, Huja S, Roberts JA (2004) Bone modeling: biomechanics, molecular mechanisms, and clinical perspectives. Semin Orthod 10(2):123–161

Blood Flow Simulation and Applications

Luisa Costa Sousa, Catarina F. Castro, and Carlos Conceição António

Abstract In the vascular system altered flow conditions, such as separation and flow-reversal zones play an important role in the development of arterial diseases. Nowadays computational biomechanics modeling is still in the research and development stage. This chapter presents a numerical computational methodology for blood flow simulation using the Finite Element method outlining field equations and approaches for numerical solutions. Due to the complexity of the vascular system simplifying assumptions for the mathematical modeling process are made. Two applications of the developed tool to describe arterial hemodynamics are presented, a flow simulation in the human carotid artery bifurcation and a search for an optimized geometry of an artificial bypass graft.

1 Introduction

Nowadays, the use of computational techniques in fluid dynamics in the study of physiological flows involving blood is an area of intensive research [1–4]. The mechanics of blood flow in arteries plays an important role in the health of individuals and its study represents a central issue of the vascular research. Arterial diseases such as wall conditions may cause blood flow disturbances leading to clinical complications in areas of complex flow like in coronary and carotid bifurcations or stenosed arteries. It is well established that once a mild stenosis is formed in the artery, biomechanical parameters resulting from the blood flow and stress distribution in the arterial wall contribute to further progression of the disease. Although blood flow is normally laminar, the periodic unsteadiness or pulsatile nature of the flow makes possible the transition to turbulence when the artery diameter decreases and velocities increase. A detailed understanding of local

L.C. Sousa (✉) • C.F. Castro • C.C. António
Faculty of Engineering, University of Porto, Porto, Portugal
e-mail: lcsousa@fe.up.pt

R.M.N. Jorge et al. (eds.), *Technologies for Medical Sciences*, Lecture Notes
in Computational Vision and Biomechanics 1, DOI 10.1007/978-94-007-4068-6_4,
© Springer Science+Business Media B.V. 2012

hemodynamic environment, influence of wall modifications on flow patterns and long-term adaptations of the vascular wall can have useful clinical applications, especially in view of reconstruction and revascularization operations [5, 6].

Flow visualization techniques and non-invasive medical imaging data acquisition such as computed tomography, angiography or magnetic resonance imaging, make feasible to construct three dimensional models of blood vessels. Measuring techniques such as Doppler ultrasound have improved to provide accurate information on the flow fields. Validated computational fluid dynamics (CFD) models using data obtained by these currently available measurement techniques [7–9] can be very valuable in the early detection of vessels at risk and prediction of future disease progression.

Hemodynamic finite element simulation studies have been frequently used to gain a better understanding of functional, diagnostic and therapeutic aspects of the blood flow. Three different issues are necessary during such study defining the following methodology:

1. Definition of suitable mathematical models - due to the complexity of the vascular system, a preliminary analysis aiming at introducing suitable simplifying assumptions in the mathematical modelling process is necessary. Obviously, different kinds of simplifications are suitable for different vascular problems;
2. Pre-processing of clinical data - the suitable treatment of clinical data is crucial for the definition of a real geometrical model, taken from a patient. This aspect demands geometrical reconstruction algorithms in order to achieve simulation in real vascular morphologies;
3. Development of appropriate numerical techniques - the geometrical complexity of the vascular system suggests the use of unstructured grids, in particular for Finite Element Method (FEM), while the strongly unsteady nature of the problem demands effective time-advancing methods.

The arterial wall is a composite of three layers, each containing different amounts of elastin, collagen, vascular smooth muscle cells and extracellular matrix. In diseased vessels which are often the subject of interest, the arteries are less compliant, wall motion is reduced and in most approximations the assumption of rigid vessel flow is reasonable.

Blood consists of formed elements suspended in plasma, an aqueous polymer solution. About 45% volume consists of formed elements and about 55% of plasma. The majority of formed elements are red blood cells (95%). In large and medium size vessels, blood is usually modelled as a Newtonian liquid. However in smaller vessels blood is a complex rheological mixture showing several non-Newtonian properties, as shear-thinning or viscoelasticity. The temperature and the presence of pathological conditions may also contribute to non-Newtonian behaviour.

For the steady flow case [10] showed that the non-Newtonian effect is small except for the peak shear stress and that for the pulsatile case the Newtonian effect in the artery is small and negligible. Perktold and co-workers examined non-Newtonian viscosity models in carotid artery bifurcation and although the Newtonian assumption yields no change in the essential flow characteristics they concluded that predicted shear stress magnitude resulted in differences on the order of 10% as compared with Newtonian models [11].

A non-Newtonian viscosity model for simulating flow in arteries is presented in this chapter. Considering blood flow an incompressible non-Newtonian flow and neglecting body forces, the fluid flow is governed by the incompressible Navier–Stokes equations. There are two potential sources of numerical instability in the Galerkin finite element solution of these equations. The first one is due to the numerical treatment of the saddle-point problem arising from the variational formulation of the incompressible flow equations. The second difficulty is related to the discretization of the nonlinear convective terms which requires the use of stabilized finite element formulations to properly treat high Reynolds number flows. Some of the approaches for the numerical solutions are presented in this study.

To demonstrate the application of the developed finite element technique for numerical simulations of blood flow in arteries, a flow simulation in the human carotid artery bifurcation and a search for an optimized geometry of an artificial bypass graft is addressed here. In medical practice, bypass grafts are commonly used as an alternative route around strongly stenosed or occluded arteries. When the arterial flow is high, artificial grafts perform well [2, 12, 13] and it has been shown over the years that they provide durable results. Su [2] investigated the complexity of blood flow in the complete model of arterial bypass. He found that flow in the bypass graft is greatly dependent on the area reduction in the host artery. As the area reduction increases, higher stress concentration and larger recirculation zones are formed bringing out the possibility of restenosis. Probst [14] concluded that computing derivatives of the flow solution (and related quantities like shear rate) with respect to viscosity could not reveal the sensitivity of the optimal graft shape to the fluid model. So, optimization should be applied to the entire framework, which would enable to actually compute the optimal shape. In the present work a multi-objective optimization framework is presented. A genetic algorithm coupled with the developed finite element methodology for blood flow simulation is considered in order to reach optimal graft geometries. Numerical results show the benefits of shape optimization in achieving design improvements before a bypass surgery, minimizing recirculation zones and flow stagnation.

2 Governing Equations

A number of important phenomena in fluid mechanics are described by the Navier–Stokes equations. They are a statement of the dynamical effect of the externally applied forces and the internal forces due to pressure and viscosity of the fluid. The time dependent flow of a viscous incompressible fluid is governed by the momentum and mass conservation equations, the Navier–Stokes equations given as:

$$\rho \left(\frac{\partial \mathbf{u}}{\partial t} + \mathbf{u}.\nabla \mathbf{u} \right) = \nabla \sigma + \mathbf{f}$$

$$\nabla.\mathbf{u} = 0 \tag{1}$$

where $\mathbf{u}$ and σ are the velocity and the stress fields, ρ the blood density and $\mathbf{f}$ the volume force per unit mass of fluid. The components of the stress tensor are defined by the Stokes' law:

$$\sigma = -p\mathbf{I} + 2\mu\boldsymbol{\varepsilon}(\mathbf{u}) \tag{2}$$

where p is the pressure, $\mathbf{I}$ the unit tensor, μ the dynamical viscosity and $\boldsymbol{\varepsilon}(u)$ the strain rate tensor. Neglecting body forces, conservation of mass and momentum (1) become:

$$\rho\left(\frac{\partial\mathbf{u}}{\partial t} + \mathbf{u}.\nabla\mathbf{u}\right) = -\nabla p + \mu\nabla\mathbf{u}$$

$$\nabla.\mathbf{u} = 0 \tag{3}$$

This equation system (3) can be solved for the velocity and the pressure given appropriate boundary and initial conditions. In this study the biochemical and mechanical interactions between blood and vascular tissue are neglected. The innermost lining of the arterial wall in contact with the blood is a layer of firmly attached endothelial cells and it appears to be reasonable to assume no slip at the interface with the rigid vessel wall; at the flow entrance Dirichelet boundary conditions for all points are considered prescribing the time dependent value $\mathbf{u}_D$ for the velocity on the portion Γ_D of the boundary:

$$\mathbf{u}(\mathbf{x}, t) = \mathbf{u}_D(\mathbf{x}, t), \quad \mathbf{x} \in \Gamma_D \tag{4}$$

At an outflow boundary Γ_N the condition describing surface traction force $\mathbf{h}$ is assumed. This can be described mathematically by the condition:

$$\left(-p\delta_{ij} + \mu\left(\frac{\partial u_i}{\partial x_j} + \frac{\partial u_j}{\partial x_j}\right)\right)n_j = h_i \quad i, j = 1, 2, 3 \quad \text{on } \Gamma_N \tag{5}$$

where n_j are the components of the outward pointing unit vector at the outflow boundary.

3 Finite Element Formulation

The finite element method is a mathematical technique for obtaining approximate numerical solution of the physical phenomena subject to initial and boundary conditions. Two different finite element models of the Navier–Stokes equations are considered in this chapter, the mixed model and the penalty finite element model.

3.1 Mixed Finite Element Model

The mixed model is a natural formulation in which the weak forms of (3) are used to construct the finite element method. The resulting finite element model is termed the velocity-pressure model or mixed model. Developing a Galerkin formulation the weak forms of (3) results in the following finite element equations:

$$\mathbf{M}\dot{\mathbf{u}}+\mathbf{C}(\mathbf{u})\mathbf{u} + \mathbf{K}\mathbf{u} - \mathbf{QP} = \mathbf{F}$$

$$- \mathbf{Q}^T\mathbf{u} = \mathbf{0} \tag{6}$$

where the superpose dot represents a time derivative. Considering N and L the element interpolation functions for the velocity and pressure, the elements of the matrices at the finite element level are defined as:

$$M_{ij} = \int_e \rho N_i N_j \, de; \quad C_{ij} = \int_e \rho N_i \left(u_x \frac{\partial N_j}{\partial x} + u_y \frac{\partial N_j}{\partial y} + u_z \frac{\partial N_j}{\partial z} \right) de$$

$$K_{ij} = \int_e \mu \left(\frac{\partial N_i}{\partial x} \frac{\partial N_j}{\partial x} + \frac{\partial N_i}{\partial y} \frac{\partial N_j}{\partial y} + \frac{\partial N_i}{\partial z} \frac{\partial N_j}{\partial z} \right) de; \quad Q_{ik}^\alpha = \int_e \frac{\partial N_i}{\partial \alpha} L_k \tag{7}$$

and the resulting equation system is:

$$\mathbf{M}\dot{\mathbf{u}}+\begin{bmatrix} \mathbf{C}+\mathbf{K} & -\mathbf{Q} \\ -\mathbf{Q}^T & 0 \end{bmatrix}\begin{Bmatrix} \mathbf{u} \\ \mathbf{P} \end{Bmatrix} = \begin{Bmatrix} \mathbf{F} \\ \mathbf{0} \end{Bmatrix} \tag{8}$$

The above partitioned system (8) with a null submatrix could in principle be solved in several ways. However, it can be asked under which conditions it can be safely solved. This problem results from the incompressibility condition. In simple terms, we want to obtain, in the linear space U of all admissible solutions, the velocity field $\mathbf{u}$ belonging to a subspace $I^h \subset U$, associated to the space of incompressible deformations. This subspace is given as:

$$I^h = \left\{ \mathbf{u}^h \in U^h : \mathbf{Q}\mathbf{u}^h = 0 \right\} \tag{9}$$

The solution I^h should then lie on the null space of $\mathbf{Q}$ that must be zero. The numerical problem described above is eliminated by proper choice for the finite element spaces of the velocity and pressure fields; in other words the evaluation of the integrals for the stiffness matrix where velocity and pressure interpolations appear must satisfy the Babuska-Brezzi compatibility condition the so called LBB condition [15–17] that states velocity and pressure spaces can not be chosen arbitrarily and a link between them is necessary.

In this chapter the numerical procedure for the transient non-Newton inelastic Navier–Stokes equations uses the Galerkin-finite element method with implicit time discretization. Considering a 3D analysis hexahedral meshes often provide the best quality solution as errors due to numerical diffusion are reduced whenever a good alignment between mesh edges and flow exists [4]; in this work a spatial discretization with isoparametric brick elements of low order with trilinear approximation for the velocity components and element constant pressure is adopted:

$$\mathbf{u}(\mathbf{x}, t) = \sum_{i=1}^{8} N_i(\mathbf{x}) u_i(t) \quad \text{and} \quad p(t) = M p_c(t) \tag{10}$$

where u_i and p_c are the unknown element velocity node values and the pressure element center value, respectively. At each time step Picard iteration is applied to linearize the non-linear convection and diffusion terms; the method is based on a pressure correction [11, 18]. The essential steps of the algorithm at a time or iteration are:

1. Calculation of an auxiliary velocity field from the equations of motion using known pressure values from the previous time step or previous iteration step;
2. Calculation of the pressure correction using lumped mass matrix;
3. Pressure updating;
4. Calculation of the divergence free velocity field;
5. Calculation of the apparent viscosity.

This method developed for obtaining a divergence-free velocity field has been based on Chorin's method [19] and validated by other authors.

3.2 Penalty Finite Element Model

The incompressibility constraint given by $\varepsilon_{ii} = 0$ is difficult to implement due to the zero divergence condition for the velocity field. The incompressible problem may be stated as a constrained minimization of a functional. The penalty function method, like the Lagrange multiplier method, allows us to reformulate a problem with constraints as one without constraints [15, 17]. Using the penalty function method proposed by Courant [20], the problem is transformed into the minimization of the unconstrained augmented functional:

$$\pi(\mathbf{u}) = \pi(\mathbf{u}) + \lambda \int_V (\varepsilon_{ii}(\mathbf{u}))^2 \, \mathrm{d}V \tag{11}$$

Considering the pseudo-constitutive relation for the incompressibility constraint the second set of (3) is replaced by:

$$\nabla \cdot \mathbf{u} = -p/\lambda \tag{12}$$

where λ is the penalty parameter. If λ is too small compressibility and pressure errors will occur and an excessively large value may result in numerical ill conditioning; generally λ is assigned to $\lambda = \beta\mu$ being β a constant of order 10^7 for double precision calculations. The second set of (3) is eliminated and the Navier–Stokes equations become:

$$\mathbf{M}\dot{\mathbf{u}} + \left(\mathbf{C} + \mathbf{K} + \mathbf{K}^\lambda\right)\mathbf{u} = \mathbf{F} \tag{13}$$

where $\mathbf{K}^\lambda$ is the so-called penalty matrix:

$$\mathbf{K}^\lambda = \lambda\mathbf{Q}\mathbf{M}^p\mathbf{Q}^t \quad \text{and} \quad \mathbf{M}^p\mathbf{P} = \lambda\mathbf{Q}^t\mathbf{u} \quad M_{ij}^p = \int_e L_i L_j \, de \tag{14}$$

Under such conditions the pressure is eliminated as a field variable since it can be recovered by the approximation of (12). If the standard Galerkin formulation is applied it is necessary to use compatible spaces for the velocity and the pressure in order to satisfy the LBB stability condition. This often excludes the use of the equal order interpolation functions for both fields. In order to avoid oscillatory results the numerical problem is eliminated by proper evaluation of the integrals for the stiffness matrix where penalty terms are calculated using a numerical integration rule of an order less than that required to integrate them exactly. This technique of under-integrating the penalty terms is known in the literature as the reduced integration.

3.3 Streamline Upwind/Petrov Galerkin Method

In a Galerkin formulation there is no doubt that the most difficult problem arises because of the nonlinear convective term in (3). In blood flow high Reynolds numbers appear and loss of unicity of solution, hydrodynamical instabilities and turbulence are caused by this apparently innocent term. The numerical scheme requires a stabilization technique in order to avoid oscillations in the numerical solution. The most appropriate technique to solve these problems is the Streamline upwind/Petrov Galerkin method, SUPG-method [21, 22]. The goal of this technique is the elimination of the instability problems of the Galerkin formulation by introducing an artificial dissipation. The method uses modified velocity shape functions, W_i, for the convective terms:

$$W_i = N_i + K_{SUPG}\frac{\mathbf{u}\nabla N_i}{\|\mathbf{u}\|} \tag{15}$$

where K_{SUPG} denotes the upwind parameter that controls the factor of upwind weighting. This parameter controls the amount of upwind weighting and is defined on an element as:

$$k_{SUPG} = \frac{1}{2}\xi_i(Pe^e)u_i^e h_i^e, \quad i = 1, 2, 3 \tag{16}$$

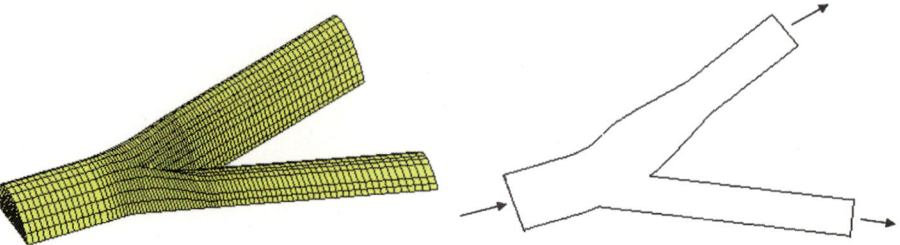

Fig. 1 Carotid artery bifurcation model

a function of u_i^e and h_i^e element velocity and length, respectively, and the grid Peclet number Pe^e. The SUPG-method produces a substantial increase in accuracy as stabilizing artificial diffusivity is added only in the direction of the streamlines and crosswind diffusion effects are avoided.

The resulting system of nonlinear equations is characterized by a non-symmetric matrix, and a special solver is adopted in order to reduce the bandwidth and the storage of the sparse system matrix; in addition the Skyline method is used to some improvement of the Gauss elimination.

3.4   Carotid Bifurcation Model

The numerical example presented here is a 3D flow simulation in the human carotid artery bifurcation. Figure 1 shows the geometrical model described by Perktold [11, 18]. The Navier–Stokes equations are solved using the Finite Element SUPG-method with implicit Euler backward differences for time derivatives and Picard iteration for nonlinear terms.

The non-Newtonian property of blood is important in the hemodynamic effect and plays a significant role in vascular biology and pathology. In this study the viscosity is empirically obtained using Casson law for the shear stress relation. Considering D_{II} the second invariant of the strain rate and c the red cell concentration, the shear stress τ given by the generalized Casson relation is:

$$\sqrt{\tau} = k_0 + k_1(c)\sqrt{2\sqrt{D_{II}}} \tag{17}$$

and the apparent dynamic viscosity $\mu = \mu(c, D_{II})$, a function of the red cell concentration,

$$\mu = \frac{1}{2\sqrt{D_{II}}}\left(k_0 + k_1(c)\sqrt{2\sqrt{D_{II}}}\right)^2 \tag{18}$$

where parameters $k_0 = 0.6125$ and $k_1 = 0.174$ were obtained fitting experimental data, considering $c = 45\%$ and plasma viscosity $\mu_0 = 0.124\,\mathrm{Pa\,s}$ [11].

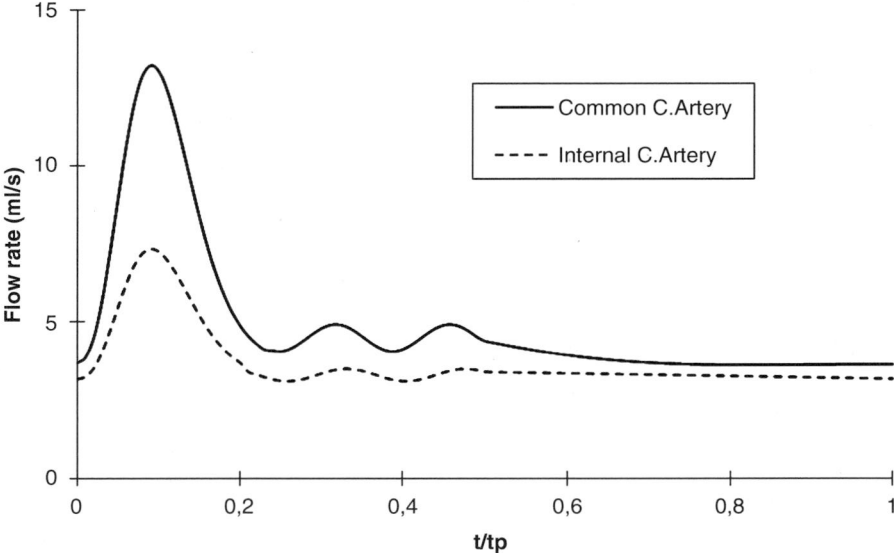

Fig. 2 Flow pulse waveform in the common carotid and in the internal carotid arteries

The computer simulation is carried out under physiological pulsatile flow conditions. The considered time dependent flow rate waveform in the common carotid and in the internal carotid arteries [11, 23] is presented in Fig. 2. The time-averaged flow rate in the common carotid is 5.1 ml/s and the mean common carotid inflow velocity is U = 169 mm/s. In this work the common carotid diameter was taken equal to D = 6.2 mm (characteristic length), the reference blood viscosity is μ = 0.0035 Pa s and the mean reference Reynolds number equal to Re = 300.

At the inflow boundary fully developed time-dependent velocity profiles are prescribed. The profiles correspond to the pulse waveform in the common carotid artery. At the rigid artery wall the no slip condition ($\mathbf{u}$ = 0) is applied. The conditions describing vanishing normal and tangential force of (5) cannot be applied simultaneously at both outflow boundaries. The flow simulation is carried out in two steps. In the first calculation step, developed flow is assumed at the internal carotid outlet according to the prescribed time-dependent flow division shown in Fig. 2 and the condition of zero surface traction force is applied at the external carotid outflow boundary. During the second calculation step, which is the actual calculation step, the condition of zero surface traction force is applied at the internal carotid outflow boundary, while at the external carotid outflow boundary the results for the velocity profiles from the first step are used.

The flow characteristics in the carotid bifurcation are presented. Figure 3 shows velocity field during the pulse cicle tp, at selected fractions of a period: t/tp = 0.05 (accelerated flow), t/tp = 0.1 (maximum flow rate) and t/tp = 0.14 (decelerated flow). At the entrance of the internal and the external carotid relatively high

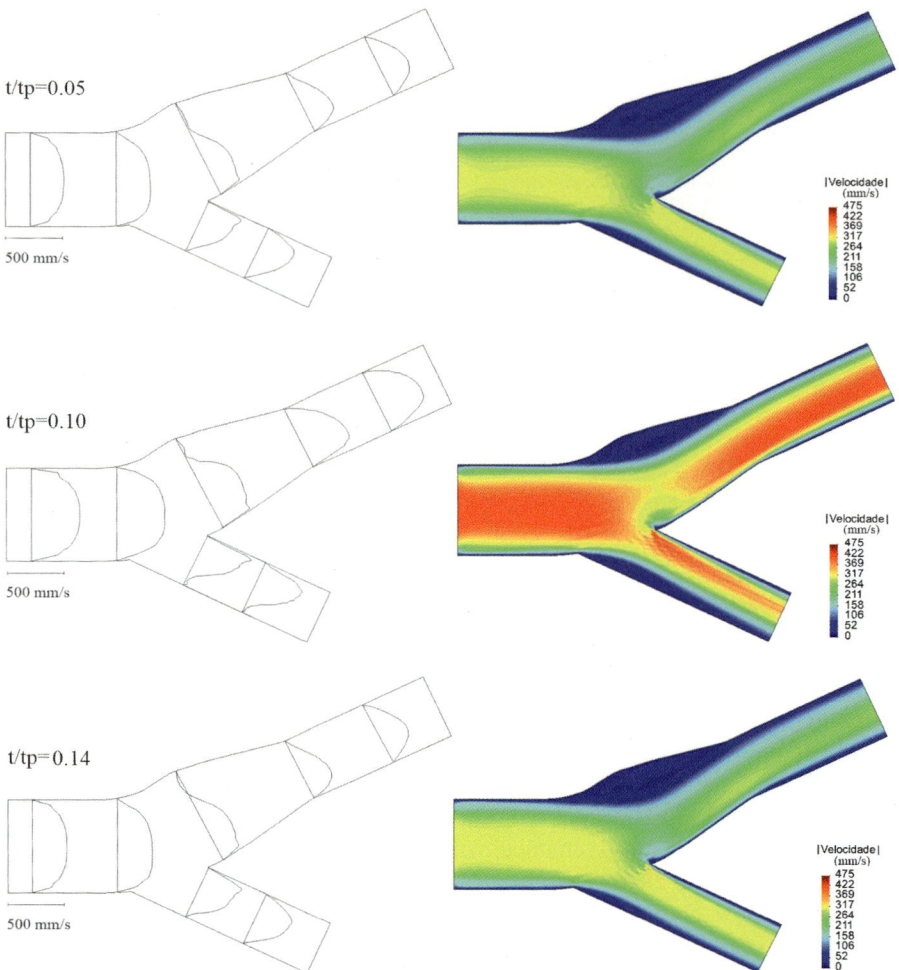

Fig. 3 Axial flow velocity profiles at the symmetry plane during the pulse cicle *tp*, at selected fractions of a period: *t/tp* = 0.05 (accelerated flow), *t/tp* = 0.1 (maximum flow rate) and *t/tp* = 0.14 (decelerated flow)

axial velocities and steep velocity gradients can be observed near the divider wall. The shifting of the mass flow to the divider wall results from the branching effect and from the curvature effect. A zone of special hemodynamic relevance is the widened segment of the internal carotid, the carotid sinus. Time-dependent stagnated and reversed flow occurs along the outer sinus wall (the wall opposite the divider wall). During systolic acceleration (*t/tp* = 0.05), only forward directed flow occurs in the sinus. At the end of flow acceleration (peak systole *t/tp* = 0.10) flow stagnation can be observed at the outer sinus wall near the entrance to the internal carotid. During systolic deceleration *(t/tp* = 0.14 where the inflow rate is the same as at $t/tp = 0.05$) significant flow separation and reversed flow appear in the sinus. The reversed flow occupies around 50% of the sinus diameter in the branching plane.

The numerical findings on flow separation near the outer sinus wall agree with previously published results. In further studies the carotid bifurcation flow field will be investigated using parameters obtained from clinical observations.

4 Optimization of an Artificial Bypass Graft

Numerical simulations of blood flow in arteries can be used to improve the understanding of vascular diseases searching efficient treatments and medical devices. A framework for graft design optimization used in a bypass surgery, which is performed to restore blood flow in stenosed arteries is described here. Coupling shape optimization to three-dimensional unsteady blood flow simulations poses several key challenges, including high computational cost, a need to handle constraints, and a need for automatic generation of parameterized vessel geometry. Instead, the applicability of the optimization framework is demonstrated considering a two-dimensional steady flow simulation. An idealized graft/artery model is parameterized with a geometry allowing the analysis of the influence of graft-to-artery angle and diameter. Search for optimized arterial bypass grafts has been presented in the literature [12, 14] always restricted to one objective function. This work represents the use of formal multi-objective optimization algorithms for surgery design.

4.1 Multi-Objective Optimization Strategy

In shape optimization, the goal is to minimize an objective function that typically depends on a state vector **u,** over a domain of design vector **b**. The state vector and the design parameters are coupled by a partial differential equation that can be written in a generic form as

$$s(\mathbf{u}, \mathbf{b}) = 0 \qquad (19)$$

This so-called state equation forms the constraint of the minimization problem

$$\text{Minimize } \Phi(\mathbf{u}, \mathbf{b})$$
$$\text{subject to } s(\mathbf{u}, \mathbf{b}) = 0 \qquad (20)$$

Furthermore, the problem can be recast using the reduced form of the objective function

$$\text{Minimize } \Phi^*(\mathbf{u}(\mathbf{b}), \mathbf{b}) \qquad (21)$$

where $\mathbf{u}(\mathbf{b})$ is the solution of (19). This form allows decoupling the solution of the state equation and the optimization problem.

A general multi-objective optimization seeks to optimize the components of a vector-valued objective function mathematically formulated as

$$\text{Minimize} \quad F(\mathbf{b}) = (f_1(\mathbf{b}), f_2(\mathbf{b}), ..., f_m(\mathbf{b}))$$

$$\text{subject to} \quad \begin{array}{l} b_i^{lower} \leq b_i \leq b_i^{upper}, \ i = 1, ..., n \\ g_k(\mathbf{b}) \qquad \leq 0, \ k = 1, ..., p \end{array} \quad (22)$$

where $\mathbf{b} = (b_1, ..., b_n)$ is the design vector, b_i^{lower} and b_i^{upper} represent the lower and upper boundary of the ith design variable b_i, $f_j(\mathbf{b})$ is the jth objective function and $g_k(\mathbf{b})$ the kth constraint. Unlike single objective optimization approaches, the solution to this problem is not a single point, but a family of points known as the Pareto-optimal set. A Pareto optimal solution is defined as one that is not dominated by any other solution of the multi-objective optimization problem. Typically, there are infinitely many Pareto optimal solutions for a multi-objective problem. Thus, it is often necessary to incorporate user preferences for various objectives in order to determine a single suitable solution.

Genetic algorithms are well suited to multi-objective optimization problems as they are fundamentally based on biological processes which are inherently multi-objective.

4.2 Genetic Search

A genetic algorithm (GA) is a stochastic search method based on evolution and genetics exploiting the concept of survival of the fittest. For a given problem or design domain there exists a multitude of possible solutions that form a solution space. In a genetic algorithm, a highly effective search of the solution space is performed, allowing a population of strings representing possible design vectors to evolve through basic genetic operators. The goal of these operators is to progressively reduce the space design driving the process into more promising regions.

Multi-objective genetic algorithms (MOGAs) were first suggested by Schaffer [24]. Since then several algorithms have been proposed on the basis of an evolutionary process searching for Pareto optimal solutions. MOGAs have been successfully applied to solve various kinds of multi-objective problems as they are not as much affected by nonlinearities and complex objective functions as mathematical programming algorithms.

One MOGA strategy consists of transferring multi-objectives to a single objective by a weighted sum approach. The weighted sum method for multi-objective optimization problems continues to be used extensively not only to provide multiple solution points by varying the weights consistently, but also to provide a single solution point that reflects preferences presumably incorporated in the selection of a single set of weights. Using the weighted sum method to solve the optimization problem given in (22) entails selecting scalar weights w_j and minimizing the following composite objective function:

$$F^*(\mathbf{b}) = \sum_{j=1,m} w_j \, f_j(\mathbf{b}) \tag{23}$$

If all of the weights are positive, as assumed in this study, then minimizing (23) provides a sufficient condition for Pareto optimality, which means that its minimum is always Pareto optimal [25]. The weighting for an individual objective can be determined by either fixed weights or random weights. A strategy of randomly assigning weights is used to search for an optimum solution through diverse directions [26, 27]. To provide decision makers with flexible and diversified solutions, this study adopts random weights calculated by using

$$w_j = \frac{r_j}{r_1 + r_2 + \dots + r_m}, \quad j = 1, \dots, m \tag{24}$$

where r_j is a random positive integer.

The genetic algorithm scheme searching for optimal solutions is based on four operators supported by an elitist strategy that always preserves a core of best individuals of the population whose genetic material is transferred into the next generations [28, 29]. A new population of solutions P^{t+1} is generated from the previous P^t using the genetic operators: Selection, Crossover, Mutation and Deletion.

The optimization scheme includes the following steps:

Coding: the design variables expressed by real numbers are converted to binary numbers, forming a string, and each binary string is looked as an individual;

Initializing: the individuals which consist of an initial population P^0 are produced randomly within each allowable interval;

Evaluation: the fitness of each individual is evaluated using the objective function given in (23), and individuals are ranked according to their fitness value;

Selection: definition of the elite group that includes individuals highly fitted. Selection of the progenitors is the mechanism that defines the process in which the chromosomes are mated before applying crossover on them. We apply a procedure that randomly chooses one parent from the best-fitted group (elite) and another from the least fitted one. Transfer of the whole population P^t to an intermediate step where they will join the offspring determined by the crossover operator;

Crossover: One offspring per each pair of selected parents is considered in the present work. The value of each gene in the offspring chromosome coincides with the value of the same gene in one of the parents depending on a given probability. The new individuals created by crossover will join the original population.

Mutation: the implemented mutation is characterized by changing a set of bits of the binary string corresponding to one variable of a randomly selected chromosome

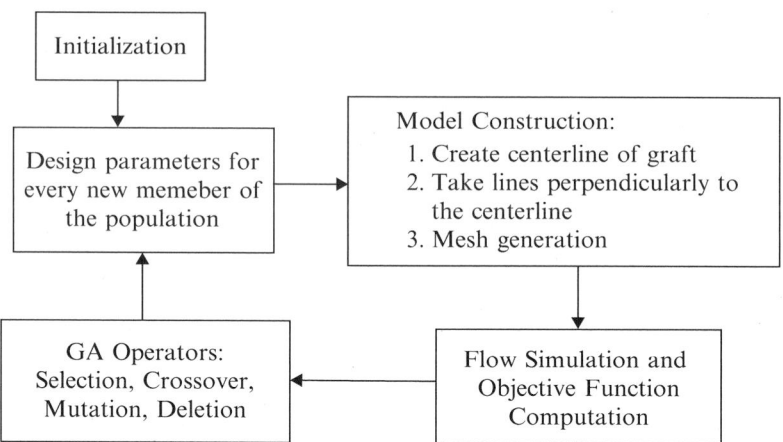

Fig. 4 Shape optimization algorithm

from the elite group making possible the exploitation of previously unmapped space design regions and guaranteeing the diversity of the generated population.

Deletion: After mutation, new ranking of the enlarged population according to their fitness. Then, it follows the deletion of the worst solutions with low fitness simulating the natural death of weak and old individuals. The original size population is recovered and the new population P^{t+1} is obtained; the evolutionary process will continue until the stopping criterion is reached.

Termination: checking the termination condition. If it is satisfied, the GA is terminated. Otherwise, the process returns to step Selection.

To fully automate the shape optimization procedure, the following sub-steps are linked in our framework: model generation, meshing, multi-objective function evaluation (flow simulation and post processing) and data transfer into the GA so that the optimization procedure does not require any user intervention. Figure 4 shows the sub-steps of the optimization procedure. The boxes and arrows in Fig. 4 form a loop that repeats until stopping criteria are satisfied.

4.3 Optimized Graft Example

Search for an optimized geometry of an idealized arterial bypass system with fully occluded host artery is addressed here. This shape optimization problem requires an efficient and accurate solver for steady flow simulation. The Navier–Stokes equations are solved using the previously described penalty finite element model. The non-Newtonian behaviour of the blood is described using Casson law given by (18).

The objective functions need to be carefully chosen to capture the physics of the underlying problem. Regarding the choice of suitable objective functions for the graft optimization problem, several different approaches have been pursued in the literature [2, 12, 14]. The most frequently considered quantities in the context of blood flow are based on either shear stress and its gradient or the flow rate. Many authors choose to minimize the integral of the squared shear rate over the entire simulated domain $\Omega(\mathbf{b})$. This integral is also called dissipation integral because it measures the dissipation of energy due to viscous effects, expressed in terms of the rate of strain tensor,

$$\frac{1}{2} \int_{\Omega(\mathbf{b})} \dot{\gamma}^2 dx \tag{25}$$

The minimization of this function is related to flow efficiency. Flow efficiency can equivalently be measured by computing the maximum pressure variation in the domain. In this project we chose to optimize the flow efficiency by minimizing the pressure variation quantified as:

$$\varphi_1(\mathbf{b}) = \Delta p = |p_{max} - p_{min}| \tag{26}$$

The second chosen objective function is related to the minimization of reversed flow and residence times along the arterial bypass system. For each idealized bypass graft geometry simulation, a domain $\Omega^*(\mathbf{b})$ has been identified indicating where reversed flow and residence times are enhanced. Then, to minimize residence times is equivalent to maximize the longitudinal velocity $\mathbf{u}_x$ in that critical domain. The following objective function is considered for the minimization problem investigated in this work,

$$\varphi_2(\mathbf{b}) = -\sum_{\Omega^*(b)} \mathbf{u}_x \tag{27}$$

The artery is simulated using a fixed diameter tube of 10 mm. Design parameters are considered for the coupled graft presenting a sinusoidal geometry. The graft mesh does not maintain the same width along its whole length. At the centre line of the graft, nodes move in the radial direction preserving their distance to the deforming centreline. The graft is properly connected to the artery always in the same region but the graft diameter will vary. Due to the sinusoidal shape, the graft artery junction is always larger than the width at the graft center line.

The developed computer program modelled blood flow in artery and graft using 2,261 nodes and 2,024 four-node linear elements for a two-dimensional finite element approximation. Figure 5 presents the geometry and finite element mesh considered for the idealized arterial bypass system simulation with the flow proceeding from left to right. The boundary conditions for the flow field are parabolic inlet velocity corresponding to a Reynolds number equal to 300, no-slip boundary conditions including the graft and a parallel flow condition at the outlet.

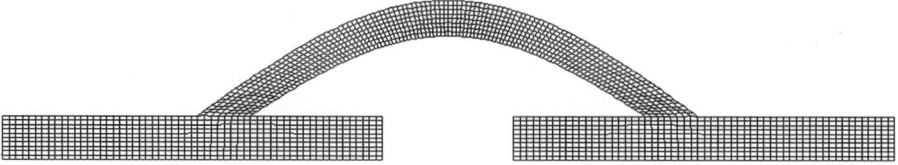

Fig. 5 Finite element mesh for the bypass optimization problem

For the optimization problem the graft/artery ratio diameter varies from 0.6 to 1.2, the height of the sinus curve varies from 10 to 20 mm and a circular anastomosis is set accordingly. Only symmetric geometries were considered since removing the symmetry constrain does not have a major effect [30]. So asymmetry is not requisite for the design of the bypass under the given flow conditions.

The search space is not known in absolute terms and simulations of 100 random possible graft designs have been conducted in order to get an indication of the objective space distribution. Figure 6 presents results for maximum pressure variation in the whole domain $\Omega(\mathbf{b})$ and for the longitudinal velocity in the critical domain $\Omega^*(\mathbf{b})$ where reversed flow and residence times are enhanced. The optimal solutions in the decision space are in general denoted as the Pareto set and its image in the objective space as Pareto front. Results shown in Fig. 6 allow identifying the likely presence of a Pareto front in the design problem. The shape optimization will allow at least a 20% decrease on the pressure variation.

Since objective values are distributed in different ranges normalizing objective values by the fittest in the generation before the weighted-sum operation has been proposed [31]. For the optimization example, (23) becomes:

$$F^*(\mathbf{b}) = w_1 \frac{\varphi_1(\mathbf{b})}{\varphi_1^*(\mathbf{b})} + w_2 \frac{\varphi_2(\mathbf{b})}{\varphi_2^*(\mathbf{b})} \tag{28}$$

where φ_1^* and φ_2^* are the fittest values for φ_1 and φ_2, respectively, in the generation. The weight parameters w_1 and w_2 are random values calculated as in (24). The fitness function to be maximized by the GA is then defined as:

$$FIT = A - F^*(\mathbf{b}) - P \tag{29}$$

being A a positive integer to ensure positiveness and P a value to penalize design vectors that do not conform with constraints. As a compromise between computer time and population diversity, parameters for the genetic algorithm were taken as $N_{pop} = 12$ and $N_e = 5$ for the population and elite group size, respectively. The number of bits in binary codifying for the design variables was $N_{bit} = 5$. Optimal bypass geometries were obtained setting the maximum number of generations as 200. One optimal graft with design parameters given as graft diameter of 11.7 mm and height 18.7 mm is discussed here. The simulated longitudinal velocity values for the optimal graft solution are given in Fig. 7. The longitudinal velocity distribution

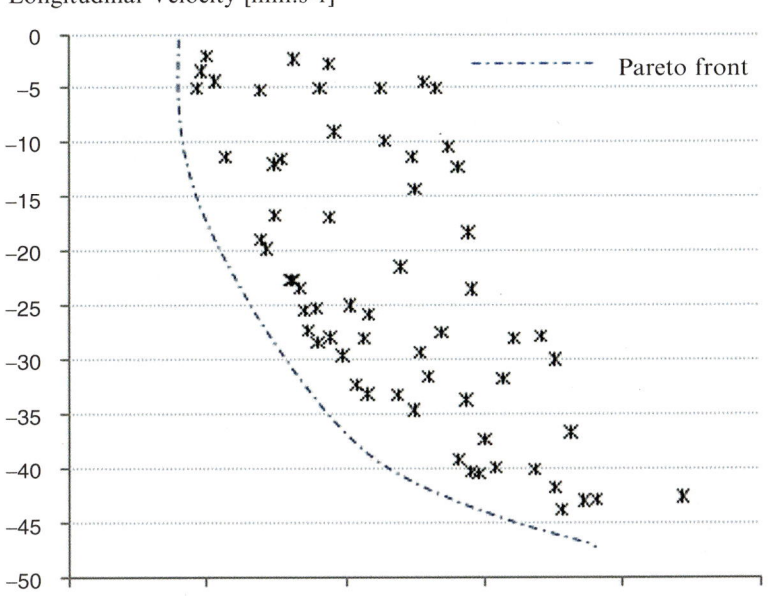

Fig. 6 Maximum pressure variation and longitudinal velocities for critical domain

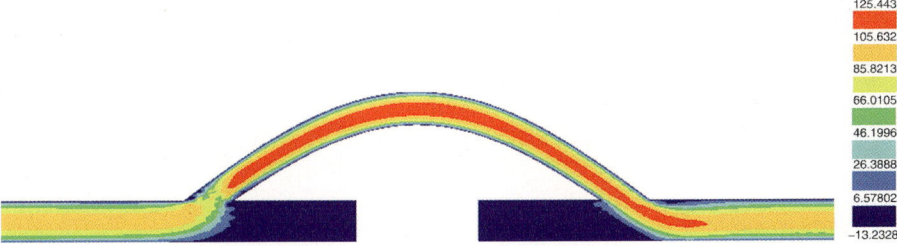

Fig. 7 Velocity distribution [mm s^{-1}] for the optimal shape

along bypass and host artery can be analysed in three parts. In the first part the flow is still undisturbed and therefore the velocity is quite uniform. In the second part the flow is within the graft area where the velocity raises as the flow moves along the graft. In the third part the flow is sufficiently far from the graft and therefore it exhibits a uniform distribution. At the exit of the graft after the artery-graft junction, the velocity values variation is rather smooth. It is interesting to notice that although the abrupt connection between artery and graft induces large velocity variations, the observable reverse flow is quite small. Long residence times usually observable immediately after the toe of the distal anastomosis are quite undetectable.

An optimal shape for idealized bypass graft geometry was obtained using a genetic search built around a developed finite element solver and adding routines evaluating objective functions. The solution exhibits the benefits of numerical shape optimization in achieving grafts inducing small gradient hemodynamic flows and minimizing reversed flow and residence times.

5 Concluding Remarks

A computational finite element model for simulating blood flow in arteries is presented. Blood flow is described by the incompressible Navier–Stokes equations and the simulation is carried out under steady and pulsatile conditions. The accuracy and efficiency of the blood simulation is tested considering two examples. In the first example the finite element method is used to simulate blood flow in a carotid artery bifurcation. Calculations of the flow field for the carotid artery are in good agreement with those reported previously in the literature. The model was able to simulate complex flow patterns in the carotid sinus like time-dependent stagnation and reversed flow along the outer sinus wall where flow separation occurs throughout the systolic deceleration phase.

The second example represents a step towards developing a formal optimization procedure for surgery design. An optimal shape for an idealized bypass is proposed. A major limitation of this study is the use of cylindrical models whereas parameterizations of patient specific models present significant challenges. Future work should also consider the influence of compliant walls and the effect of uncertainties in simulation parameters. Robust optimization that accounts for uncertainties could identify solutions that are less sensitive to small changes in design parameters, thus allowing a hospital surgical implementation.

Further studies will consider experimental data collected in clinical practice.

Acknowledgments This work was partially done in the scope of project PTDC/SAU-BEB/102547/2008, "Blood flow simulation in arterial networks towards application at hospital", financially supported by *FCT – Fundação para a Ciência e a Tecnologia* from Portugal.

References

1. Pedrizzetti G, Perktold K (2003) Cardiovascular fluid mechanics. Springer, New York
2. Su CM, Lee D, Tran-Son-Tay R, Shyy W (2005) Fluid flow structure in arterial bypass anastomosis. J Biomech Eng 127:611–618
3. Maurits NM, Loots GE, Veldman AEP (2007) The influence of vessel elaticity and peripheral resistance on the carotid artery flow wave form: a CFD model compared to in vivo ultrasound measurements. J Biomech 40:427–436
4. De Santis G, Mortier P, De Beule M, Segers P, Verdonck P, Verhegghe B (2010) Patient-specific computational fluid dynamics: structured mesh generation from coronary angiography. Med Biol Eng Comput 48(4):371–380

5. Taylor CA, Hughes TJR, Zarins CK (1998) Finite element modeling of blood flow in arteries. Comput Meth Appl Mech Eng 158:155–196

6. Quarteroni A, Tuveri M, Veneziani A (2003) Computational vascular fluid dynamics: problems, models and methods. Comput Vis Sci 2:163–197

7. Leuprecht A, Kozerke S, Peter Boesiger P, Perktold K (2003) Blood flow in the human ascending aorta: a combined MRI and CFD study. J Eng Math 47(3):387–404

8. Kaazempur-Mofrad MR, Isasi AG, Younis HF, Chan RC, Hinton DP, Sukhova G, LaMuraglia GM, Lee RT, Kamm RD (2004) Characterization of the atherosclerotic carotid bifurcation using MRI, finite element modeling and histology. Ann Biomed Eng 32(7):932–946

9. Schumann C, Neugebauer M, Bade R, Preim B, Peitgen H-O (2008) Implicit vessel surface reconstruction for visualization and CFD simulation. Int J Comput Assist Radiol Surg 2:275–286

10. Himeno R (2003) Blood flow simulation toward actual application at hospital. In: The 5th Asian computational fluid dynamics, Korea

11. Perktold K, Resch M, Florian H (1991) Pulsatile non-Newtonian flow characteristics in a three-dimensional human carotid bifurcation model. ASME J Biomech Eng 113:463–475

12. Abraham F, Behr M, Heinkenschloss M (2005) Shape optimization in steady blood flow: a numerical study of non-Newtonian effects. Comput Meth Biomech Biomed Eng 8(2):127–137

13. Huang H, Modi VJ, Seymour BR (1995) Fluid mechanics of stenosed arteries. Int J Eng Sci 33:815–828

14. Probst M, Lülfesmann M, Bücker HM, Behr M, Bischof CH (2010) Sensitivity of shear rate in artificial grafts using automatic differentiation. Int J Numer Meth Fluids 62:1047–1062

15. Babuska I (1973) The finite element method with Lagrangian multipliers. Numer Math 20:179–192

16. Brezzi F (1974) on the existence, uniqueness and approximation of saddle-point problems ar sing from Lagrangian multipliers. RAIRO Anal Numér 8(R2):129–151

17. Babuska I, Osborn J, Pitkaranta J (1980) Analysis of mixed methods using, mesh dependent norms. Math Comp 35:1039–1062

18. Perktold K, Rappitsch G (1995) Mathematical modeling of local arterial flow and vessel mechanics. In: Crolet J, Ohayon R (eds) Computational methods for fluid structure interaction, vol 306, Pitman research notes in mathematics. Harlow, Longman, pp 230–245

19. Chorin AJ (1968) Numerical solution of the Navier-Stokes equations. Math Comp 22:745–762

20. Courant R (1943) Variational methods for the solution of problems of equilibrium and vibration. Bull Amer Math Soc 49:1–23

21. Hughes TJR, Franca LP, Balestra M (1986) A new finite element method for computational fluid dynamics: V. Circumventing the Babuska-Brezzi condition: a stable Petrov-Galerkin formulation of the Stokes problem accommodating equal order interpolations. Comput Meth Appl Mech Eng 59:85–99

22. Hughes TJR, Franca LP, Hulbert GM (1989) A new finite element method for computational fluid dynamics: VIII the Galerkin/least squares method for advective diffusive equations. Comput Meth Appl Mech Eng 73:173–189

23. Ku DN, Giddens DP, Zarins CZ, Glagov S (1985) Pulsatile flow and atherosclerosis in the human carotid bifurcation. Arteriosclerosis 5:293–302

24. Schaffer JD (1985) Multi-objective optimization with vector evaluated genetic algorithms. In: Proceedings of the 1st international conference of genetic algorithms, pp 93–100

25. Marler RT, Arora JS (2009) The weighted sum method for multi-objective optimization: new insights. Struct Multidisc Optim. doi:10.1007/s00158-009-0460-7

26. Kim IY, de Weck OL (2006) Adaptive weighted sum method for multiobjective optimization: a new method for Pareto. Struct Multidiscip Optim 31:105–116

27. Coello CAC, Lamont GB, Veldhuizen DAV (2007) Evolutionary algorithms for solving multi-objective problems. Springer, New York

28. António CC, Castro CF, Sousa LC (2005) Eliminating forging defects using genetic algorithms. Mater Manuf Process 20:509–522

29. Castro CF, António CAC, Sousa LC (2004) Optimisation of shape and process parameters in metal forging using genetic algorithms. J Mater Process Technol 146:356–364
30. Probst M, Lülfesmann M, Nicolai M, Bücker HM, Behr M, Bischof CH (2010) Sensitivity of optimal shapes of artificial grafts with respect to flow parameters. Comput Meth Appl Mech Eng 199:997–1005
31. Cochran JK, Horng S, Fowler JW (2003) A multi-population genetic algorithm to solve multi-objective scheduling problems for parallel machines. Comput Oper Res 30:1087–1102

Measuring Biomechanics of the Vision Process, Sensory Fusion and Image Observation Features

Jaroslav Dušek and Tomáš Jindra

1 Introduction

Study of the vision process biomechanics is an important part of the vision care. We acquire more than 90% of information by vision system, thus the system is the most important for our quality of life. Physicians focus their attention on care about the eyesight especially on infants. In this period the vision system develops and any disturbance can affect the development process and cause a pathological progress. The focus of our research is in measuring biomechanics of the vision process, sensory fusion and image observation features especially in infants with strabismus to support the diagnose and treatment. But in this text we will talk about methods and present results in normal (health) children.

1.1 Anatomy, Physiology and the Vision Process

1.1.1 Anatomy and Physiology of Eye

The eye is a paired organ situated in an orbit. Front part of eyeball, the cornea, is interface between the air outside and the aqueous humour on the inner side, which raises its refractive index (n = 1.37). The cornea's dioptric value is about 42 D. The aqueous humour is clear colourless liquid (similar to water) with a refractive

J. Dušek (✉)
Institute of Biophysics and Informatics, Charles University in Prague, Prague, Czech Republic
e-mail: jaroslav.dusek@lf1.cuni.cz

T. Jindra
Department of Radioelectronics, Faculty of Electrical Engineering, Czech Technical University in Prague, Prague, Czech Republic
e-mail: jindrto3@fel.cvut.cz

R.M.N. Jorge et al. (eds.), *Technologies for Medical Sciences*, Lecture Notes in Computational Vision and Biomechanics 1, DOI 10.1007/978-94-007-4068-6_5, © Springer Science+Business Media B.V. 2012

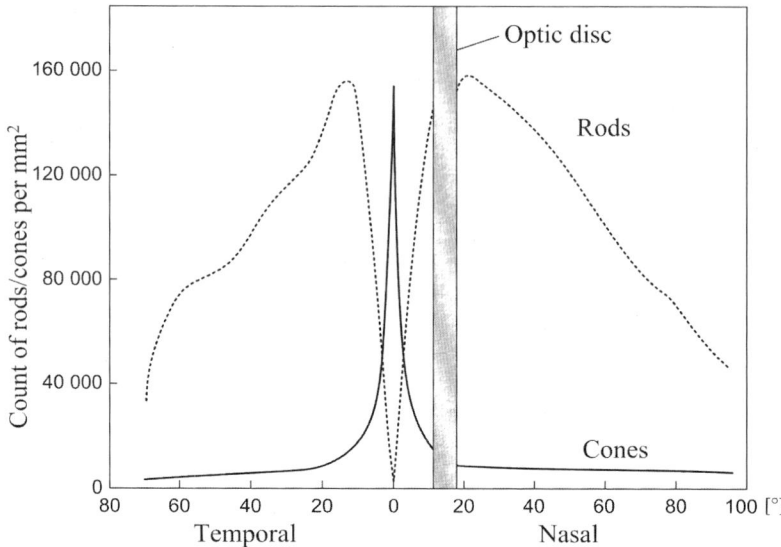

Fig. 1 Distribution of rods and cones in retina

index of n = 1.33. It contains a small amount of proteins providing nutrient for the cornea and lens. The iris is a circular structure in front of the lens. Its function is to control the diameter of the pupil and corrects optical aberration of the lens. Pupil diameter is reflexively controlled depending on the amount of incident light on the retina. The lens is a transparent elastic biconvex structure with a refractive index of n = 1.42. Its shape (and thereby focal length) is changed by contracting and relaxing the ciliary muscle. This process is called accommodation and is driven reflexively. The vitreous humour (n = 1.33) fills the inner space of the vitreous chamber. Its composition is similar to the aqueous humour and, in addition, contains vitrein accounting for the gel-like state of the vitreous humour. The sensory part of the eye is the retina located at the rear of the eyeball. Photoreceptors in the retina are the first of the four neurons in the visual pathway, but they are spatially located as the last layer of retina. There are two types of photoreceptors – cones and rods. Cones are chromatic photoreceptors suitable for photopic vision. Their greatest concentration is in the fovea centralis (150,000 per mm^2), which is the point of sharpest vision. The total number of cones is about 6–7 millions. Rods are achromatic sensors designed for scotopic vision. The approximate number of rods is 120 million with the greatest concentration in a circle of 5–6 mm diameter around the fovea centralis and concentration decreases towards the periphery (Fig. 1). More information can be found in e.g. [1].

   The next two neurons of the visual pathway are also located in the retina – bipolar and ganglion cells [1]. The axons of the ganglion cells transmit impulses around the inner perimeter of the eyeball and converge on the nervus opticus. Axons go through the chiasma opticum where part of the fibres cross to the opposite nervous fascicle (left and right tractus opticus). A small part of the tractus opticus fibres are separated

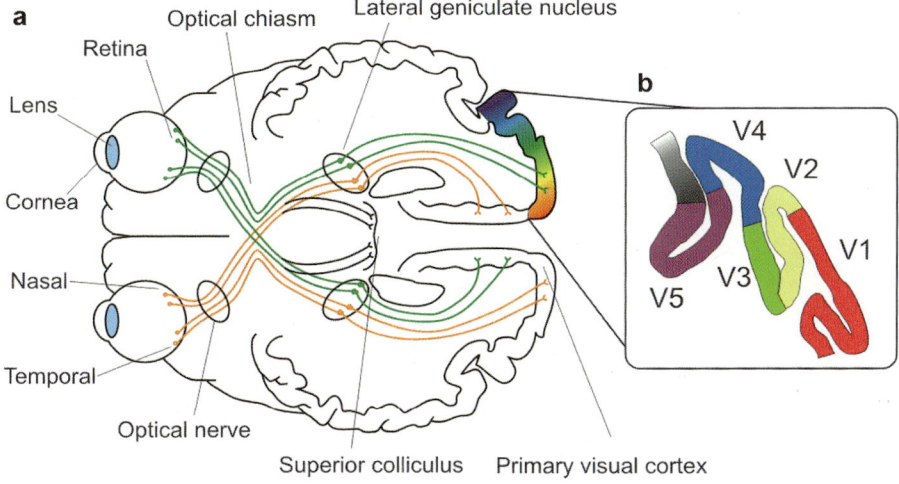

Fig. 2 Visual pathway (**a**) with the detailed visual cortex topography (**b**)

as radix optica mesencephalica and other fibres end in the lateral geniculate nucleus. Here the axons of the ganglion cells connect to the last neuron of the visual pathway (Fig. 2a). The axons of the fourth neuron constitute the tractus geniculocorticalis and terminate in the occipital lobe cortex (visual cortex) where they form the cortical image of the external world. The visual cortex is divided by its function into five smaller areas called V1-V5 (Fig. 2b). V1 area is the most studied part of the visual cortex from the point of image processing. It is divided into six main layers. V1 cells are similar with circle symmetry to retinal ganglion cells or lateral geniculate nucleus cells. They have receptive fields divided into inhibit and exhibit areas. These areas are not radial symmetric but they have oriented receptive fields with reaction to the specific space oriented stimulus (edge orientation, spatial frequencies, space locations, time frequencies and their combinations) [2]. From the V1 area is the image information send to the higher layers V2-V5 that are responsible for the complicated task of the vision process. These areas are still in the centre of the research. It is known e.g. that V4 is responsible for color vision and V5 for temporal vision. More in [1–7].

1.1.2 Eye Movements

Eye movements are a result of contracting and relaxing six ocular muscles. In physiological conditions multiple muscles are activated during eye movement, thus, muscles have more functions depending on the initial eye position. The movement of only one eye is called duction; the movement of both eyes with the same direction is version (dextroversion, levoversion, supraversion, infraversion). The opposite movement of the eyes is called vergence (convergence is medial

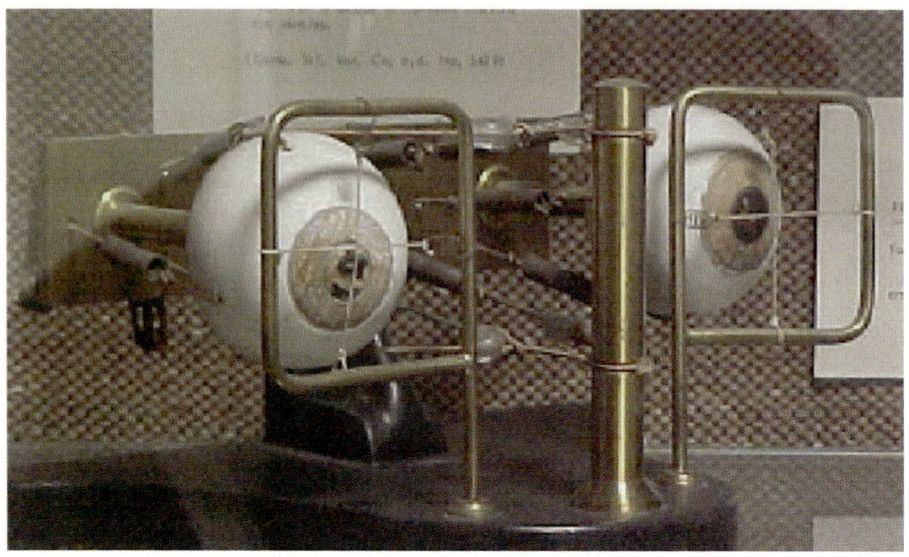

Fig. 3 Sherington's model of binocular balance (University Laboratory of Physiology, Oxford University, Oxford, UK)

movement, divergence is lateral movement). Multiple muscles in both eyes are used for directional eye movement. Every muscle has its antagonist in the same eye and synergist and antagonist in the opposite eye. Antagonist muscles work in the opposite direction, synergists in the same direction. The coordination and fluency of pair movements is driven in accordance with Hering's [8] and Sherrington's law [9]. According to Hering's law the innervation impulse for eye movement from the motor centre of the brain cortex is equally divided between the synergists of both eyes. In this case the synergist acts like a single organ. The same is true of antagonists in the reverse sense. Sherrinton's law describes reciprocal innervation of the muscles. Contraction of synergists has to be supplied by relaxing their antagonists. Movement Sherington's balance was practically modelled (Fig. 3). Ocular muscles are driven by three cranial nerves: n. III (n. oculomotorius), n. IV (n. trochlearis) and n. IV (n. abducens). Their motor kernels are situated in the rear of the brainstem and are connected with each other. Eye movements are driven by three brain centres. The first is occipital brain centre that governs eye-conditioned reflex movements (optomotorical) – accommodation, convergence, fusion, fixation and the blink reflex. The second centre is in the frontal brain lobe that drives volitional movements. The third centre is represented by statokinetical reflexes that are driven by the motor centre on the vestibular apparatus. Head and body position changes are aligned by this centre. These reflexes are congenital and are preserved even with blindness. Sensor fusion is essential for coordinating correct eye movements.

1.1.3   Binocular and Stereoscopic Vision

One of the most important functions of the human visual system is binocular vision. This enables us space perception and orientation.

The development of human binocular vision has two phases. In the first phase, it is the development of monocular vision. After birth components of the child's vision system mature. A newborn is capable of short-term monocular fixation, the squint in the other eye is physiological (strabismus spurius). Fixation becomes active from the beginning of the 2nd month, the child observes persons and moving objects. However, tracking movements aren't continual. The immaturity of brain centres causes low visual acuity. From the beginning of the 5th week, the child is capable of foveolar fixation. The critical phase of visual development sensitivity occurs in the 2nd and 3rd months. Visual acuity rapidly improves. Any pathological states in this period could affect visual development and lead to a disorder of the brain's vision centre and the development of amblyopia. There is a second phase after achieving a sufficient state of monocular vision. The afferent visual pathway connects to binocular cortical cells sensitive to stimulation of both eyes and to monocular cells sensitive to stimulation of one of the eyes. Binocular cortical cells are present in a newborn. The utilization of these cells depends on the anatomical and physiological condition of the eyes as well as on retinal stimulation and the parallel position of the eyes, which changes with age. Binocular vision progresses along with the development of optomotorical coordination. Visual development becomes pathological when any disturbance during normal development occurs. The visual centre is suppressed and amblyopia, strabismus, anomal retinal correspondence or alternating vision could evolve.

The development of normal visual development can be arrested by:

1. Optical obstruction – refractive disorder, cataract, unsuitable optical correction, eye occlusion
2. Neural obstruction – retinal or visual pathway disorders
3. Congenital deviation – skull, orbit or a tumour
4. CNS disorder – during brain dysfunction

Single binocular vision conditions:

– Motor

  1. Free eye movements in all directions
  2. Normal function of motor pathways and coordination centres for accommodation and convergence
  3. Parallel eye position for distance vision

– Sensory

  1. Normal vision of both eyes
  2. Foveal fixation of both eyes
  3. Approximately identical size of retinal images
  4. Normal retinal correspondence
  5. Regular binocular reflexes

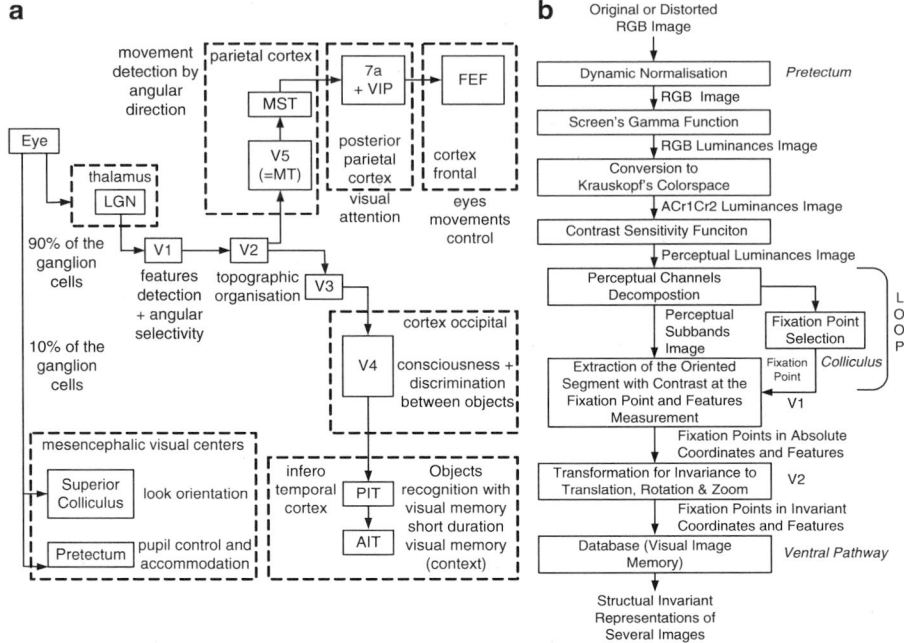

Fig. 4 Model of human vision process [14] – block scheme of the human vision process (**a**) and modeled mathematical algorithm of the human vision process (**b**)

It is very important to monitor these conditions in childhood to prevent abnormal vision. Automated methods for observing visual functions that are suitable for screening have been developed [17, 18, 26–28].

1.1.4 Vision Models – HVS (Human Vision Models)

Above mentioned anatomy and physiology features and process of vision are very often mathematically modelled [7, 10–14]. Example of complex model is presented in the Fig. 4a. There is shown whole process of vision. This model was performed by Carneca, Calleta and Barby [14]. Its mathematical algorithm is presented in the Fig. 4b.

1.2 Measuring Accommodation and Eye Movements

Important part of the vision process is coordination of accommodation with eye movements. We developed two unique measurement systems E.M.AN and Ir.M.A. that are described in this part. First who has been interested in measuring of

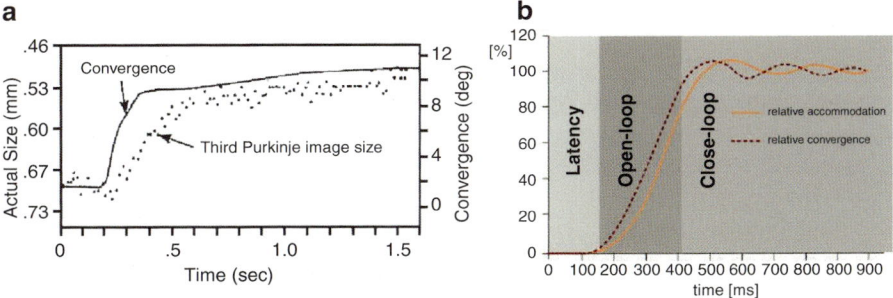

Fig. 5 Allen's results of measuring accommodation and vergence (**a**), expected course of the accommodation and vergence (**b**)

accommodation and vergence was M. J. Allen in 1949 [15]. His results shows Fig. 5a. On the Fig. 5b there is a theoretically setup curve of accommodation and vergence. First latency period is the time between the retinal stimulus and the start of the reaction (accommodation, vergence). Second pre-programmed period is the Open-loop initiative phase of accommodation or vergence. It is similar to saccadic movements. The third is the Close-loop phase and it is tune of the reaction conducted by the nervous feedback.

1.2.1 E.M.AN. – Eye Movement ANalyser (2D stimulation)

E.M.AN. is a videometric device for analysing eye movement and accommodation it is intended for measuring accommodation vergence synkinesis in small children [25]. The characteristics of the oculomotoric system are ascertained during step changes in the distance of a fixation images. Instant accommodation and vergence values are obtained by measurements using videometric apparatus and the subsequent offline software analyses of the image sequences. To detect the eye's horizontal position the Hirschberg test is used in conjunction with Purkinje images; the eccentric photorefraction method is used to obtain information about the dioptric power of the lens. Instant values of both parameters are contained in every measured image, thus it is possible to subsequently reconstruct the temporal changes of these parameters during measurement.

1.2.2 Principles and Methods

Purkinje images arise when light falling on the interface of the eye tissues is reflected. Purkinje described four types of image [16] (Fig. 6). The first of these (1st PI) arises on the interface between the air and the outer surface of the cornea and it is bright and erect. Thanks to the great difference in refraction indices, it has the greatest intensity. The second PI is formed by the reflection on the inner surface

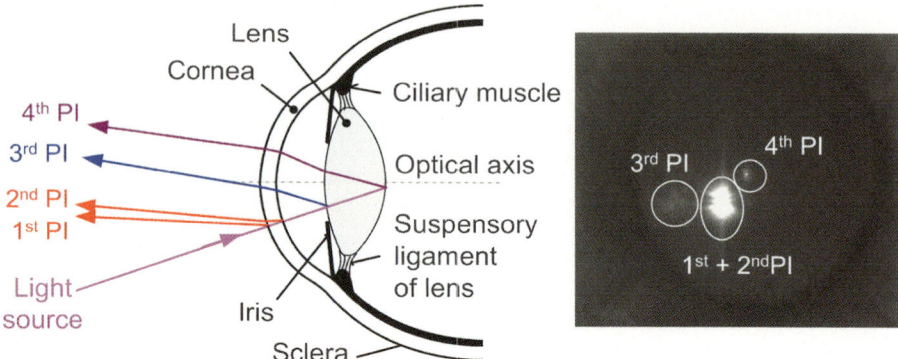

Fig. 6 Purkinje images

of the cornea and the aqueous humour. It is bright and erect, though less bright than the 1st PI often merging with it. The third image (3rd PI) arises on the interface of the aqueous humour and the anterior surface of the lens. The difference in the refraction indices is small (about $\Delta n = 0.09$), thus the intensity of 3rd PI is very low. Similar to the others this image is bright and upright. Its size depends on the curvature of the anterior surface of the lens, thus it can be used to detect the eye's accommodation. The 4th PI, which is formed on the interface of the posterior surface of the lens and the vitreous humour, is real and inverted. Several optometric methods were elaborated on the basis of knowledge about the Purkinje images based on analysis of their position or size in relation to the stationary point source of the measuring light. The instant position of the eye is ascertained using the Hirschberg test [19].

On the recorded image, the centre of the pupil is determined and compared with the position of the 1st PI, which is immobile with regards to the stationary light source. The eyes' position can also be measured from the disparity of 1st PI and 4th PI [17,18]. An analysis of the position and size of 3rd and 4th PI can be used to determine the radius of curvature of the anterior and posterior surface of the lens [17,18]. The problem with this method, however, is that the automated detection of 3rd PI is difficult. The image arising on the interface with a small difference in the refraction indices is blurred and it has a low intensity. An alternative to ascertaining the eye's accommodation using 3rd PI can be the eccentric photorefraction method, which has been used in these experiments.

The eccentric photorefraction method [19] is based on modifying and recording light that passes through the eye. A special diaphragm is placed on the lens of the recording equipment (camera, video-camera) (Fig. 7), which is eccentric to the measuring light source.

The measuring light passes through the eye's optic system and the part of it reflected from the retina returns. The light direction and intensity change depending on the dioptric power of the lens. The modified measuring light falls on the eccentric diaphragm and part of it enters the lens of the recording equipment. Using this

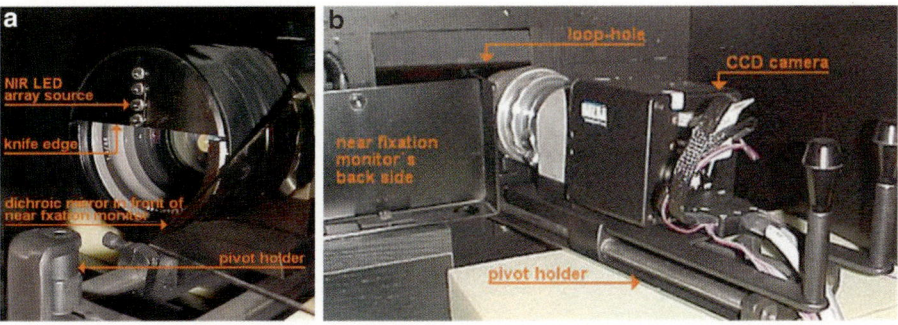

Fig. 7 Videometric part – pivot holder (**a**) and detail of eccentric diaphragm (**b**)

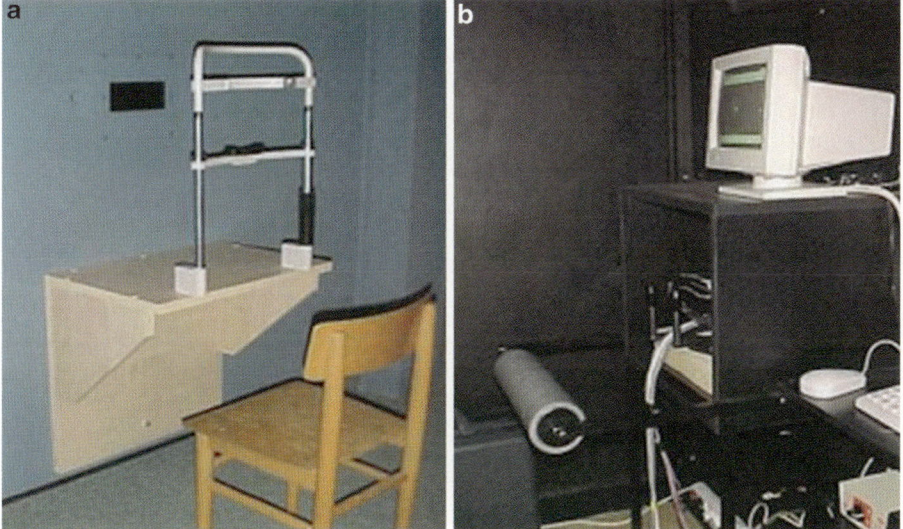

Fig. 8 Scheme of the image analysis

procedure a vertically variable brightness profile arises in the pupil image and its gradient corresponding to the immediate accommodation state of the eye (recorded image shown in Fig. 8).

The source of the measuring light beam is made up of four luminescent diodes stacked on one another (Fig. 7a). The wavelength is chosen from the invisible part of the light spectrum ($\lambda = 850$ nm), so there is no physiological miosis of the pupil and the patient's attention is not distracted. At the same time, the measuring light source is used for creating Purkinje images. Both measured artefacts are thus created by one wavelength and gained from one image.

A standardised stepped change in the distance of a fixed image stimulates a change in the accommodation and vergence of the eye apparatus. This is displayed to the patient on two fixation monitors. The distant monitor is 3.17 m from the patient's

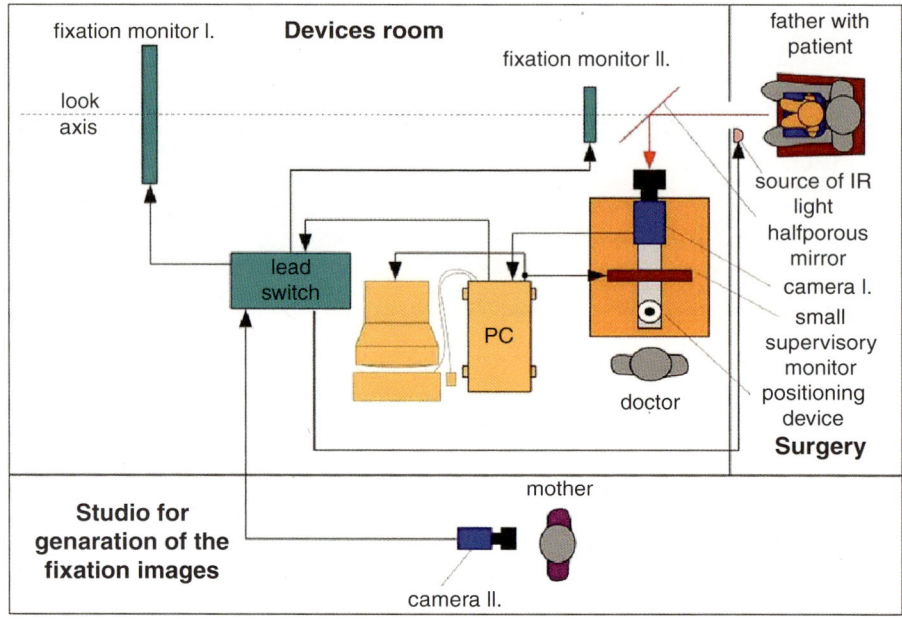

Fig. 9 Block scheme of E.M.AN system

eyes the close one is 0.37 m. From the patient's point of view, they have the same angular size. The monitors are displayed using a beam-splitter so that they have a common optical axis and approximately the same brightness. The fixed image is the face of the child's mother, who is captured on video in another room. The mother has feedback in the form of another video camera that records the child's face giving them visual communication.

1.3 Measuring System E.M.AN

Block scheme of the E.M.AN. system is presented in Fig. 9. The child, with its head fixed in the head-rest, sits in the first room (Fig. 10a). The mother's face is shown on the monitors. She sits in a separate room and is filmed and has another video camera to communicate visually with the child. The measuring apparatus, fixed monitors and a control station are in the measuring room (Fig. 10b). The child's eye is filmed separately.

An eccentric diaphragm with a NIR measuring ray source for invoking Purkinje images and a retinal reflex is placed in front of the lens of the measuring camera (Fig. 7a). Before measuring, the physician in the service room sets the camera position (Fig. 7b) and starts measuring. A digital monochromatic camera DALSA

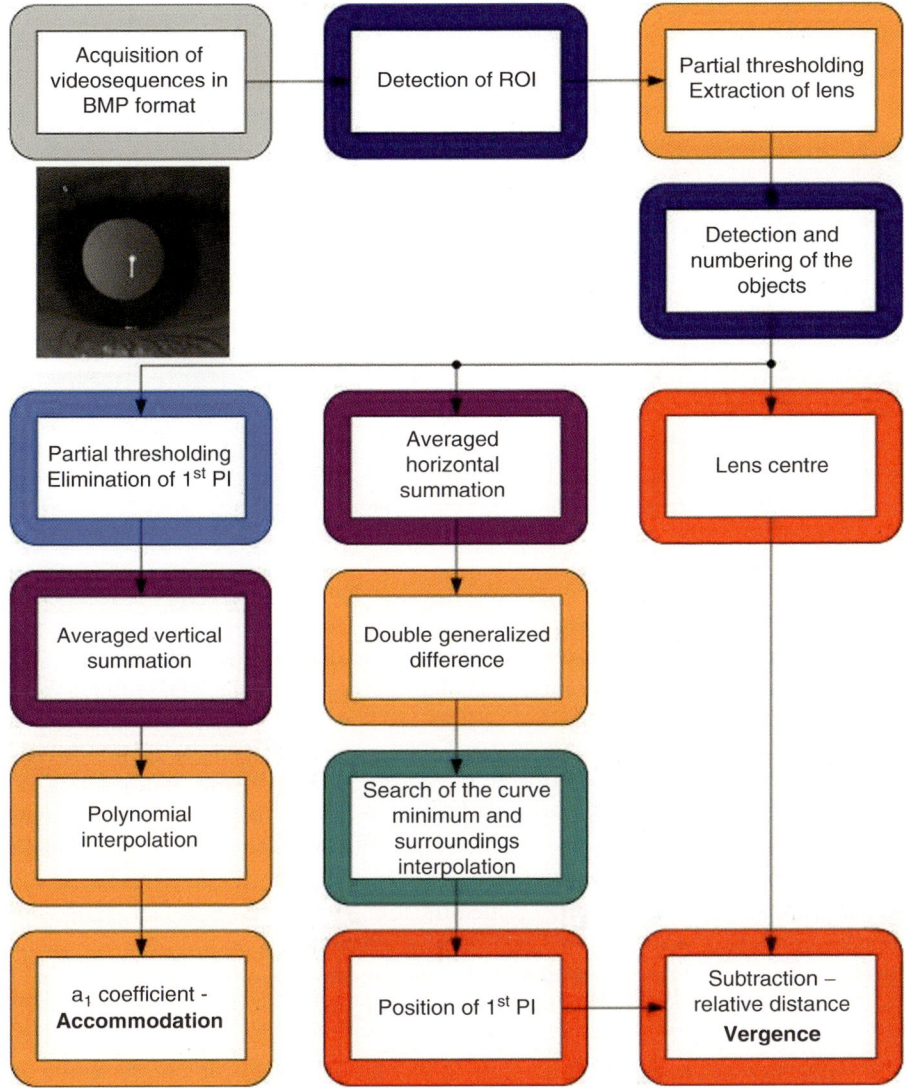

Fig. 10 Real photos of E.M.AN. – patient's room (**a**), measuring room (**b**) (details in Fig. 7)

CA-DI-0256A was used for the measurements. The maximum spectral sensitivity of the DALSA IA-DA image sensor is at the wavelength $\lambda = 825$ nm, the sensor's spatial resolution is low 128×128 pixels (256×256 with used binning). The camera speed is 360 fps with regards to the velocity of reaction in hundreds of ms. Only one eye is recorded to achieve sufficient resolution.

This image analysis is the same for each pictures of the grabbed sequence. First step of our image analysis is choice of a region of interest (ROI) that eliminates

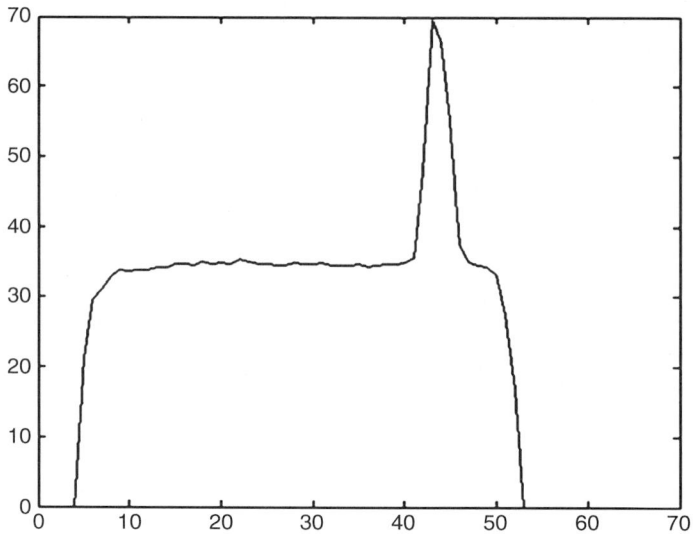

Fig. 11 Average vertical summation

amount of image data (comprises only lens and necessary surroundings). For next image analysis, only necessary image data left that is rectangular ROI with lens and part of iris (see Fig. 8).

Second step of image analysis is determination of threshold for partial thresholding [20]. For automatic setting of the threshold we choose another smaller rectangular ROI on the border of lens and iris. In this ROI, program finds minimum and maximum value and computes the average value that is set as threshold. Finally partial thersholding for ROI is applied.

The third step is 8-neighborhood identification (for more details see [20]) that controls and labels shapes in ROI and remove any possible undesirable objects or areas except lens because of head and eye movements. Then the image analysis is divided into two ways. The fist one is for convergence and the second one is for accommodation.

For convergence analysis is necessary to find horizontal position of the center of lens by following equation:

$$x_t = \frac{1}{n} \sum_{j,k} x_j (j,k),$$

where n is number of pixels, x_j is value j – position (j,k) pixel of the shape in the picture, n is number of pixels in object, x_t is co-ordinate of the centre of lens (COL). Next step determinates horizontal position of the 1st PI. First, we do average vertical summation (Fig. 11) that is vertical summation in pixel columns devided by number of nonzero pixels in the same column. Then general difference with weighting window that eliminates local extremes is applied twice:

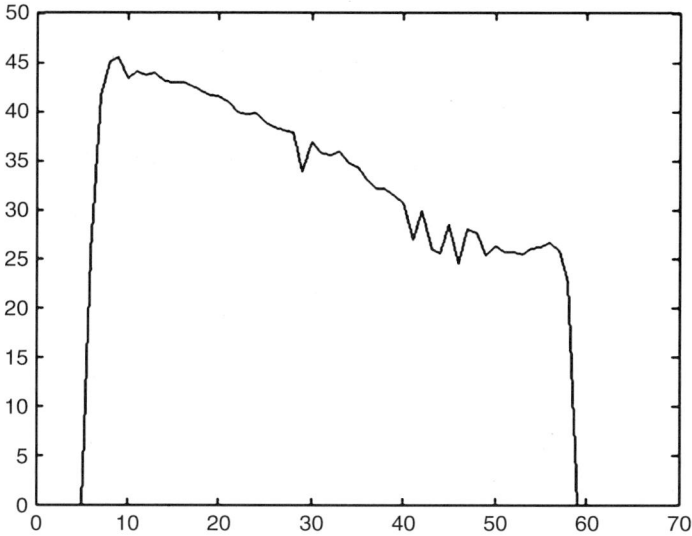

Fig. 12 Average horizontal summation

$$d(x) = \frac{\displaystyle\sum_{k=-L}^{L} k.f\,(x + k)}{\displaystyle\sum_{k=-L}^{L} k^2},$$

where x is point where the general difference is computed, $d(x)$ is the value of the general difference in point x, L is half of the width of the weighting window, k is point of the surroundings and it's weight.

Then, we minimum find zero crossing point in first difference and in second difference that of this curve that represented maximum of the original curve – global extreme. To gain high precision we interpolate surroundings of this extreme. Result is the horizontal position of the 1st PI.

For convergence analysis we subtract 1st PI and x_j, that represents distance between 1st PI and COL and show us time demanding process of convergence.

First step of accommodation analysis is to remove the 1st PI from thresholded ROI by a new partial thresholding. New threshold is set in 70% of dynamic range and it eliminates higher values of brightness that represent 1st PI. Then average horizontal summation (the same as in convergence analysis but in horizontal direction) is presented in Fig. 12. This is the horizontal summation in pixel rows devided by number of nonzero pixels in the same row. By fitting middle part of this curve we get polynomial of the first order:

$$y = a_0 + a_1 x.$$

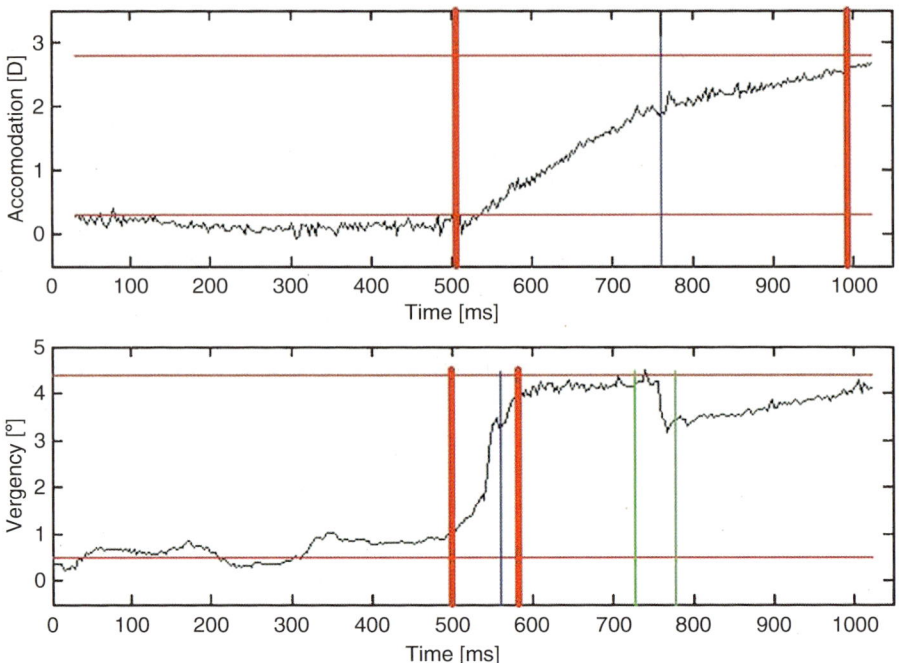

Fig. 13 Graph of the courses of accommodation and vergence

For accommodation analysis we use coefficient by second root a_1 that represents slope of the curve.

Last step involves calibration of both curves to corresponding units (dioptre and degrees of movement). This calibration depends on geometrical position of both monitors and patient. For calibration of accommodation we use distances of the fixation monitors that represents relative defocus and start dioptric power that is computed as average of first 25 values of the $a1$ (before accommodation starts, fixation on the first monitor).

Calibration of convergence is angle transformation between view axis of the eye and camera and it is individual for each eye. Range of convergence is given by position of the fixation monitors. Start angel is computed as average of first 25 values of relative distance between PI and COL (before convergence starts – fixation on the first monitor). Results of analysis are graphs of accommodation and vergence in dependence of time (Fig. 13). Thin horizontal lines represent the theoretical start- and end-point of the reactions (see below). The two thick vertical lines divide curves to three segments (the first line corresponds to latency period; the second line divides initial and post-initial segments of responses). The thin vertical lines determinate fragments in segments mentioned below.

First step of the signal analysis is to eliminate noise oscillations by averaging convolution with two-sided one neighbour window. Generalized difference (see

Table 1 Analysis of the accommodation and vergence curves from the Fig. 13

Accomodation	Vergence
Latency: 507 ms	Latency: 501 ms
Duration initial segment: 489 ms	Duration initial segment: 82 ms
Velocity of initial segment: 4.84 D/s	Velocity of initial segment: 36.9°/s
Time constant of initial segment: 225 ms	Time constant of initial segment: 49 ms
Peak velocity in initial segment: 29.7 D/s	Peak velocity in initial segment: 306°/s
Number of fragments in initial segment: 2	Number of fragments in initial segment: 2
1. fragment – contribution: 64%	1. fragment – contribution: 67%
1. fragment – velocity: 6.46 D/s	1. fragment – velocity: 38.3°/s
2. fragment – contribution: 28%	2. fragment – contribution: 20%
2. fragment – velocity: 3.07 D/s	2. fragment – velocity: 33.1 D/s
Proportion of theoretical dynamic range: 93%	Proportion of theoretical dynamic range: 88%
	Saccadic trajectory: 88%
	Saccadic contribution: 67%

above) with weighting window is used for finding maximum changes in acceleration profile of the signals. The two maximum values of this difference divide three main segments in signal (latent, initial and post-initial) in accordance with theoretical hypothesis Fig. 5b. Numerical parameters describing initial segment: latency, duration, percentage contribution to whole reaction, velocity, peak velocity and time constant (time when signal reach 60% of the maximum of the initial segment). The determination of fragments in initial and post-initial segments is performed by searching zero crosses of the first and the second generalized difference of the signal. Then is computed percetage contribution and mean velocity of fragments in initial segment. In post-initial segment the parameter of instability (represents ratio of reverse reaction in this segment) is calculated. If any fragment of the vergence reaction reaches peak velocity higher than 20°/s then saccadic parameters of the reaction are computed. They are: saccadic trajectory and saccadic contribution. Saccadic trajectory is defined as sum of all absolute contributions to total vergence reaction added by saccadic fragments. Saccadic contribution is defined as sum of all contributions to total vergence reaction added by saccadic fragments. The examples of the curve analysis from Fig. 13 give Table 1.

1.4 Ir.M.A. – Infrared Measurement of Accommodation (3D stimulation)

The Ir.M.A. (Infrared Measurement of Accommodation) measuring system is the second generation system for accommodation – vergence synkinesis analysis (Fig. 14) [29, 30].

Measuring methods result from experiences with the E.M.AN. measuring system. For determining relative vergence, the Hirschbeg's test is also used. The relative refractive power of the eye lens is measured by the eccentric photorefraction

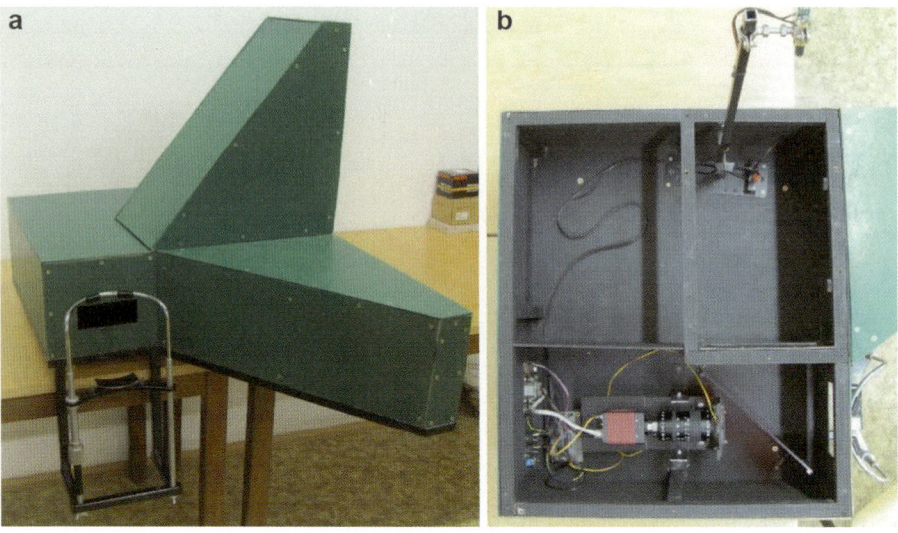

Fig. 14 Experimental measuring system Ir.M.A. (**a**), inner ordering of the system (**b**)

method as before. The main difference compared to the first generation is the use of a camera AVT Prosilica GE-680B with higher resolution (640 × 240 with double vertical binning) that preserves image capture speed 200 fps. The second change is in the method of fixating image projection. The unique system of 3D stimulation holograms is used. Fig. 13 gives the scheme for the Ir.M.A. system. The observer is situated in front of the input aperture of the instrument with the head fixated in a headrest. Thanks to higher camera resolution it is possible to observe both eyes simultaneously (in contrast to E.M.AN.). Therefore, it is possible to obtain information about the eyes' cooperation during a fixation point distance change. The eccentric photorefraction diaphragm and infrared measuring beam source are fixed on the lens of a high speed camera in the measuring part. Two prismatic lenses in front of the camera lens remove an insignificant central part of the image (nose root), shift edges to the centre and thereby allow higher resolution to be maintained in the region of the pupils. A beam splitter located in front of the measuring part separates the measuring and stimulating part. The transitivity of the beam-splitter has to be maximal for the wavelength of the measuring beam and reflexivity has to be maximal for the wavelength of the fixating images (Fig. 15).

The patient's sight is fixated by laser reconstructed 3D holograms. Holography allows a spatial object to be recorded on the surface of a photosensitive medium. The situation is similar to classic photography. The object beams go through an optical system and fall on a sensitive layer. Information about the intensity of each particular beam is recorded in this sensitive layer. However, information about the beam phase, the holder of spatial information, is lost. It is possible to record both beam properties (intensity and phase) through the interference of light beams on the sensitive medium. Fine grain photosensitive emulsion (about 10 μm) on a glass

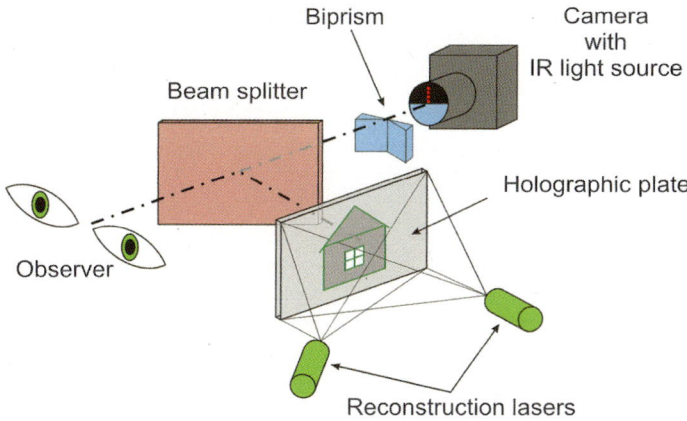

Fig. 15 Scheme of Ir.M.A. system

plate is able to record fine interference images. An important condition for hologram recording and reconstruction is the monochromatic and coherent character of the light source for maintaining a high quality hologram.

If the image is recorded in the sensitive layer without a reference beam, it is only a brightness image similar to a photo. The beam phase is recorded by the interference of the object beam with the reference beam. The resulting interference patterns represent the intensity and phase component of the object beam. The holographic object is reconstructed by illuminating the holographic plate with a monochromatic reconstruction beam with the same geometrical position as the reference beam. This makes it possible to reconstruct the virtual object at the original distance from the holographic plate as with the recording. In addition, holography enables several different objects to be registered on one plate. If two objects at different distances were to be recorded on a holographic plate, then each object's distance will be recorded separately. Through reconstruction, the sources are situated in the same geometrical position as the reference sources recorded. By changing the reconstruction sources, it is possible to display two separate objects with the stepped change of virtual distance.

In the case of stimulating the patients' visual apparatus, the distance difference is in range of metres (for E.M.AN. it is 2.75 m, for Ir.M.A. 1.81 m). Therefore, space requirements make it impossible to be used in the usual conditions of ophthalmologist's office. Holographical stimulation used in Ir.M.A. allows space requirements to be minimised for virtual stimulating objects. Figure 16 gives an example of reconstructed holographic objects. The real distance between the holographic plate and the reconstruction beam source is 0.6 m.

A further goal of research is realising a system with moving stimulating objects. A few objects positioned in the near and far planes will be sequentially reconstructed to give the impression of moving objects. A moving fixation object will be more

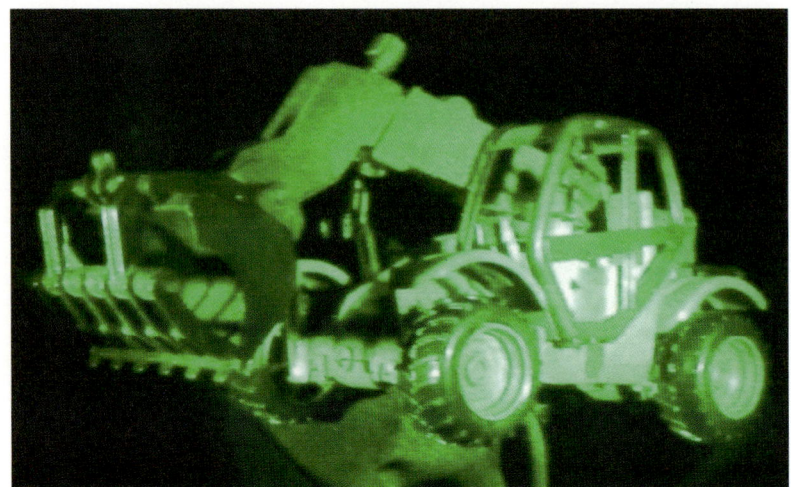

Fig. 16 Reconstructed used holographic image

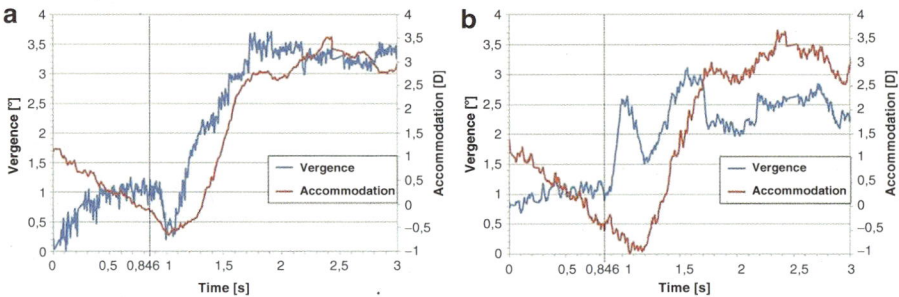

Fig. 17 Graph of accommodation and vergence measured on *left* (**a**) and *right* (**b**) eye by Ir.M.A. device

interesting for a young patient than a static one. The moving part of an object fixes the patient's attention onto a small area without vision movements affecting measurement.

Image analysis of videosequences gained by Ir.M.A. system is similar to analysis of E.M.AN. videosequences with modification in method for determining centre of pupil and 1st PI. On the videosequences the both eyes are recorded, therefore analysis has to be performed twice. Result of analysis of one eye accommodation and vergence is in the Fig. 17.

In initial part of graph (0–0.846 s) the analysing algorithm is calibrated. Change of distance of the fixation object performs in 0.846 s. After that follows phase of latency (about 200 ms) and Open-loop initiative phase of accomodation and vergence (vergence is followed by the accommodation). Last phase of nervous feedback, Close-loop, begins approximately in time 2 s. Course of the vergence-accommodation synkinesis corresponds with theoretically setup curve presented in Fig. 5b.

2 Vision Psychology

Vision psychology is very important part of vision (perception) process. The image attraction plays very important role in the vision process. We measure eye movement during the image observation on different types of scene that is presented below. And during the process of HVS modelling we set up a criterion of picture activity (*PA*) that corresponds with an attraction of the image information [21].

2.1 Measuring Eye Movement During Image Observation

For studying visual system function a small experiment was conducted. This experiment used E.M.AN. for image recording and its modified image analysis.

For this purpose only the distant monitor (PAL television at 3.12 m – given by the device's construction) was used to stimulate the visual apparatus. It showed images of the testing scenes. Before the testing scene, the initial shot with the sequence's serial number was shown for 5 s. The subject focussed on the centre of this image. After changing the scene on the analysed image, eye movement was recorded after the scene. The observation period was about 6 s.

Another modification to the equipment took place in the analysis software part (block scheme of the original image analysis is in Fig. 8). Analysis of accommodation was left out and the assessment of the eye's horizontal movement was also used in an analogous manner for assessing vertical movement. The next step analysed the shot sequence and assessed eye movement after the observed scene. The result was a two row matrix with horizontal and vertical vergence values for the given shot. The result of the analysis was related to the originally observed centre of the image. A calculation of the trajectory to the monitored image is then made from the geometric distance of the monitor and the eye. The eye position values were plotted onto the original fixed image and connected by lines to represent individual trajectories. Results eye movements during the observation of selected scenes are in Fig. 18.

The first point of the eye trajectory is in the middle at the top for the SQUARE image (marked by the red arrow) followed by movement in the direction of the lamp and then to the crowd, the church and back to the crowd. In the PORTRAIT image the situation is different. Observation starts on the left with the hair, followed by an analysis of the woman's face details then moving to the right analyzing the hair, part of the sweater and finishing with the face. Between the measured points (given by a camera frame rate of 360 fps) the saccadic movements are shown, which often goes very quickly through the areas of constant texture (the background with low image activity – frequency). It seems from both images that for the observer the quality of the edges together with sensitivity to face colour (skin tone) play an important role. Edges often represent areas with high frequencies. If they are low-quality (blurred) it very often results in poor image quality, more so than distortion

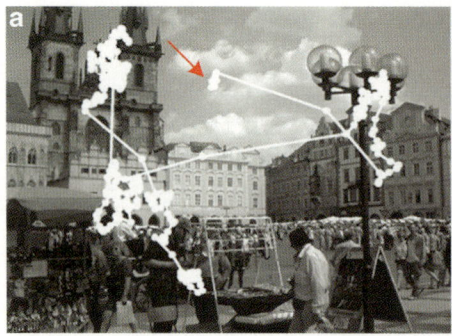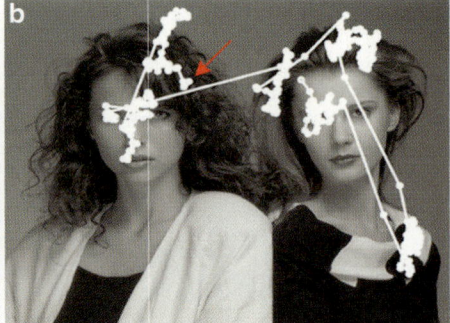

Fig. 18 Scene square and portrait – eye movement over the observed images during first 6s, *red arrows* identify initial observing point

caused by noise. The next important factor is the faithfulness of skin tone. The next important factor that plays an important role is the content of the image for the observer, this increases the attraction of the image observed. An attempt was made to mathematically express this feature as a criterion of image activity, which is defined as follows:

$$PA = \frac{1}{N} \cdot \sum_{i=1}^{N} |o_i - f_i|,$$

where N represents number of the image pixels, o_i is original image and f_i is original image filtered by median filter with kernel 8×8 pixels. *PA* describes local activities in the image thereby categorize image from the size of the areas with the same color. This criterion (*PA*) is dependent on the image content and partially correspondent with human visual features. Presented scenes (Fig. 18) PORTRAIT ($PA = 4.83$) a SQUARE ($PA = 12.07$) represents images with high and low picture activity. At the images with high *PA* there are less eye saccadic movements during the observation than at the images with low *PA*. This can be evaluated for example with parameter saccadic trajectory that summing length of saccadic movements with velocity higher than $20°/s$ [22, 23]. More about PA can be found in [21].

Thus an important finding from this experiment can be discussed. The test sequences show that during an analysis of a "quality" image the human eye first analyses the areas of high frequencies and favours skin tone. Hence, for assessing the quality of an image, quality edges in the image and the faithfulness of the skin tone are of prime importance. In compressed images, the edges generally get less distinct and therefore the relevant quality is assessed as worse. It is the same for skin tone, though with compression it is not very distorted. This phenomenon of distorting the tone is known, for instance, in analogue television systems NTSC (distorting the differential phase).

2.2   Fusion of Binocular Vision – Normal 3D Vision

Fusion is the neuropsychic mechanism that normal binocular vision is based on. It is prerequisite for normal 3D binocular vision. All disorders of the binocular functions disrupt this mechanism. The response is fusion adapting to the sub-normal mechanism (abnormal retinal correspondence) or it decays (suppression). This innate ability of fusion is the base for pleoptic and orthoptic therapy. However, an objective assessment of the efficacy of fusion is almost impossible in clinical conditions.

Dichoptic masking [24] is a complicated suppression process that removes a monocular object with poor contrast from the binocular processing. A monocular stimulus with better contrast resolution uses this physiological mechanism to prevent the perception of a two-sided stimulus with lesser contrast. Contrast rivality is the basis of the complicated suppression phenomenon. A basic condition for dichoptic masking is normal binocular vision.

It is assumed that a more robust fusion retains an image with worse resolution of contrasts in the binocular visual awareness, whilst a weaker fusion mechanism will suppress this image. This methodology is based on discovering how big the degradation in contrast of the retinal image must be for dichoptic masking. For testing the dynamics of the masking mechanism, a variable burden was chosen in the form of a forced unadaptable relative vergence.

A special computer haploscope was developed comprises two identical 17″ LCD monitors placed on two independent brackets. The testing images displayed on both monitors are viewed separately by the left and right eye through + 2.75 D converging lenses that place the monitors at optical infinity. The person being tested has their head stabilised in an adjustable headrest. Figure 19 shows the set up of this computer haploscope.

The image sequence for measuring the dichoptic masking effect was set up from a number of modified test images with a growing level of degradation in the image information (see Fig. 20).

The degradation of the initial image was carried as a low pass filtering of the image. The degradation of the images was calibrated in line with the fusion cover test (FCT) with 10° scale (which is clinically applied). The cut-off values for the frequency filter were set up empirically. Their logarithmic regression with regards to the FCT scale was confirmation of their correct determination, which allowed interpolation of the degradation in quarter of degrees. The measuring sequence of the progressively degraded images according to previous interpolation (by the FCT scale) was form 1 to 5 degraded by ¼ (1, 1.25, 1.5 ... 4.75) and from 5 to 6 by ½ (5, 5.5, 6). The duration of images was 2 s (0.5 fps). The indicator of the onset of the dichoptic masking effect (suppression of the degraded image) was the eye deviating from the forced vergence position to a phoric position. Subjectively this moment was indicated by removing the red line from the red measuring box (see in Fig. 21).

The measuring box had a width of 1 Δ of the fixation disparity to the exodeviation, i.e. to the esodeviation and was placed in the image for the dominant eye. The measuring sequence with the measuring line was presented to the non-dominant eye (ocular dominance was established using the Dolman method hole-in-the-card).

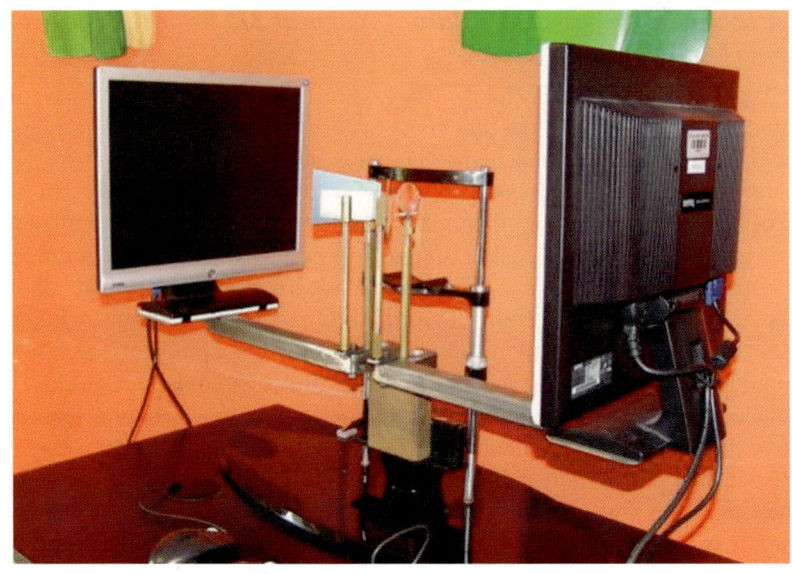

Fig. 19 Experimental arrangement of the computer haploscope

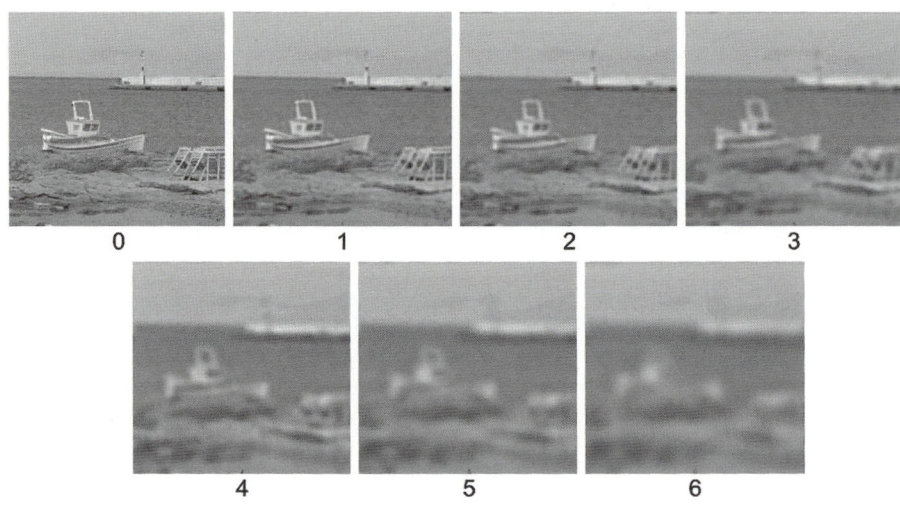

Fig. 20 Degradation of the fixation image according to the FCT scale

The sequence measuring the dichoptic masking effect was presented at the end of the burden sequences inducing a relative vergence burden (starts at position as it shown in Fig. 21c). During these sequences, the haploscopic fixation images moved counter to one another on the monitors (Fig. 21b). Measurements were made at relative convergence burdens of 5, 10, 15, 20 and 25 Δ BT (temporal) and at

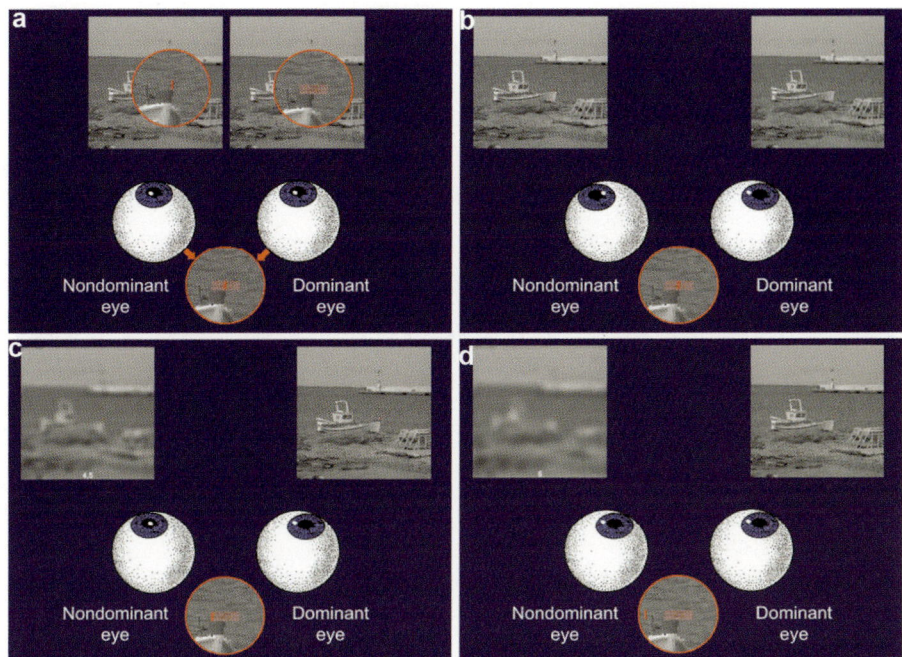

Fig. 21 Scheme of the measuring process with indicator box. (**a**) start position of the experiment nondegraded images in the same position (**b**) first process moving of the nondegraded images to the vergence load (both eye must fixate image – goes to squint) (**c**) in the maximal fixation position given by step b the degradation of the image on nondomimant eye is applied (**d**) when the red line is observed outside box the patient's fusion is disturbed and nondominat eye goes to the undefined position

relative divergence burdens of 2.5, 5.0, 7.5, 10.0 and 12.5 Δ BN (nasal). The relative vergence burden started at zero and increased by 2.5 Δ for convergence and 1.25 Δ for divergence. The image speed was 0.33 fps (i.e. image changed after 3 s). Whole process clearly illustrates Fig. 21. For the speed of the growth in the forced vergence and for zeroing it before another measurement there could not have been adaptation to this burden and this was thus labelled as unadaptable.

Four people underwent the experiment ranging in age from 16 to 32. All were orthotropic with exophorie 0–4 Δ BT, without any other clinically detectable deviations from normal binocularity. The central visual acuity of all eyes was 1.0. Statistical analysis was made by Student's t-test.

The average threshold value for the degradation of a one-sided image (in the FCT scale) necessary for the dichoptic masking effect for individual values of forced relative vergence is given in Fig. 22. It is clear that with increasing unadaptable burden a lesser degree of degradation of the one-sided image is necessary for its suppression. This trend is roughly three times more distinct during a burden on relative divergence.

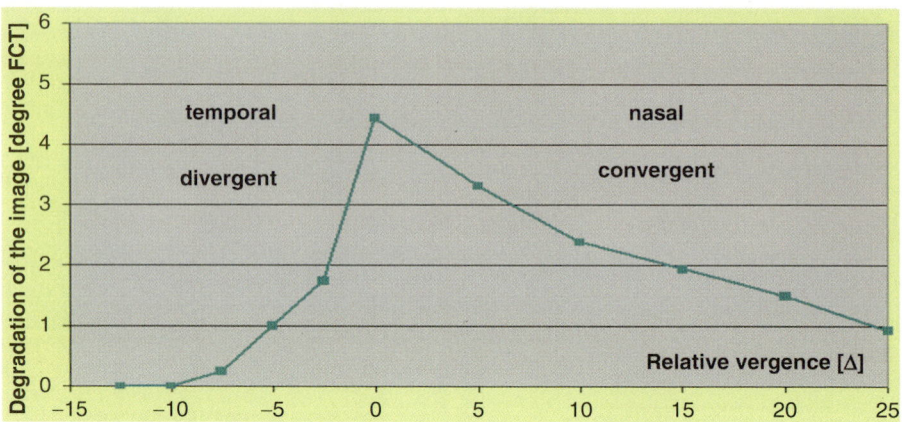

Fig. 22 Dependence of dichoptic masking on forced unadaptable relative vergence (average from four subjects)

Dichoptic masking could be used for measuring the robustness (strength) of the fusion mechanism. It is likely a part of the fusion mechanism, it processes dichoptic visual inputs in parallel and the threshold value of masking is easily detected.

This study also proved that there is good agreement between threshold values for experimental masking under unburdened conditions (zero vergence burdens under natural conditions) with the empirical experience when using the fusion cover test (FCT) in healthy children.

3   Conclusions

Correct anatomical and physiological functions are basic for a human binocular vision. In case of any obstruction in these functions isn't possible the development of the simple binocular vision. Described methods for measuring of the eye ver-gence and accommodation and eye movements during image observation was developed to improve care about the eyesight and measure theoretical hypothesis of physiological and biomechanical processes of vision perception.

Content of observed scene (image activity) has also significant influence to whole vision process and its features. These parameters aren't measured in general practice but could be applied in diagnostics of functional vision disorders.

Application of videometric systems provides non-invasive simplicity and quickness of measuring.

References

1. Cornsweet TN (1970) Visual perception. Academic, New York, p 475
2. De Valois RL, De Valois K (1988) Spatial vision. Oxford University Press, New York
3. Cronly-Dillon JR (1991) Vision and visual dysfunction. In: Regan D (ed) Spatial vision, vol 10. CRC Press, Ontario/Boca Raton, p 311
4. Dowling J (1987) The retina: an approachable part of the brain. Harvard University Press, Cambridge MA
5. Hubel DH, Diesel TN (1959) Receptive fields of single neurones in the cat's striate cortex. J Physiol 148:574–591
6. Hubel DH (1988) Eye, brain and vision. Scientific American Library, New York
7. Wu HR, Rao KR (2005) Digital video image quality and perceptual coding, Marcel Dekker series in signal processing and communications. CRC Tailor & Francis, Boca Raton, p 600
8. Hering E, Stark L, Bridgeman B (1977) The theory of binocular vision. Plenum Press, New York. ISBN ISBN 0-306-31016-3
9. Wright K (1995) Pediatric ophthalmology and strabismus. Mosby, St.Louis, p 902. ISBN ISBN 0-8151-9359-9
10. Watson AB (1987) The cortex transform: rapid computation of simulated neural images. Comput Vis Graph Image Process 39:311–327
11. Lambrecht CJvdB (2001) Vision models and applications to image and video processing. Kluwer, Dordrecht, p 229
12. Lubin J (1997) Sarnoff JND vision model, IEEE subcommitte D-2.1.6, Sarnoff Corporation, Priceton, p 3
13. Osberger W (1999) Perceptual vision models for picture quality assessment and compression applications. Queensland University of Technology, Brisbane, p 268
14. Carnec M, Callet P, Barba D (2003) Full reference and reduced reference metrics for image quality assessment. In: Seventh international symposium on signal processing and its applications, SuviSoft Oy, Paris/Tampere
15. Allen MJ (1949) An objective high speed photographic technique for simultaneously recording changes in accommodation and convergence. Am J Optom Arch Am Acad Optom 26:279–289
16. Purkyně JE (1823) Commentatio de examine physiologico organi visus et systematis cutanei, Breslau, Prussia, University of Breslau Press
17. Dušek J, Dostálek M (2002) Eye movement analyzer. In: Biomedical engineering and education. CTU, Prague, pp 85–87. ISBN ISBN 80-01-02499-7
18. Dušek J, Hozman J, Hromádka Z, Dostálek M (2003) Automatická detekce horizontální polohy Purkyňových obrazů (automatic detection of Purkinje images' horizontal coordinates). Physician Technol 34(2):47–59, ISSN 0301-5491
19. Schaeffel F, Farkas L, Holand HC (1987) Infrared photoretinoscope. Appl Opt 26(1987):1505–1509
20. Šonka M, Hlaváč V, Boyle R (2008) Image processing, analysis, and machine vision. Thomson Learning, Toronto, 829 stran. ISBN ISBN-13 978-0-495-08252-1
21. Dušek J (2008) Objektivní hodnocení subjektivní kvality obrazu na základě modelu (Objective evaluation of subjective image quality based on HVS model). Doctoral thesis, Faculty of electrical engineering, Czech Technical University in Prague, p 181
22. Dušek J, Baxa V, Dostálek M (2004) Extraction of Selected Parameters of the Eye Reactions. In: 8th international student conference on electrical engineering, POSTER 2004, CTU, Prague, p NS7
23. Dušek J, Dostálek M, Baxa V (2004) Extraction of selected parameters of the vergence-accommodation synkinesys of eyes. In: Analysis of biomedical signals and images. Brno University, Brno, pp 208–210
24. Abadi RV (1976) Introduction masking – a study of some inhibitory interactions during dichoptic viewing. Vision Res 16:269–275

25. Dostalek M, Dusek J (2004) E.M.A.N. (eye movement and accommodation analyzer) device for vergence accommodation synkinesis recording and analysis. In: de Faber J-T(ed) Transactions, 28th European strabismological association meeting, Taylor & Francis, London/New York, pp 357–361
26. Hromádka Z (2001) Diplomová práce E.M.AN. (eye movement analyzer) – hardwarové řešení, Czech Technical University in Prague, Prague, Czech Republic, p 78
27. Dušek J (2001) Diplomová práce E.M.AN. (eye movement analyzer) – softwarové řešení, Czech Technical Univeristy in Prague, Prague, Czech Republic, p 66
28. Jindra T (2009) Infrared measurement of accommodation and eye movements – hardware design. Charles University in Prague, Prague, p 43
29. Dušek J, Jindra T, Dostálek M (2011) Measurement system of eye vergence and accommodation with 3D hologram stimulation. In: R.M.N. Jorge, J.M.R.S. Tavares, M.P. Barbosa and A.P. Slade. *Technology and medical sciences: 6th international conference on technology and medical sciences (TMSi).* 1. vyd. London: CRC press Taylor & Francis Group, s. 15–17. ISBN 978-0-415-66822-4
30. Dušek J, Jindra T, Dostálek M (2010) Infračervené měření dynamiky akomodace a vergence s holografickou stimulací. In: Zborník príspevkov 18th annual conference proceedings of technical computing, RT Systems s.r.o./CDROM, Bratislava, pp 1–4, ISBN 978-80-970519-0-7

Motion Correction in Conventional Nuclear Medicine Imaging

Francisco J. Caramelo and Nuno C. Ferreira

1 Introduction

In an imaging technique, it makes sense to address the issue of motion correction only if the relation between the frame rate of the image acquisition and the speed of the motion is such that there is an impact on the acquired image. When the acquisition frame rate is much higher than the speed of motion of the object, the harmful effects on the acquired images can usually be neglected. However, the opposite has dramatic consequences on the images, requiring specific procedures to correct for the motion effects.

Emission imaging techniques, such as SPECT (Single Photon Emission Computed Tomography) and PET (Positron Emission Tomography), require relatively long periods of data acquisition (typically, 10 min), during which the patient must remain still. These long periods are due to the nature of the techniques, which are based on the detection of gamma photons. Motion is thus a critical problem in SPECT and PET, especially with non-collaborative subjects such as patients with movement disorders and young children. To avoid this problem, subjects are often sedated or, if collaborative, can be held by the technicians and restrained by belts. Even so, most of the times, motion has to be corrected after the exam. Motion correction algorithms that rely solely on SPECT/PET data tend to have low effectiveness, since its accuracy depends on the use of high acquisition rates, which are limited by noise considerations. Other solutions separate motion detection from SPECT/PET data which in turn makes more difficult the acquisition.

In this chapter we intend to discuss the consequences of motion in the acquired images as well as the strategies to minimize these effects. For a better understanding

F.J. Caramelo (✉) • N.C. Ferreira
Institute of Biomedical Research on Light and Image – IBILI, Faculty of Medicine of the University of Coimbra, Portugal
e-mail: fcaramelo@ibili.uc.pt

R.M.N. Jorge et al. (eds.), *Technologies for Medical Sciences*, Lecture Notes in Computational Vision and Biomechanics 1, DOI 10.1007/978-94-007-4068-6_6, © Springer Science+Business Media B.V. 2012

of the subject we start with a brief explanation of the operation of SPECT and PET scanners, addressing later the specific problem of motion in these imaging techniques.

2   Basic Principles of the Nuclear Medicine Imaging

Nuclear medicine images can be obtained either by detecting photons that are emitted from atomic nuclei or by positron annihilation that results in two photons whose opposite trajectories are (almost) collinear.

When the radioisotopes are gamma emitters, a special collimated detector system is used to obtain the images. This detector system is known as the gamma camera and the overall process of imaging is usually called planar scintigraphy or simply scintigraphy.

The gamma camera can rotate around the subject of study, allowing the acquisition of multiple views from different angles, which after filtering, are used in the reconstruction algorithm to obtain tomographic images. In this case, the technique is known as SPECT. For positron emitters, the detector (also of gamma radiation) does not need a physical collimator because collimation can be performed electronically, by detecting in coincidence the two 511 keV annihilation photons that result from the positron annihilation in matter. When these photons, emitted in opposite directions, are detected in coincidence (within a certain time interval) they define a line of response (LOR). This technique is called PET and the detector is known as a PET scanner.

The versatility of these two techniques is based on the combination of specific radioactive emitters with an appropriate detector which allows the reconstruction of two or three dimensional images that provide functional information.

Both the gamma camera and the PET scanner can be regarded as passive devices since the radiation is emitted by radioactive isotopes that are administered to patients.

Labeling different molecules of biological interest, i.e. molecules that play an active role in the physiological processes, is a powerful procedure that enables obtaining important information regarding the various functions of the human body.

In general terms, the nuclear imaging technique involves the administration to the patient of an adequate radiopharmaceutical and the detection of the gamma photons that are emitted directly by the radioisotope or that result from the annihilation of positrons. Thus, the image reveals objectively the spatial distribution of the radiopharmaceutical to which the doctor lends clinical significance.

There are several technical challenges in nuclear medicine imaging. On one hand, there are important issues regarding the detection of radiation, namely: the correlation between the location of the detection and the actual position of the emission of the photon, the efficiency of the detection, the energy resolution, and the spatial and temporal resolution. On the other hand, it is crucial to improve the aspects related to the signal source, which implies the development of new and more efficient ways of labeling biological molecules with radioactive isotopes. These biological molecules are usually composed of elements of low atomic number (Z), which limit the choice of possible radioisotopes. This limitation arises from the fact that conventional nuclear medicine requires gamma emitters, usually of much larger Z and with suitable periods for diagnosis purposes. Consequently, there was (and still exists) the need to develop ways of labeling biological molecules with gamma emitters of high Z that do not induce substantial changes in the physiological behavior of these molecules. Another issue is the process of image reconstruction where the research on faster and more accurate algorithms has been a constant.

Hence, there are several aspects that may worsen the final image and, in practice, there is almost a corresponding discipline dedicated the improvement of each of these factors (e.g. overall efficiency of the detector, radiopharmacy, ...). One of the factors that impair the quality of the image, and consequently the clinical information, is the movement of the subject during the image acquisition.

2.1 The Signal Source

Gamma photon or positron emission is considered the signal used for nuclear imaging, which when combined with the capacity of labeling numerous biological molecules significantly enhances the ability to study several physiological processes. Hence, whenever a relevant process has to be inspected, a specific molecule is chosen and labeled with a proper radionuclide, seeking to map the entire process and attempting to achieve all the necessary information. One of the most important eligibility conditions for the target molecule is to be present with high concentration, in order to enhance the signal to noise ratio even when it exists only at infinitesimal quantities. Nonetheless, the possibility to visualize the structures considering the spatial resolution of the scanner should also be taken into account [1]. It is also critical for the success of the technique that the tracer molecule reaches the compartment of interest which depends both on the abundance in blood plasma and on the permeability of the biological interfaces. Actually, in order to the free molecule be in sufficient quantity and at the right time in the compartment, not only the molecule availability in plasma is of extreme importance but also the nature and the kinetic of the chemical bond while the molecule is transported by the blood. On the other hand, the transport across biological membranes depends either on a specific transport mechanism or on an adequate nature of the substance that allows to be passively transported. Once at the compartment, the radionuclide labeled molecule connects not only with the target of interest (specific binding) but also with other structures (non-specific binding). Consequently, the SNR depends on the ratio between the specific and non-specific binding, and generally this is the parameter that is quantified in molecular imaging. Since the specific and non-specific binding naturally depend on the kinetics and on the extent of reaction, the signals due to each of the bindings may be temporally separable. That's why in some cases there is a time delay between the administration of the radiopharmaceutical and the image acquisition.

One of the objectives pursued in the radiolabeling is the preservation of the physical and chemical characteristics of the molecule, in order to maintain the physiological behaviour. Therefore the isotopic substitution of an atom or a chemical group comes out as an obvious solution. However, if this is accessible to PET technology that makes use of positron emitters that are isotopes of biological elements such as Carbon, Oxygen and Nitrogen, it is practically infeasible for SPECT that employs gamma emitters such as Technitium or Thalium. Contributing to the choice of a particular radionuclide, the half-life period, the energy, its decay mode and its production process are also of importance. However, the radionuclides of low atomic number that are gamma emitters and that can be employed in the above-mentioned isotopic substitution are not suitable since the half-life periods are much too long for use in conventional nuclear medicine. This problem does not exist in PET, since the isotopes are positrons emitters and, frequently, present adequate features for clinical purposes. Note that very short half-life periods could hinder the radiolabeling and long half-life periods have adverse dosimetric effects.

Regarding the gamma photon energy, it must lie between 70 and 250 keV in order to maximize the efficiency of the gamma camera. In PET, the energy of the annihilation photons is constant and equal to 511 keV.

Gamma photons with low energy will produce a very small number of photo-electrons when they interact with the detector's scintillator crystal. Since this is a random process governed by Poisson statistics, it generates a large uncertainty in the amplitude of the electric signals that are produced in the photomultiplier tubes, with consequent degradation of the image contrast.

On the other hand, high-energy photons are more likely to penetrate the collimator, corrupting the SPECT image quality and degrading spatial resolution and contrast.

The importance of the decay mode is mainly related with dosimetric aspects (except for the loss of spatial resolution due to the path of the positrons before thermalization), since the emission of particles prior to the gamma radiation increases the dose in patients without any benefit for the formation of the image.

The most commonly used radionuclide in conventional nuclear medicine is technetium-99 m (^{99m}Tc), whereas for PET it is fluorodeoxyglucose (18 F-FDG). Technetium is the lightest chemical element (Z = 43) with no stable isotope; none of the technetium isotopes has a longer half-life of more than 4.2 million years and therefore it is not surprising that technetium is found in nature only in trace amounts. Although predicted by Mendeliev and named as *ekamanganese*, its name has changed in 1937 to Technetium (from Greek τεχνητός which means artificial) after the synthesis of the isotope 97. The ^{99m}Tc is a radioactive metastable isotope that emits gamma radiation with 140 keV with a half-life of 6.01 h. These features, combined with the fact that there are commercial kits available for production, make it the preferred radionuclide in conventional nuclear medicine. There are several examples of radiotracers used in clinical routine based on ^{99m}Tc, some of them are shown in Table 1.

Table 1 Examples of radiotracers labeled with ^{99m}Tc (SPECT) and ^{18}F (PET)

Name	Application
^{99m}Tc − DTPA	Kidney, lung (aerosol)
^{99m}Tc − DMSA	Kidney, tumors
^{99m}Tc − HMPAO	Cerebral perfusion, infection/inflammation
^{99m}Tc − FPCIT	Basal ganglia
^{99m}Tc − Sestamibi	Parathyroid, myocardial perfusion, thyroid tumors and breast cancer
^{99m}Tc − Technegas	Pulmonary ventilation
^{99m}Tc − MAG3	Kidney
^{99m}Tc − Tetrofosmina	Parathyroid, myocardial perfusion
^{18}F-Fluorodeoxyglucose (FDG)	Glucose metabolism
^{18}F-Fluorothymidine	Cell proliferation
^{18}F-Fluoromisonidazole	Hypoxia

2.2 Interaction of Radiation with Matter

The typical gamma photon energy used in nuclear imaging ranges from 70 to 511 keV. In fact, for PET technology, which makes use of positron emitters, all the photons resulting from positron annihilation have energies equal to 511 keV. For this range of energies, the two predominant effects of radiation with matter interaction are the photoelectric and the Compton effect. It also occurs Rayleigh effect, even though the occurrence probability is much smaller than the other two cases. Only for higher energies (>1,022 keV) there is pair production, and photonuclear interaction only becomes significant for energies above a few MeV.

When a photon interacts with an electron and there is a deviation of the photon and simultaneously recoil of the electron, a process called Compton effect or Compton scattering occurs.

Applying the law of conservation of energy and the principle of conservation of momentum to the scattering, we get the relation between the energy of the incident photon, E_i, and the energy of the scattered photon, E_d, which is:

$$E_d = \frac{E_i}{1 + \frac{E_i}{m_e c^2} (1 - \cos\alpha)}, \tag{1}$$

where $m_e c^2$ is the energy of the electron at rest (=511 keV).

Despite the representation depicted in Fig. 1 may indicate that the deflection angle is fixed or there is an equal probability of deflection, this is not what occurs. In fact, the probability of a photon to be deflected into a certain angle is not constant and is given by the differential cross section, $d\sigma/d\Omega$, which is the probability of a photon being scattered into the solid angle, $d\Omega$. The relation that defines the

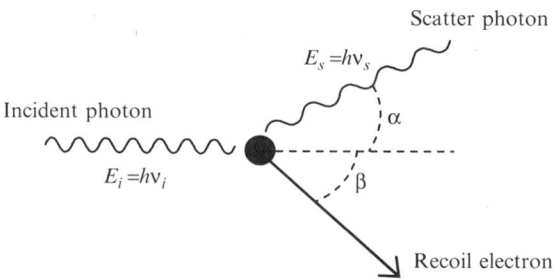

Fig. 1 Schematic representation of the Compton effect. The incident photon with energy E_i interacts with an electron: the photon is deflected (represented by angle α) and the electron recoils (at an angle β) because of the energy given by the incident photon. Consequently the scattered photon has less energy (longer wavelength) than the incident photon

differential cross section for the Compton effect suffered by X and gamma radiation was introduced by Klein and Nishina [2] in 1928 and is generally known as Klein-Nishina formula:

$$\frac{d\sigma}{d\Omega} = \frac{r_0^2}{2}\left(P_{E_i,\alpha} - P_{E_i,\alpha}^2\ \text{sen}^2\left(\alpha\right) + P_{E_i,\alpha}^3\right), \tag{2}$$

where $r_0\ \left(= e^2 \big/ \left(4\pi\ \varepsilon_0\ m_0 c^2\right) = 2{,}817 \times 10^{-15}\text{m}\right)$ represents the classical electron radius and $P_{E_i,\alpha}$ is the ratio between the energies before and after the Compton effect, which is given by:

$$P_{E_i,\alpha} = \frac{E_d}{E_i} = \frac{1}{1 + \frac{E_i}{m_0 c^2}\left(1 - \cos\alpha\right)}. \tag{3}$$

While in the Compton effect the incident photon transfers only part of his energy, in the photoelectric effect the photon gives all its energy to an electron of an atom, causing the ejection of the electron with an energy equal to the difference of photon energy and the binding energy.

$$E_{\text{c. electron}} = h\ \upsilon_{\text{incident photon}} - E_{\text{binding}} \tag{4}$$

The ionization created by the electron ejection has short duration and the gap is filled by another electron. This process is accompanied by the emission of a photon (fluorescence) or an Auger electron.

In Rayleight scattering, the photon is deflected without loosing energy to the electron. Therefore, the conservation of the kinetic energy holds and the scattering is elastic. The differential cross section per electron for a photon that is scattered into the solid angle α is given by:

$$\frac{d\sigma_e}{d\Omega} = \frac{r_0^2}{2}\left(1 + \cos^2\alpha\right), \tag{5}$$

where r_0 is, as before, the "classical radius" of the electron.

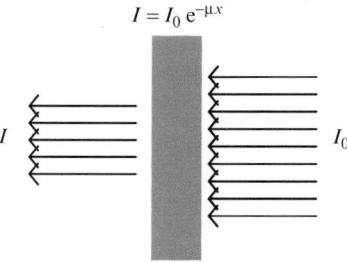

$$I = I_0\, e^{-\mu x}$$

Fig. 2 Representation of the interaction that a monoenergetic beam of photons suffer when passes through an object of thickness x. I_0 is the intensity of the incident beam. I represents the intensity of the emerging beam. The intensity of the incident beam is reduced by a fraction equal to $e^{-\mu x}$ where μ is the linear attenuation coefficient of the medium

From (5) it can be concluded that there is a symmetry plane (front/rear) and, as a corollary, that the cross section has the same value for $\alpha = 0°$ and $\alpha = 180°$, which is the maximum.

Note that for low energies, the Klein-Nishina formula (2) reduces to the Rayleigh formulation (5). For this circumstance, $P_{E,\alpha}$ can be considered equal to the unity and after replacing this condition in (2) the conclusion is direct. When a high energy photon ($>1,022$ keV) produces an electron-positron pair by interacting with the nucleus, the process is known by pair production. Since it only takes place for very high energies, this process is not likely to occur in the range of energies used in nuclear medicine.

The probability of occurrence of photoelectric effect is higher than for Compton effect for low energy photons. On the contrary, for average energies, such as those used in nuclear medicine, the likelihood of Compton effect occurring is higher than for the photoelectric effect. For higher energies, pair production is the dominant process (Fig. 3).

As a result of the interaction of radiation with matter, when a photon beam with intensity I (energy per unit area) is incident on an object of thickness x, it suffers attenuation. That is, the beam intensity is reduced by a factor that depends on the material and on the thickness of the object and, also, on the energy of the photons. The relation between the intensities of the incident beam (I_0) and emerging beam (I), is described by the exponential equation:

$$I = I_0\, e^{-\mu x} \tag{6}$$

The attenuation is often due to a multiple process where several and successive interactions occur until the photon energy is completely transformed (Fig. 2).

Figure 3 shows the variation of the attenuation coefficient for each of the interaction mechanisms as a function of the energy of the incident photons. The attenuation coefficient is presented normalized to the total attenuation. The attenuation coefficient shown is relative to the water, which is the main constituent of the human body and, therefore, generally considered as the biological equivalent.

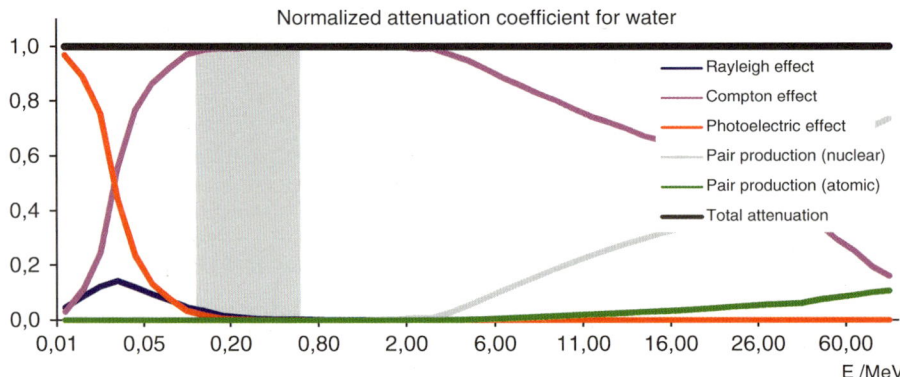

Fig. 3 Variation of attenuation coefficient due to various effects normalized to total attenuation. The shaded area represents the energy range used in nuclear medicine (Data obtained from [3])

As can be observed in Fig. 3, the Compton effect is predominant at the energy range of nuclear medicine (100–511 keV – shaded area), unfortunately contributing to the degradation of image quality.

2.3 Gamma Camera

In order to detect the gamma photons, they must interact within the detector and the deposited energy should be directly related with his characteristics. Therefore, gamma radiation interacts with the detector by one of the mechanisms described above, leading to the collection of charge which is, generally, proportional to the energy of radiation.

The gamma camera is the detector that has been adopted in conventional nuclear medicine. Its configuration, due to Hal Anger [4], has been improved and at the present is close to the maximum ratio efficiency/cost. The main components of the gamma camera are the collimator, the scintillation crystal, the optical contact, the photomultipliers and the electronics needed for the signal processing (Fig. 4).

The collimator is a device, made usually of lead, which is interposed between the crystal and the object and whose function is to absorb the scattered rays that can not be used for the image formation. It is a circular or rectangular plate ($\phi \approx 50$ cm) with thousands of tiny holes that are evenly distributed, forming a regular lattice. The direction of these holes determines the function and designation of collimators, such as the parallel holes, convergent and divergent collimators. Due to the impossibility of refraction of the gamma photons, the collimators are essential for forming the image since they can establish a spatial correlation between the detection point and the place of emission. However, the impact on sensitivity is very

Fig. 4 Components of a gamma camera

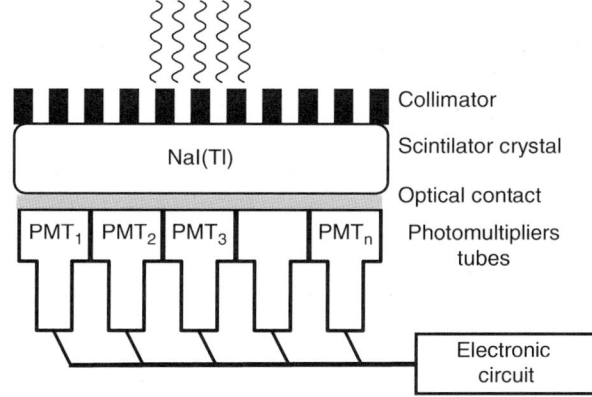

Fig. 5 Source point seen by a gamma camera. The geometric relationships between the distance of spatial resolution (d), the characteristics of the septa and the distance to the source (f) can be derived directly from the figure

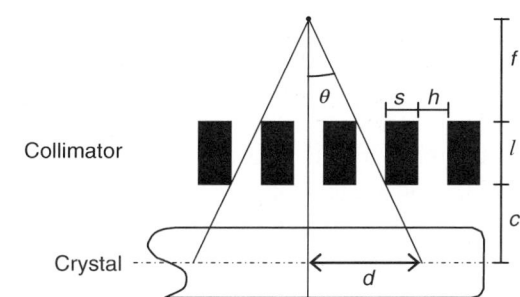

important since only a fraction less than 1% of the photons cross the collimator and reaches the crystal [5]. This collimator is not necessary in PET (because electronic collimation is used instead) and is the main reason why PET is a technique with much higher sensitivity. Another interesting aspect associated with the collimators is its direct influence on the spatial resolution of the system. These geometric relationships are well known and can easily be established from Fig. 5.

Figure 5 shows a point source viewed by a gamma camera located at a distance f from the collimator. The width of the septa[1] is s and the height is ℓ. The width of the holes is represented by h and c is the distance between the collimator and the crystal. Applying the rules of similar triangles to Fig. 5, we get:

$$d = \frac{h}{\ell}(c + \ell + f).\tag{7}$$

The capacity of discriminating two distinct points (spatial resolution) is inversely related to the resolution distance, d, which in turn is directly proportional to the distance, f, between the collimator and the source. Since, in general, the distance, f, to the source is larger than the height of the septa, ℓ, and larger than the distance, c, from the collimator to the crystal, the resolution depends significantly on the

---

[1] Septa are the walls that confine a hole of the collimator.

distance of the gamma camera to the subject. Hence the gamma camera is always placed as near as possible to the patient. Moreover, (7) also shows that the lower the quotient between the width of the hole, h, and the septa height, ℓ, the greater the capacity for discriminating thin structures. However, the decrease of the hole area necessarily implies a reduction of the sensitivity, requiring the adoption of compromise solutions.

The scintillator crystal is essential as a means of transforming the energy of the gamma photons into visible light which in turn is converted into an electrical signal by photomultiplier tubes. The gamma photons interact within the crystal either by photoelectric or by Compton effect. Secondary interactions can occur, causing scintillations (emission of visible light) that are then amplified and converted into electrical signal in the photomultipliers tubes.

The most common material used to manufacture the crystal scintillator of the gamma camera is sodium iodide activated with thallium (NaI(Tl)), whose characteristics make it a good choice. Despite presenting a poor energy resolution, a relatively long response time and hygroscopic properties, it still remains the most frequent crystal used in the construction of the gamma cameras. This choice is mainly due to the fact that sodium iodide presents a good photoelectric fraction,[2] good light yield and an advantageous cost. For the higher photon energies used in PET (511 keV), other crystals have to be used, with higher attenuation coefficient, such as Luthetium-oxyorthosilicate (LSO), that is also dense and luminous. An ideal crystal should have a small attenuation length, high light yield and photoelectric fraction and small decay constant [7]. The attenuation length is defined as the length necessary to absorb 63% of the incident photons. It is common to impose a minimum thickness of the crystal of two attenuation lengths, therefore the shorter the attenuation length the thinner the crystal can be. Moreover, the intrinsic spatial resolution depends on the thickness of the crystal, which is an additional reason for using detecting materials with a short attenuation length. The photoelectric fraction is directly related to the possibility of the energy be deposited in a unique location, which benefits the spatial resolution, in contrast to interactions by Compton effect whose deposition is multiple and spatially spread. Finally, the decay constant is directly associated with the time resolution of the detector.

Photomultiplier tubes (PMTs) (Fig. 6) are extremely sensitive detectors particularly suited for near infrared, visible and ultraviolet light. PMTs combine a high gain and low noise which makes them a good choice for detecting the scintillation light originated at the crystal. The process for converting the scintillation light into an electrical signal follows a simple process of avalanche amplification [8]. Light from the crystal strikes the PMT's photocathode causing the ejection of electrons that are accelerated, by an electric field, onto the first dynode. The electrons that reach the first dynode cause the release of more electrons multiplying the charge. From the first to the second dynode, the process repeats: more electrons are accelerated

---

[2]The photoelectric fration, ε, is given by $-\varepsilon = \sigma_F/(\sigma_F + \sigma_C)$ - which is the relation between the photoelectric scattering cross section, σ_F and the Compton scattering cross section σ_C [6].

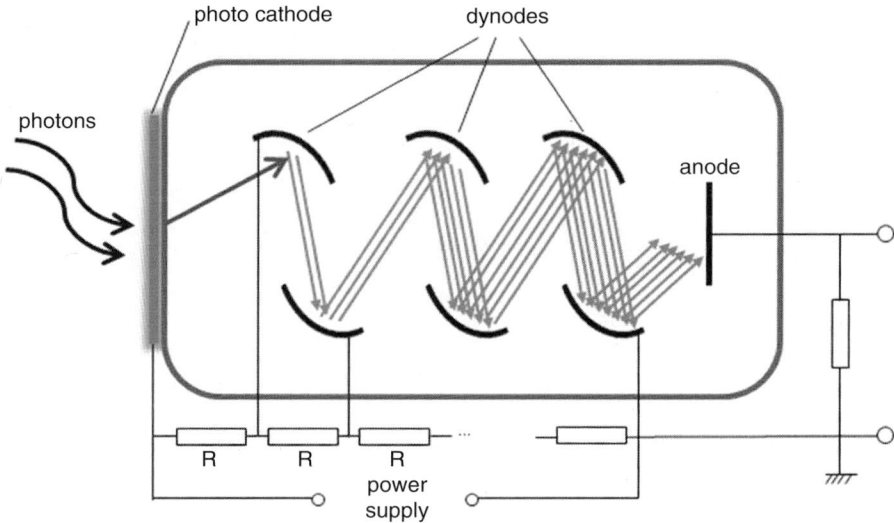

Fig. 6 Schematic of a photomultiplier tube (PMT). Photoelectrons are ejected from the photocathode and accelerated onto the 1st dynode after scintillation photons have reached the photomultiplier window. The charge multiplication occurs along the dynode chain where more electrons are successively ejected

causing the ejection of even more electrons in the second dynode. At each dynode the process is repeated successively, thus producing an avalanche of electrons (from 10^7 to 10^{10} electrons) that are collected at the anode originating an electrical signal.

The photomultiplier output is a short duration ($\sim$microseconds) current pulse which, after being amplified, is analyzed by a pulse height analyzer. This circuit allows the discrimination of the photon energy because there is proportionality between the amplitude of the generated signal and the energy of radiation incident on the photocathode, which is also directly related to the energy of radiation incident on the crystal. The detected pulses can then be counted and associated to a particular spatial position that is determined using the Anger logic [9].

In PET systems, PMTs have been used in block detectors, which consist of an array of several dozen crystals coupled to a small number of photomultipliers (typically 4). The signals from the photomultipliers are integrated for a certain period of time so that their amplitudes are analysed, allowing to determine the photon energy and the instant of detection. Since this time information will be used to determine if two 511 keV photons were detected in coincidence (called a true coincidence), small and fast photodetectors are necessary (given the small sizes of the crystals used in PET, which are directly related with spatial resolution). For these reasons, alternative photodetectors based on semiconductors are replacing the use of conventional PMTs in PET, such as Avalanche Photodiodes (APDs) and Silicon Photomultipliers (SiPMTs).

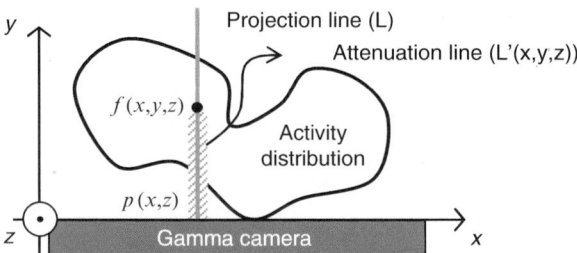

Fig. 7 Representation of the data acquisition by a gamma camera with a parallel hole collimator. The administration of the radionuclide originates the distribution $f(x, y, z)$ within the body. A point (x, y) of the distribution emits in all directions but (ideally) only the direction ($p(r)$: projection line) orthogonal to the gamma camera is detected. On the path, before reaching the detector, the emission is attenuated

2.4 Image Formation

For the emission imaging technology a compound, labeled with a suitable radionuclide, is introduced into the patient's body and forms an emitter density $f(x, y, z)$. In the case of gamma photon emitters (planar scintigraphy and SPECT), the photons cross the patient's body and are detected at the gamma camera. During the path they may suffer interaction which eventually may prevent their detection by the gamma camera (Fig. 7).

The emission of photons at any point (x, y, z) is assumed isotropic, meaning that there is not a privileged direction. However, because of the collimator (parallel holes), less than $1\%^3$ of the emitted photons will be detected: only the photons orthogonal to the crystal surface. During the path along the line, L, the photons interact with matter suffering attenuation. Therefore, taking into account (6) and neglecting the noise, we can write the following relationship between the radionuclide distribution and a measure of the emission (the projection, $p(x, z)$ [10]):

$$p(x, z) = k \int_L f(x, y, z) \, e^{-\int_{L'(x,y,z)} \mu(x,y,z) \, dy'} \, dy, \qquad (8)$$

where k is the proportionality factor between the concentration of radionuclide and the detected signal and $\mu(x, y, z)$ is the linear attenuation coefficient map.

The collection of all line integrals (8), along x and z, corresponds to a planar imaging (scintigraphy). The obtained image is an orthogonal projection of the object.

---

[3] In fact, other photons whose path is slightly tilted to perpendicular will also be detected which causes image blurring and loss of spatial resolution. (Fig. 5).

As for the case of SPECT, the gamma camera rotates around the patient obtaining a series of projections taken at different angles which are then combined to form a tri-dimensional image. Considering now a tomographic acquisition which implies rotation of the detector, then for a particular projection line it must take into account the angle, θ. Thus, (8) generalizes according to:

$$p\,(x,z,\theta) = k \int_{L_\theta} f\,(x,y,z)\, e^{\displaystyle -\int_{L'_\theta(x,y,z)} \mu(x,y,z)\,ds'}\, ds. \qquad (9)$$

The problem of determining the radionuclide distribution, $f\,(x,y,z)$, from the projections, $p\,(x,z,\theta)$, is known as the image reconstruction problem. In scintigraphy, there is not enough data to determine the radionuclide distribution. Consequently, the image reconstruction refers only to tomography.

Note that for a given value z, the set of projections $p\,(x,\theta)$ is the (attenuated) Radon transform of the object. However, it is common in certain clinical applications, to assume that attenuation is constant (usually zero), and (9) takes a simpler form:

$$p\,(x,z,\theta) = k \int_{L_\theta} f\,(x,y,z)\, ds, \qquad (10)$$

which constitutes the Radon integral.

Despite (10) is only a crude approximation of the measurement process involved in emission imaging, it is widely applied in SPECT reconstruction methods used in clinical routine. The images obtained are not quantitatively exact, but qualitatively they are good enough to permit accurate diagnosis. The problem of quantification in SPECT is complex since it implies that the attenuation map have to be considered in the reconstruction step. The method for correcting the attenuation most used in clinic, because it is easy to apply, was proposed by Chang [11] and consists on the correction of the estimates of the radionuclide distribution slice by slice, according to the equation:

$$f_{\text{corrected}}\,(x,y)|_z = k\,(x,y) \times f_{\text{estimate}}\,(x,y)|_z. \qquad (11)$$

The map of the weighting, $k\,(x,y)$, is the inverse of the average attenuation considered in all the projection lines that contain the point (x,y). Other more accurate methods such as analytical and iterative techniques produce better results but are less used in clinical routine since they are slower. Analytical methods are generally based on the analytic inversion of the attenuated Radon transform [12–14]. On the other hand, iterative methods allow to include the attenuation correction into the model itself.

Regarding the image reconstruction methods, it is usual to distinguish between analytical and iterative methods.

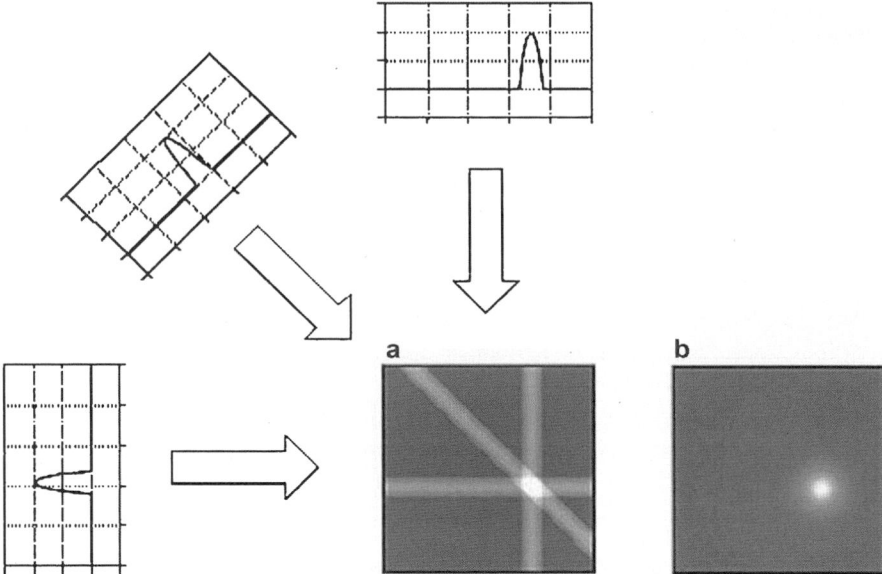

Fig. 8 Representation of the simple backprojection method. The value of a given projection is uniformly distributed on the image that are being calculated. (**a**) Represents the process for only three views; (**b**) the same process for a large number of views (Adapted from [16])

Analytical methods can be classified into three groups: simple backprojection, filter of the backprojection and backprojection of filtered projections [15]. The iterative methods can be divided into statistical and non-statistical methods. Statistical methods do not make assumptions about the nature of the noise presented in the data. Conversely, statistical methods assume that noise contaminating the data follows either a Gaussian or a Poisson distribution, resulting from there a logical division within the statistical methods.

In the simple backprojection the measurements are uniformly distributed along the line of projection. Proceeding similarly for all projections at different angles an estimate of the activity distribution will be obtained.

Although being a fairly simple process, the results are not accurate, as can be observed in Fig. 8 where the reconstructed image of a point source appears blurred. The filtered backprojection (FBP) corrects this problem by filtering the projections before backprojection [17] (Fig. 9).

Although in clinical practice the analytical methods are usually preferred, the iterative methods have characteristics that make them more attractive to those who are looking for accuracy and versatility (even at the expense of more processing time). Iterative methods allow incorporating models that are more realistic and therefore correct several effects that occurred during data acquisition.

In general, iterative methods involve four basic steps, outlined in Fig. 10.

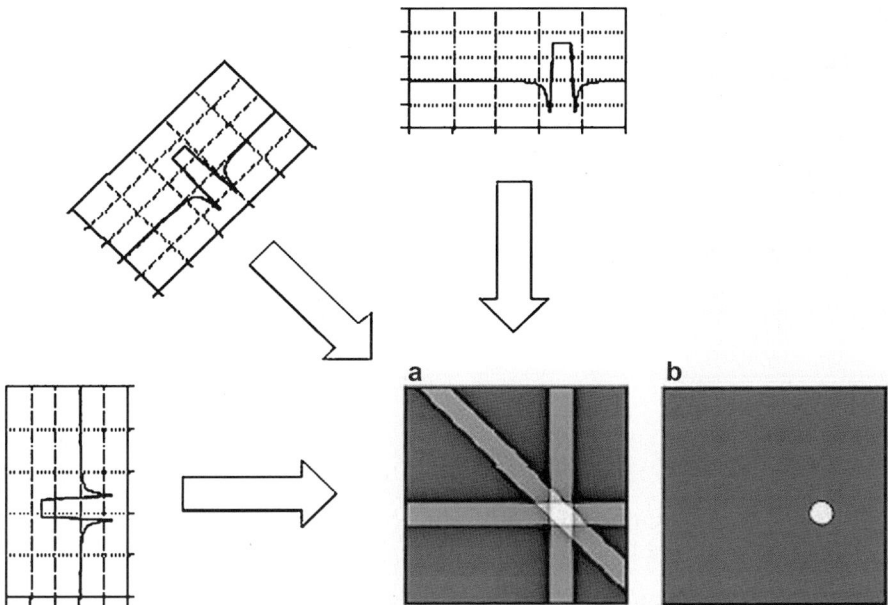

Fig. 9 Representation of the filtered backprojection method. Each view is first filtered or convoluted with an appropriate function. (**a**) Represents the process for only three views; (**b**) the same process for a large number of views (Adapted from [16])

Fig. 10 Overview of iterative methods for image reconstruction

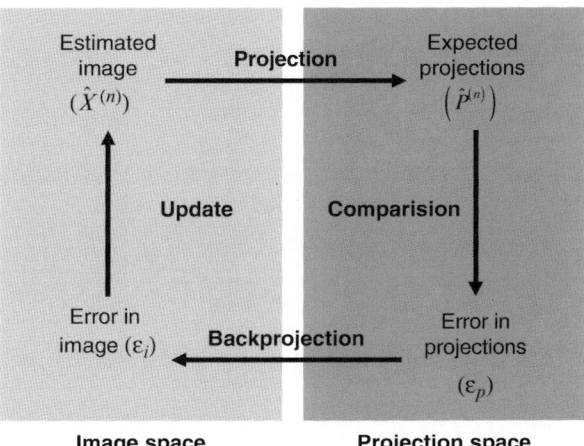

1. The process starts with an estimate initial image, $\hat{X}^{(n)}$, which is projected obtaining the set of projections, $\hat{P}^{(n)}$, which would be the expected projections if $\hat{X}^{(n)}$ were the true picture.
2. The projections $\hat{P}^{(n)}$ are then compared with the measured projections P, obtaining a set of errors, ε_p, in the space of projections.

Fig. 11 Illustration of the basic model used in iterative methods of reconstruction. The line of projection, p_i, is originated by the sum of the contributions of the pixels, f_j (voxels in 3D case) that are crossed by the line. The values a_{ij} represent the fraction that the pixel j contributes to the line of projection i

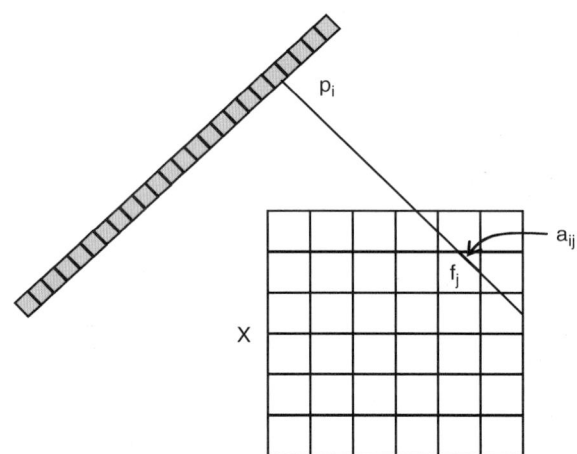

3. The errors are backprojected to the image space resulting in the set ε_i;
4. Finally, the errors in the image space are used to update the image, $X^{(n)}$;

From the mathematical point of view, the reconstruction can be analyzed with the help of Fig. 11. Initially, a voxelized space is established (or pixelated, in the 2D case) in which each projection line crosses certain voxels (or pixels). Therefore, each measurement is originated by the weighted sum of the intensity values of the voxels (pixels) that are over the line of projection and the noise associated to the process.

Thus, the projection, p_i, is defined by

$$p_i = \sum_j a_{ij} \, f_j, \tag{12}$$

where a_{ij} represent the fraction that pixel j contributes to the line of projection i. The backprojection, on the other hand, will be:

$$f_j = \sum_i a_{ij} \, p_i, \tag{13}$$

The reconstruction can then be more generally presented as a matrix problem:

$$P = A \, X + R, \tag{14}$$

where P represents the set of all projections, p_i, (measurements), A is the matrix of elements a_{ij}, called the system matrix that links the projections with the unknown values X, and R represents the noise.

If the noise was known and the matrix A invertible, the solution would be direct. However, neither the noise is known nor the matrix is generally invertible, thus it is usually necessary to employ other methods.

The algorithm ART (*Algebraic Reconstruction Technique*) was proposed in 1970 [18] and is one of the simplest iterative methods of reconstruction. In this method the estimates under a given line are compared with the measured projection and corrected using a simple subtraction. The process follows projection after projection iterating a certain number of times. With a suitable choice of the over-relaxation parameters, it has been shown that this algorithm is capable of producing high quality images [19].

In a Bayesian approach, the reconstruction (14) is seen as an optimization problem where the values X are the ones that better explain the observable data, meaning that the reconstruction algorithm is guided to determine the most likely values of the image, X, given its projections, P, or to maximizing the conditional probability, $P[X|P]$, which is the probability of occurring X given P [10]. According to Bayes' formula, we can rewrite the conditional probability as follows:

$$P[X|P] = \frac{P[P|X]\ P[X]}{P[P]}. \tag{15}$$

As the denominator in (15) is constant, maximizing $P[X|P]$ is equivalent to maximizing only the numerator. The term $P[P|X]$ is called likelihood and signifies how close the data and the image are or, again, the probability of P given X. In the reconstruction by maximum likelihood the probability $P[P|X]$ is maximized.

In the case a Poisson model is considered for the emission, the conditional probability is given by

$$P[P|X] = \prod_i \frac{e^{-\sum a_{ij} f_j}\left(\sum a_{ij} f_j\right)^{p_i}}{p_i!}. \tag{16}$$

Applying logarithms to (16) and maximizing it:

$$\ln(P[P|X]) = \sum_i \left\{ p_i \sum a_{ij} f_j - \sum a_{ij} f_j - \ln(p_i!) \right\}. \tag{17}$$

Although there are several methods to maximize the likelihood (16) the most used is expectation maximization [20]. This method (ML-EM) involves an iterative technique whose convergence is guaranteed [21]. The method follows the general procedure explained above (Fig. 10) and can be summarized by the following equation:

$$f_j^{(n+1)} = \frac{f_j^{(n)}}{\sum_\ell a_{\ell j}} \sum_i a_{ij} \frac{p_i}{\sum_k a_{ik} f_k^{(n)}}. \tag{18}$$

One of the most important variants of the ML-EM algorithm is the OSEM algorithm (Ordered Subset Expectation Maximization) [22], which converges faster than its predecessor, however, there is no proof that OSEM converges to the same solution of MLEM [23]. The basic idea of this method is to use data blocks that are successively employed to calculate the estimates of the image. One iteration is divided into several steps that requires less data but sufficient to update the estimated image. Hence, at the end of an iteration, which corresponds to the use of all available data, the image was already updated as many times as the number of groups utilized, allowing a significant acceleration of the process.

3   Motion Correction

One of the vital problems during the acquisition of biomedical images is to ensure that the object is still relatively to the camera, to avoid image degradation. This is particularly important in children or patients who have movement disorders. Although patients are instructed to remain still during the scan, it is not always possible and sometimes it is necessary to use restraints systems. This problem gets worse on techniques that require long acquisition times, typically nuclear imaging techniques such as PET and SPECT. Movement promotes significant reduction in resolution, severe augmentation of partial volume effects, reducing the accuracy of quantitative methods, alters the pattern definition of metabolic abnormalities and impacts negatively on patient management. Consequently, motion correction techniques become essential.

3.1   Effect of Motion in Emission Imaging

The effect usually attributed to motion is blurring of the moving objects, which implies spread of the activity and loss of edge definition. These effects result both in the appearance of artifacts and in the reduction of the detectability of small lesions.

Figure 12 illustrates the effect of the motion of a point source. The emission is made from different points over time, which due to the temporal resolution of the gamma detector, are impossible to discriminate. As a result the source is seen as a larger source with less activity.

Another important aspect to consider is the relationship between the amplitude of motion and the spatial resolution of the detector, since, for situations where the amplitude is much smaller than the resolution distance, the movement will have a negligible effect

Murase et al. [24] were the first to study systematically the impact of motion in SPECT. They evaluated by simulation and with real tests, using adequate phantoms, the impact of respiratory motion in SPECT imaging and concluded that for an amplitude of 14 mm the contrast in lesions with 2 cm diameter decreased approximately 20% when compared to the situation without motion.

Currently, it is well established that respiratory movements can cause artifacts in myocardial perfusion SPECT exams with direct implications for the diagnosis [25–33]. Concerning this result, Matsumoto et al. concluded that the artifacts created

Fig. 12 Illustration of the image blurring caused by movement of a point source. (**a**) Acquisition of a static point source. (**b**) Hypothetical situation of a point source with a given periodic translation movement

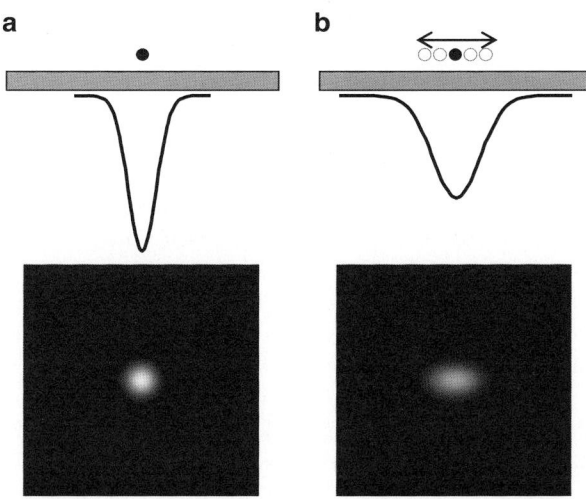

depended on the time and nature of the motion and also on the number of camera heads used, e.g.: for deviations of less than 1 pixel no perfusion defects were detected (assessed by QPS[4]), but for the deviations of 3 pixels the defects detected corresponded to 8.1% for a camera of one head and 11.8% for a camera with two heads.

Regarding PET, Osman et al. investigated the effect of motion in PET/CT studies finding deviations between PET and CT in the localization of lesions. According to this study, the localization deviations between the two techniques, which are afterwards fused, can result in some cases (2%) in gross lesions localization errors. Moreover, the need for attenuation correction in PET from the CT images cause several artifacts when there is patient motion [34–36]. It was also shown that respiratory motion causes a reduction in the accuracy on the determination of volume and activity of lung lesions when examined with ^{18}F-FDG PET [37, 38].

Studies performed in other areas [39–42], particularly in radiotherapy, report an increase of the volume and errors in the localization of tumors that lead to inadequate planning.

3.2 Methods for Detecting Motion

Motion detection is the precursor of the correction and is a key step for the success of any technique to compensate for motion effects. There are numerous forms to detect motion that could be classified into two groups: techniques that use directly the scintigraphic images (data driven) and techniques that utilize external sensors to detect the motion.

---

[4]Quantitative Perfusion SPECT.

3.2.1 Data Driven Methods

The way to quantify the movement that involves the least interference with clinical protocols and usually do not require additional hardware is the one that uses the clinical images that are acquired. This is the primarily reason why these methods are attractive and preferred in the clinical setting.

In the 70s, some methods for determining the movement of translation were proposed: for liver scintigraphy, based on the centroid of the image or, in more simplified versions, just based on the centroid of the coordinate yy of the gamma camera [43–45]. Also for scintigraphic images, the use of two external sources attached to the patient's body was proposed. The images of the sources allow an easy detection of motion [46].

The detection for tomographic images becomes more complex. Several different processes have been suggested which can be classified into five groups. The methods can then be classified as: cross-correlation (CC) [47–49], diverging squares [50], two-dimensional fit (2DF) [51], external radioactive markers (EM) [28, 52] and optical flow (OF) [53].

All these methods try to estimate motion from the projections which, in the case of SPECT, are the planar images.

CC between two data vectors, V and V', is based on the equation:

$$CC(i) = \sum_{j=1}^{m} V(j) \times V'(j+i), \tag{19}$$

where m represents the number of existing values in each vector. Variable i is the deviation (in pixels) to be determined and it is usual to consider $-10 \leq i \leq 10$.

The movement is then calculated by considering the CC between vectors obtained from consecutive images. Generally, for defining the vectors horizontal and/or vertical profiles are used, which are chosen either from a region of the image [47] or from the entire image [48].

The DS algorithm was developed for application to myocardial perfusion tomographic imaging. Initially, in the first projection image the user defines a rectangle of 10 x 10 pixels inside the left ventricle. Four new rectangles of 11×11 pixels are defined such that each square contains the initial rectangle and also one of the four possible adjacent rows and columns. From these four rectangles, it is chosen the one that has the highest number of counts. Following the same criteria used previously, four new rectangles of 12×12 pixels are defined. The process goes on until reaching a square of 20×20 pixels. The center of this square is considered the "center of the heart" for the first projection. For the remaining projections center of the heart is determined following the same procedure. Finally, the motion is computed taking into account the geometry associated to the rotation of the gamma camera.

The 2DF method was also developed specifically for cardiac SPECT images. The user defines in the 45° image projection (left anterior oblique projection) a circular region of interest containing all the activity of the myocardium. Pixels contained in the circular region are compared with the adjacent image (next projection) using the sum of squared differences, defined by:

$$SSD_{i\,j} = \sum_k \sum_\ell \left(I_{x-k;\,y-\ell} - I'_{i-k;\,j-\ell}\right)^2, \tag{20}$$

(x, y) are the coordinates of the circular region center, (k, ℓ) are in the range of pixels in the region of interest, I is the original image and I' the adjacent image. The minimum of the function SSD_{ij} is calculated by a parabolic interpolating and the coordinates of the minimum and $(\Delta x, \Delta y)$ are the translation values that align the image I' with the image I. The center of the circular region is then placed in the adjacent image, I' at the coordinates $(x + \Delta x, y + \Delta y)$ and the process repeats for a new adjacent image. At the end all images will be aligned.

ME techniques are perhaps the most straightforward since motion is computed from the deviations of the external markers centroid seen in different projection images.

Motion in the OF algorithm is obtained by optical flow (movement of an intensity pattern on the image caused by the movement of the scene or the camera) considering two consecutive projections. For a faster calculation optical flow is generally determined on a region of interest. This option permits also to reduce the possible effects of motion on the determination of optical flow since it is assumed that these effects are global.

In addition to the methods mentioned before, the visualization of the projection images consecutively as if it were a film enable to detect sudden movements.

Several studies comparing [51–55] the various methods were carried out but there are no agreement in the conclusions and it seems that there is not a method that performed better than all the others.

3.2.2 Motion Detection Using External Devices

Motion tracking is technically possible with various types of transducers, however the requirements demanded at the clinical setting significantly limits the available solutions. Therefore, video cameras working either in the visible [56–58] or in the near-infrared range [59–61] have been the most frequent option. The basic idea of these methods is to place markers on the patient's body that could be seen by various cameras and that could be tracked three-dimensionally. Following the marker's positions it is possible to measure the motion of the body which they are linked to. Cameras working in near-infrared range allow to operate with dark conditions that are advantageous for some neurological examinations, and also allow better markers identification since the signal to noise ratio is higher. On the other hand, the use of cameras working in the visible range allows a reduction of costs and the use of a large number of markers.

In the case of respiratory movements (PET), it is common to use external devices that generate a *trigger* signal for protocols based on gated acquisition [62]. Some of these devices are the pressure sensors, spirometers, temperature sensors and also dedicated video cameras.

3.3   Strategies for Motion Correction

The techniques that aimed at reducing the effects of movement were formerly categorized by Baimel et al. in three groups [43]: *gating* techniques, computational techniques and analog circuit techniques. The analog circuit techniques include those that apply electronic circuits to the outputs of the position of the gamma camera and correct the detected events based on a centroid calculation [43, 44]. With the development of computers, these techniques were naturally replaced by others that were more efficient.

Currently, the gating and the computational techniques continue to be considered, though new categories have been proposed to better classify the correction algorithms that have been devised.

Gating methods should not be considered as a motion compensation technique in the strict sense, since in fact, it is assumed the presence of a particular class of motion which is inevitable but trackable. Generally, the motion is periodic such as the heartbeat. Hence, instead of trying to devise a way of eliminating the motion (with post processing computation), the acquisition is performed at precise instants allowing to obtain images at different phases of movement. The drawback that has to be overcome is the small number of counts (due to dosimetric considerations) that are usually obtained for each image. To solve this situation the motion cycle is divided in a certain number of intervals and data is accumulated on each of these intervals cycle after cycle (Fig. 13). It is, therefore, indispensable the existence of a way to trigger each new cycle - in the case of cardiac imaging it is used the R wave of electrocardiogram.

One of the most common forms of performing motion compensation in clinical routine (for dynamic acquisitions) is to detect motion by visualization of the images and then to remove the images with motion. Despite being quick and easy to perform implies a loss of number of counts per pixel which increases noise. An efficient alternative to the image elimination is the manual alignment of images which will ensure an improvement of the final image [63]. However, this technique is time consuming, cumbersome and user dependent and is therefore worse than others.

In the case of planar scintigraphy (e.g. renogram [64]) the motion correction is performed after the detection of movement, by aligning the images with proper interpolation methods. This simple approach allows only the correction of either translational movements that occur in the projection plane or rotation about a perpendicular axis to the plane of projection.

Tomography requires more complex methods that involve the techniques of image reconstruction. The refinement of the methods is clear in the literature: firstly

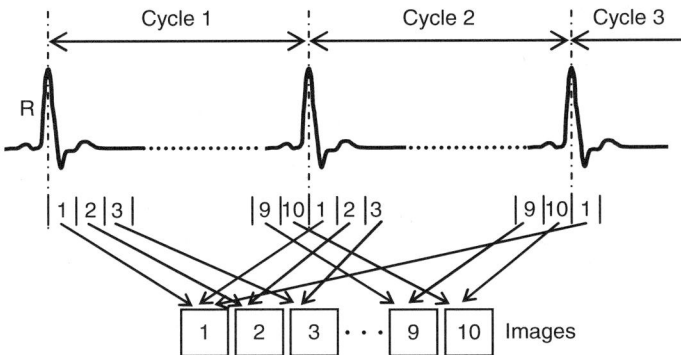

Fig. 13 Scheme of a cardiac gating acquisition. The R wave is used as a trigger signal – on the rising-edge starts a new cycle that ends up in the new transition. During this period several acquisitions (10 in the picture) are made. At each new cycle the images are updated

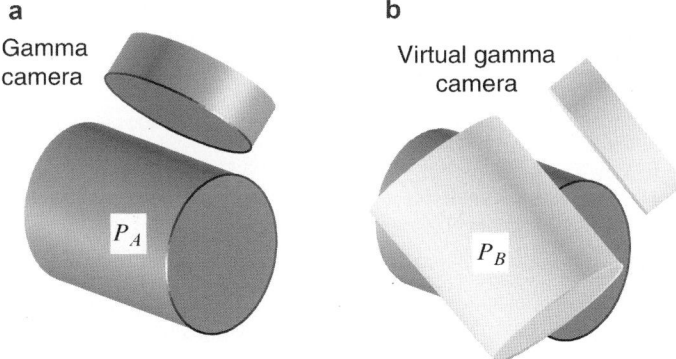

Fig. 14 Representation of the cylinder associated to the movement of the gamma camera during a tomographic acquisition. (**a**) Without motion of the patient; (**b**) situation where the patient moves – a virtual cylinder is generated and associated with it the set of projections P_B

the correction began to be made in each projection and the reconstruction step carried out later [47, 48, 50, 54]. Later, Fulton et al. presented a new approach for the correction of motion with application to SPECT brain imaging. This new strategy treated the movement of the patient as a new virtual position of the gamma camera, thus generating a new projection. In the absence of motion of the patient the gamma camera describes a cylinder, whose set of projections can be designed by P_A (Fig. 14). When the patient moves, a new set of projections, P_B, may be introduced by creating a virtual cylinder that is rotated relative to the original [65].

The image reconstruction is then performed using an iterative method (OSEM), which is applied in two-dimensional form using the sets of projections in each sub-iteration. Between each sub-iteration it is necessary to apply a rigid transformation to the reconstructed object in order to put it in the original position and orientation. This operation is intended to avoid a three-dimensional reconstruction (*fully* 3D) that was tested later by the same author [66].

Another form of correcting motion is to perform a list mode acquisition and to detect externally the motion using video cameras [67]. The list mode acquisition generates a list of all detected events. The information saved for each event is the position, the photon energy and the instant of time. Motion compensation is performed by correcting spatially each event using the information of the motion detected by the video cameras. Once spatially corrected, the events transform naturally in the projections and the reconstruction is performed. Recently, the same group also generalized the procedure enabling correction of deformable movements [68].

References

1. Prata MI, Abrunhosa A (2008) Física em Medicina Nuclear: Temas e Aplicações. Imprensa da Universidade de Coimbra
2. Klein O, Nishina Y (1928) The scattering of light by free electrons according to dirac's new relativistic dynamics. Nature 122:398–399
3. http://physics.nist.gov/PhysRefData/Xcom/html/xcom1.html
4. Anger HO (1964) Scintillation camera with multichannel collimators. J Nucl Med 5:515–531
5. Ricard M (2004) Imaging of gamma emitters using scintillation cameras. Nucl Instrum Methods Phys Res, Sect A 527(1–2):124–129
6. Derenzo SE, Moses WW, Weber MJ, West AC (1994) Methods for a systematic, comprehensive search for fast, heavy scintillator materials. In: Materials research society symposium - proceedings, vol 348, Lawrence Berkeley Lab, Berkeley, pp 39–49
7. Moses W, Gayshan V, Gektin A (2006) The evolution of SPECT from anger to today and beyond. In: Radiation detectors for medical applications, pp. 37–80
8. Knoll GF (1979) Radiation detection and measurement. Wiley, New York
9. Links JM, Prince JL (2006) Medical imaging signals and systems. Pearson Prentice-Hall Bioengineering, New Jersey
10. Wernick MN, Aarsvold JN (eds) (2004) Emission tomography - the fundamentals of PET and SPECT. Elsevier Academic Press, San Diego, CA
11. Lee-Tzuu C (1978) A method for attenuation correction in radionuclide computed tomography. IEEE Trans Nucl Sci 25(1):638–643
12. Novikov R (2002) An inversion formula for the attenuated x-ray transformation. Arkiv för Matematik 40(1):145–167
13. Sidky EY, Pan X (2002) Variable sinograms and redundant information in single-photon emission computed tomography with non-uniform attenuation. Inverse Probl 18(6):1483–1497
14. Markoe A (1984) Fourier inversion of the attenuated x-ray transform. SIAM J Math Anal 15(4):718–722
15. Frey EC, Tsui BMW (2006) Quantitative analysis in nuclear medicine imaging. Springer, New York
16. http://www.dspguide.com/ch25/5.htm
17. Bruyant PP (2002) Analytic and iterative reconstruction algorithms in spect. J Nucl Med 43(10):1343–1358
18. Gordon R, Bender R, Herman GT (1970) Algebraic reconstruction techniques (art) for three-dimensional electron microscopy and x-ray photography. J Theor Biol 29(3):471–481
19. Herman GT, Meyer LB (1993) Algebraic reconstruction techniques can be made computationally efficient [positron emission tomography application]. IEEE Trans Med Imaging 12(3):600–609

20. Dempster AP, Laird NM, Rubin DB (1977) Maximum likelihood from incomplete data via the em algorithm. J R Stat Soc 39:1–38
21. Shepp LA, Vardi Y (1982) Maximum likelihood reconstruction for emission tomography. IEEE Trans Med Imaging 1(2):113–122
22. Hudson HM, Larkin RS (1994) Accelerated image reconstruction using ordered subsets of projection data. IEEE Trans Med Imaging 13(4):601–609
23. Zaidi H, Hutton BF, Nuyts J (2006) Quantitative analysis in nuclear medicine imaging. Springer, New York
24. Murase K, Ishine M, Kataoka M, Itoh H, Mogami H, Iio A, Hamamoto K (1987) Simulation and experimental study of respiratory motion effect on image quality of single photon emission computed tomography (spect). Eur J Nucl Med 13(5):244–249
25. Botvinick EH, Zhu YY, O'Connell WJ, Dae MW (1993) A quantitative assessment of patient motion and its effect on myocardial perfusion spect images. J Nucl Med 34(2):303–310
26. Cooper JA, Neumann PH, McCandless BK (1992) Effect of patient motion on tomographic myocardial perfusion imaging. J Nucl Med 33(8):1566–1571
27. Eisner R, Churchwell A, Noever T, Nowak D, Cloninger K, Dunn D, Carlson W, Oates J, Jones J, Morris D (1988) Quantitative analysis of the tomographic thallium-201 myocardial bullseye display: critical role of correcting for patient motion. J Nucl Med 29(1):91–97
28. Friedman J, Berman DS, Van Train K, Garcia EV, Bietendorf J, Prigent F, Rozanski A, Waxman A, Maddahi J (1988) Patient motion in thallium-201 myocardial spect imaging. an easily identified frequent source of artifactual defect. Clin Nucl Med 13(5):321–324
29. Friedman J, Van Train K, Maddahi J, Rozanski A, Prigent F, Bietendorf J, Waxman A, Berman DS (1989) "upward creep" of the heart: a frequent source of false-positive reversible defects during thallium-201 stress-redistribution spect. J Nucl Med 30(10):1718–1722
30. Germano G, Kavanagh PB, Kiat H, Van Train K, Berman DS (1994) Temporal image fractionation: rejection of motion artifacts in myocardial spect. J Nucl Med 35(7):1193–1197
31. Ter-Pogossian MM, Bergmann SR, Sobel BE (1982) Influence of cardiac and respiratory motion on tomographic reconstructions of the heart: implications for quantitative nuclear cardiology. J Comput Assist Tomogr 6(6):1148–1155
32. Tsui BMW, Segars WP, Lalush DS (2000) Effects of upward creep and respiratory motion in myocardial spect. IEEE Trans Nucl Sci 47(3):1192–1195
33. Wheat JM, Currie GM (2004) Impact of patient motion on myocardial perfusion spect diagnostic integrity: part 2. J Nucl Med Technol 32(3):158–163
34. Erdi YE, Nehmeh SA, Pan T, Pevsner A, Rosenzweig KE, Mageras G, Yorke ED, Schoder H, Hsiao W, Squire OD, Vernon P, Ashman JB, Mostafavi H, Larson SM, Humm JL (2004) The ct motion quantitation of lung lesions and its impact on pet-measured suvs. J Nucl Med 45(8):1287–1292
35. Goerres GW, Kamel E, Heidelberg T-NH, Schwitter MR, Burger C, von Schulthess GK (2002) Pet-ct image co-registration in the thorax: influence of respiration. Eur J Nucl Med Mol Imaging 29(3):351–360
36. Visvikis D, Barret O, Fryer TD, Lamare F, Turzo A, Bizais Y, Le Rest C.C (2004) Evaluation of respiratory motion effects in comparison with other parameters affecting pet image quality. In: Nuclear science symposium conference record, 2004 IEEE, vol 6, pp 3668–3672
37. Boucher L, Rodrigue S, Lecomte R, Bénard F (2004) Respiratory gating for 3-dimensional pet of the thorax: feasibility and initial results. J Nucl Med 45(2):214–219
38. Nehmeh SA, Erdi YE, Ling CC, Rosenzweig KE, Squire OD, Braban LE, Ford E, Sidhu K, Mageras GS, Larson SM, Humm JL (2002) Effect of respiratory gating on reducing lung motion artifacts in pet imaging of lung cancer. Med Phys 29(3):366–371
39. Balter JM, Ten Haken RK, Lawrence TS, Lam KL, Robertson JM (1996) Uncertainties in ct-based radiation therapy treatment planning associated with patient breathing. Int J Radiat Oncol Biol Phys 36(1):167–174
40. Hugo GD, Agazaryan N, Solberg TD (2003) The effects of tumor motion on planning and delivery of respiratory-gated imrt. Med Phys 30(6):1052–1066

41. Seppenwoolde Y, Shirato H, Kitamura K, Shimizu S, van Herk M, Lebesque JV, Miyasaka K (2002) Precise and real-time measurement of 3d tumor motion in lung due to breathing and heartbeat, measured during radiotherapy. Int J Radiat Oncol Biol Phys 53(4):822–834

42. Shimizu S, Shirato H, Kagei K, Nishioka T, Bo X, Dosaka-Akita H, Hashimoto S, Aoyama H, Tsuchiya K, Miyasaka K (2000) Impact of respiratory movement on the computed tomographic images of small lung tumors in three-dimensional (3d) radiotherapy. Int J Radiat Oncol Biol Phys 46(5):1127–1133

43. Baimel NH, Bronskill MJ (1978) Optimization of analog-circuit motion correction for liver scintigraphy. J Nucl Med 19(9):1059–1066

44. Elings VB, Martin CB, Pollock IG, McClintock JT (1974) Electronic device corrects for motion in gamma camera images. J Nucl Med 15(1):36–37

45. Oppenheim BE (1971) A method using a digital computer for reducing respiratory artifact on liver scans made with a camera. J Nucl Med 12(9):625–628

46. Fleming JS (1984) A technique for motion correction in dynamic scintigraphy. Eur J Nucl Med 9(9):397–402

47. Britten AJ, Jamali F, Gane JN, Joseph AE (1998) Motion detection and correction using multi-rotation 180 degrees single-photon emission tomography for thallium myocardial imaging. Eur J Nucl Med 25(11):1524–1530

48. Eisner RL, Noever T, Nowak D, Carlson W, Dunn D, Oates J, Cloninger K, Liberman HA, Patterson RE (1987) Use of cross-correlation function to detect patient motion during spect imaging. J Nucl Med 28(1):97–101

49. Pellot-Barakat C, Ivanovic M, Weber DA, Herment A, Shelton DK (1998) Motion detection in triple scan spect imaging. IEEE Trans Nucl Sci 45(4):2238–2244

50. Geckle WJ, Frank TL, Links JM, Becker LC (1988) Correction for patient and organ movement in spect: application to exercise thallium-201 cardiac imaging. J Nucl Med 29(4):441–450

51. Cooper JA, Neumann PH, McCandless BK (1993) Detection of patient motion during tomographic myocardial perfusion imaging. J Nucl Med 34(8):1341–1348

52. Germano G, Chua T, Kavanagh PB, Kiat H, Berman DS (1993) Detection and correction of patient motion in dynamic and static myocardial spect using a multi-detector camera. J Nucl Med 34(8):1349–1355

53. Noumeir R, Mailloux GE, Lemieux R (1996) Detection of motion during tomographic acquisition by an optical flow algorithm. Comput Biomed Res 29(1):1–15

54. Leslie WD, Dupont JO, McDonald D, Peterdy AE (1997) Comparison of motion correction algorithms for cardiac spect. J Nucl Med 38(5):785–790

55. O'Connor MK, Kanal KM, Gebhard MW, Rossman PJ (1998) Comparison of four motion correction techniques in spect imaging of the heart: a cardiac phantom study. J Nucl Med 39(12):2027–2034

56. Bloomfield PM, Spinks TJ, Reed J, Schnorr L, Westrip AM, Livieratos L, Fulton R, Jones T (2003) The design and implementation of a motion correction scheme for neurological pet. Phys Med Biol 48(8):959–978

57. Bruyant PP, Nadella S, Gennert MA, King MA (2005) Quality control of the stereo calibration of a visual tracking system (vts) for patient motion detection in spect. In: IEEE nuclear science symposium conference record, vol 5, pp 2599–2602

58. Gennert MA, Bruyant PP, Narayanan MV, King MA (2002) Assessing a system to detect patient motion in spect imaging using stereo optical cameras. In: IEEE nuclear science symposium conference record, vol 3, pp 1567–1570

59. Goddard JS, Gleason SS, Paulus MJ, Majewski S, Popov V, Smith M, Weisenberger A, Welch B, Wojcik R (2002) Real-time landmark-based unrestrained animal tracking system for motion-corrected pet/spect imaging. In: IEEE nuclear science symposium conference record, vol 3, pp 1534–1537

60. Weisenberger AG, Gleason SS, Goddard J, Kross B, Majewski S, Meikle SR, Paulus MJ, Pomper M, Popov V, Smith MF, Welch BL, Wojcik R (2005) A restraint-free small animal spect imaging system with motion tracking. IEEE Trans Nucl Sci 52(3):638–644

61. Weisenberger AG, Kross B, Gleason SS, Goddard J, Majewski S, Meikle SR, Paulus MJ, Pomper M, Popov V, Smith MF, Welch BL, Wojcik R (2003) Development and testing of a restraint free small animal spect imaging system with infrared based motion tracking. In: IEEE nuclear science symposium conference record, vol 3, pp 2090–2094
62. Nehmeh SA, Erdi YE (2008) Respiratory motion in positron emission tomography/computed tomography: a review. Semin Nucl Med 38(3):167–176
63. Fitzgerald J, Danias PG (2001) Effect of motion on cardiac spect imaging: recognition and motion correction. J Nucl Cardiol 8(6):701–706
64. De Agostini A, Moretti R, Belletti S, Maira G, Magri GC, Bestagno M (1992) A motion correction algorithm for an image realignment programme useful for sequential radionuclide renography. Eur J Nucl Med 19(7):476–483
65. Fulton RR, Hutton BF, Braun M, Ardekani B, Larkin R (1994) Use of 3d reconstruction to correct for patient motion in spect. Phys Med Biol 39(3):563–574
66. Fulton RR, Eberl S, Meikle SR, Hutton BF, Braun M (1999) A practical 3d tomographic method for correcting patient head motion in clinical spect. IEEE Tran Nucl Sci 46(3):667–672
67. Ma L, Gu S, Nadella S, Bruyant PP, King MA, Gennert MA (2005) A practical rebinning-based method for patient motion compensation in spect imaging. In: Proceedings of international conference on computer graphics, imaging and vision: new trends, pp 209–214
68. Songxiang Gu, McNamara JE, Mitra J, Gifford HC, Johnson K, Gennert MA, King M.A (2007) Body deformation correction for spect imaging. In: IEEE nuclear science symposium conference record NSS'07, vol 4, pp 2708–2714

OCT Noise Despeckling Using 3D Nonlinear Complex Diffusion Filter

C. Maduro, P. Serranho, T. Santos, P. Rodrigues, J. Cunha-Vaz, and R. Bernardes

Abstract An improved despeckling method, based on complex diffusion filtering, is herein presented to enhance structure segmentation in high-definition spectral domain optical coherence tomography (OCT) data. We propose to extend the traditional nonlinear complex diffusion filter concept propose by Gilboa (IEEE Trans Pattern Anal Mach Intell 26:1020–1036, 2004) from 2- to 3-dimensions, taking into account the consistency of noise along the entire 3D data volume. Moreover we also propose the extension to 3D of an improved complex diffusion filter (Bernardes et al. Opt Express 18:24,048–24,059, 2010), that was specially built for retinal tissue signal preservation in OCT data and that takes into account an adaptive optimized time step for the finite difference discretization. The extension to 3D of the traditional method compares favorably to existing methods reducing speckle noise and preserving edges and features. As expected, the improved 3D version has better performance than the traditional one. Numerical simulations show the feasibility of the method.

C. Maduro (✉) • T. Santos • P. Rodrigues • J. Cunha-Vaz
Association for Innovation and Biomedical Research on Light and Image (AIBILI),
Coimbra, Portugal
e-mail: cmaduro@aibili.pt; torcato@aibili.pt; prodrigues@aibili.pt; cunhavaz@aibili.pt

P. Serranho
Institute of Biomedical Research on Light and Image (IBILI), Faculty of Medicine,
University of Coimbra, Coimbra, Portugal
e-mail: pserranho@fmed.uc.pt

R. Bernardes
Association for Innovation and Biomedical Research on Light and Image (AIBILI),

Institute of Biomedical Research on Light and Image (IBILI), Faculty of Medicine,
University of Coimbra, Coimbra, Portugal
e-mail: rcb@aibili.pt

R.M.N. Jorge et al. (eds.), *Technologies for Medical Sciences*, Lecture Notes
in Computational Vision and Biomechanics 1, DOI 10.1007/978-94-007-4068-6_7,
© Springer Science+Business Media B.V. 2012

1 Introduction

Optical coherence tomography (OCT) is a non-invasive imaging modality with several applications. It provides in vivo high-resolution cross-sectional imaging of the retinal tissue through light scattering. However, as any imaging technique that has his image formation based on coherent waves, OCT images suffer from speckle noise which reduce its quality [9].

Speckle noise is a random phenomenon generated by interference of waves with random phases [10], being a common problem to other imaging modalities as ultrasound, synthetic-aperture radar (SAR) or laser imaging, leading to research and resulting on many speckling reduction techniques [10].

It creates a grainy appearance that can mask diagnostically significant image features and reduces the accuracy of segmentation and pattern recognition algorithms [10, 26, 28]. Please refer to [10, 31] for a further description of the speckle in OCT characteristics.

The statistical mechanism of laser speckle formation was first presented by Goodman [14]. Besides the theoretical results, this study also supports the idea that speckle noise could be rejected by linear filtering. On the other hand, Wagner et al. [35], Burckhardt et al. [8] and Abbott et al. [1] conclude that linear filtering, the way it was presented in [14], suppresses the noise at the cost of smoothing out image details.

Schmitt et al. [29] described the first OCT speckle suppression technique where a compounded image was formed from the sum of the signals from a quadrant photodiode detection system. A similar angular compounding approach was also used by Bashkansky and Reintjes [5] and by Iftimia et al. [16].

Like angular compounding there were also developed other speckle reducing methods applied before image formation (physical techniques), such as frequency compounding or spatial compounding.

A frequency compounding technique has been used by Skankar [33] and by Pircher et al. [25], where the contrast was increased and the quality image improved without loss of resolution.

Kim et al. [18] presented a space diversity speckle reduction technique, reporting a substantial reduction of speckle despite the reduced transverse resolution.

Yung et al. [38] described a zero-adjustment procedure (ZAP) to OCT which was first applied by Healey et al. [15] in medical ultrasound.

The requirements on modifying the hardware led to the development of post-processing methods, being the CLEAN algorithm one of the first image processing techniques for OCT despeckling [30]. Among these are the median filtering [7], homomorphic Wiener filtering [12], enhanced Lee filter (ELEE) [22], symmetric nearest neighbor (SNN) filter, adaptive smoothing [20], multiresolution wavelet analysis [37], filtering techniques based on rotating kernel transformations [27], Kuwahara filter [21] and anisotropic diffusion filtering [24, 28].

The median filter calculates for each pixel its median value in a local neighborhood. Koozekanani et al. [19] applied it to reduce the speckle of the OCT images to a posterior measurement of the retinal thickness. On the other hand, Ishikawa et al. [17], with the same purpose of measuring the retinal thickness, used a modified mean filter to reduce the noise. The Gaussian filter is another filter applied on the retinal segmentation algorithms [3,4,32,34]. In the adaptive filtering the algorithm is modified locally based on the pixel's neighborhood, combining an effective noise reduction and an ability to preserve the image edges. The Lee filter is one of this adaptive filters that was successfully applied to OCT images. Ozcan et al. [23] compare the performance of different filters (an enhanced Lee filter, two *à trous* wavelet-transform-based filters, a hybrid median filter, a symmetric nearest-neighbor filter, a Kuwahara filter and an adaptive Wiener filter), when applied independently or when applied in association, to reduce the speckling present on an OCT tomogram of a bovine retina [26]. A fuzzy thresholding algorithm in the wavelet domain was proposed by Puvanathasan [26] to remove the speckle noise in OCT images of a human finger tip.

Fernández et al. [11] and Salinas et al. [28] have shown that a nonlinear complex diffusion filter can be successfully applied to remove OCT speckle noise while preserving image features. Recently, [6] proposed an improvement to these approaches, suggesting an adaptive time step and a particular choice of parameters to be more conservative in the diffusion of signal within retinal tissue, therefore taking a specific approach for OCT data despeckling that can be generalized for similar medical images.

Current despeckling methods applied to process noisy optical coherence tomography data take into consideration each B-scan individually, therefore looking to the 3D data as a set of individual 2D images [23,26,28]. In this way, the consistency of noise along the entire 3D data volume is not taken into account.

In the work herewith presented, we have extended the application of complex diffusion filters [28] and [6] from 2- to 3-dimensions therefore considering the entire volume as a single entity and not as a set of aggregated 2D entities.

As a proof-of-concept, the proposed method will be compared resorting to quantitative measures with filtering methods from the literature.

2 Material and Methods

2.1 Optical Coherence Tomography

The OCT working principle is similar to ultrasound and adopted some of its terminology from that field.

The volumetric OCT information is composed of a set of A-scans (depth-wise information on refractive index changes) (Fig. 1). The scanning is performed along a series of parallel lines covering the 20° field-of-view of the eye fundus and allows users access to an unprecedented detail of the retina structures from in vivo subjects.

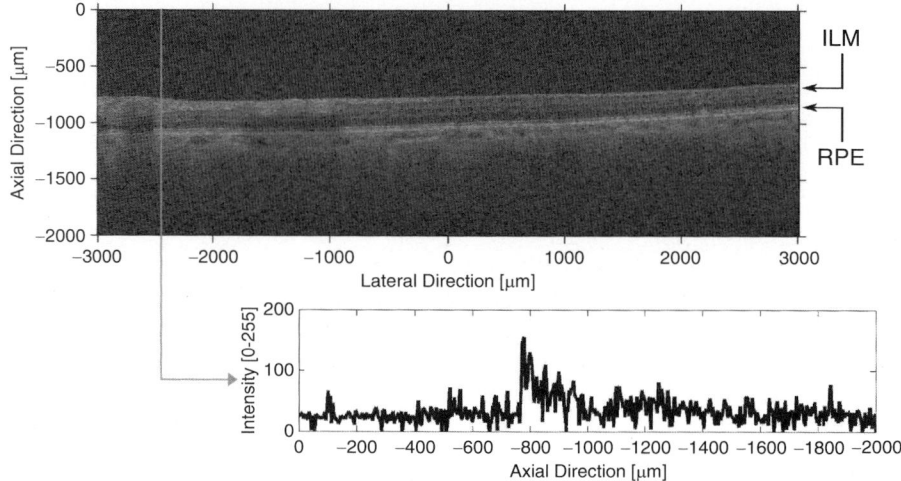

Fig. 1 Optical coherence tomography example of a B-scan (*top*) and an A-scan profile (*bottom*)

Fig. 2 Volumetric OCT data shown over an eye fundus reference

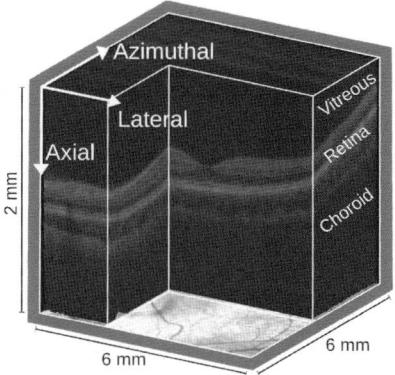

In this work the high-definition spectral domain Cirrus OCT (Carl Zeiss Meditec, Dublin, CA, USA) was used.

This retinal imaging system allows for an acquisition scan of $200 \times 200 \times 1{,}024$ or $512 \times 128 \times 1{,}024$ voxels for the lateral, azimuthal and axial directions, respectively, with a depth and lateral resolutions of 5 and $20\,\mu m$ in tissue, respectively. This volumetric data is obtained from a $6{,}000 \times 6{,}000 \times 2{,}000\,\mu m^3$ volume of the human macula (Fig. 2).

OCT readings result from reflections and/or light scattering due to refractive index changes along the light path and are therefore dependent on the content and structure organization of the eye.

OCT has been used to assess structural information from the eye fundus, in vivo, allowing to identify and compare retinal changes in different instants of time.

2.2   3D-Nonlinear Complex Diffusion Filter

The application of diffusion filters to image processing is based on the analogy to physical diffusion processes, the rationale being to balance different concentrations without creation or destruction of mass/energy [36].

Here, the concentration becomes the image intensity and the diffusion equation becomes:

$$\frac{\partial I}{\partial t} = \nabla \cdot (D \, \nabla I), \tag{1}$$

where the initial condition is given by the original image ($I_{t=0} = I_0$), D is the diffusion coefficient, ∇ is the gradient operator and $\nabla \cdot$ is the divergence operator.

Commonly, the diffusion coefficient is chosen to be dependent on the image gradient [24], hence

$$D = d(|\nabla I|), \tag{2}$$

where $|\cdot|$ denotes the magnitude.

Fernández et al. [11] and Salinas et al. [28] shown that a nonlinear complex diffusion filter can be successfully applied to remove the OCT speckle noise while preserving image features. Both defined the diffusion coefficient as

$$d(\mathrm{Im}(I)) = \frac{e^{i\theta}}{1 + \left(\dfrac{\mathrm{Im}(I)}{k\theta}\right)^2}, \tag{3}$$

where $\mathrm{Im}(\cdot)$ is the imaginary value, $i = \sqrt{-1}$, k a threshold parameter and θ a phase angle [28].

This choice relies on the fact that for small θ the imaginary part can be considered as a smoothed second derivative of the initial signal factored by θ and time (t) [13]

$$\lim_{\theta \to 0} \frac{Im(I)}{\theta} = t \Delta g * I_0, \tag{4}$$

where Δ is the laplacian, g is a gaussian and $*$ the convolution operator.

This formulation does not require to compute expressly derivatives of the image, thus avoiding the numerical instabilities due to noise at early stages and is a good choice regarding edge preservation.

In the work herewith presented we extended this application from 2- to 3-dimensions taking advantage of the volumetric information provided by the Cirrus HD-OCT.

The extension to 3D is proposed by implementing a forward in time and centered in space (FTCS) finite difference scheme, being the iterative update given by

$$I_{l,j,m}^{(n+1)} = I_{l,j,m}^{(n)} + \Delta t \left(\bar{D}_{l,j,m}^{(n)} \Delta_h I_{l,j,m}^{(n)} + \nabla_h D_{l,j,m}^{(n)} \cdot \nabla_h I_{l,j,m}^{(n)} \right), \tag{5}$$

where Δ_h and ∇_h are, respectively, the discrete second order laplacian and gradient operators, Δt is the step in time, l, j and m are the indexes for the voxels of I and $\bar{D}$ is given by

$$\bar{D}_{l,j,m}^{(n)} = \frac{6D_{l,j,m}^{(n)} + D_{l\pm1,j,m}^{(n)} + D_{l,j\pm1,m}^{(n)} + D_{l,j,m\pm1}^{(n)}}{12}. \tag{6}$$

As shown in [2] this explicit method is stable if

$$\Delta t \leq \frac{1}{\alpha} \cos\theta \min_{l,j,m} \left(1 + \left(\frac{\mathrm{Im}(I)}{k\theta} \right)^2 \right), \tag{7}$$

where $\alpha = 4$ in 2D and $\alpha = 6$ in 3D.

2.3   Improved Adaptive 3D NCDF

In the previous analysis, the parameter k is left constant. However, it can be adaptively used to improve the despeckling method's performance in the case of OCT data. The diffusion coefficient can be approximated by

$$D \approx \frac{1}{1 + (\Delta I/k)^2}. \tag{8}$$

As motivation for these kind of functions, this expression can be seen as a Lorentzian function (9) modified to have its maximum equal to 1 and $w = k/2$.

$$L(x) = \frac{2Aw}{\pi \left(w^2 + 4(x - x_c)^2 \right)}. \tag{9}$$

In this way, a family of curves can be generated from (8) as shown in Fig. 3, simply by modifying the value of k.

The choice for the k parameter (3) is therefore important, as it modulates the spread of the diffusion coefficient in the vicinity of its maximum, that is, at edges and homogeneous areas, where the image laplacian vanishes. From the plot, it becomes clear the difference in D for ΔI constant from low- (higher k) to high-intensity areas (lower k), thus increasing the diffusion for low-intensity areas and decreasing it for higher-intensity ones.

Fig. 3 Family of curves from
the diffusion coefficient as a
function of k (8)

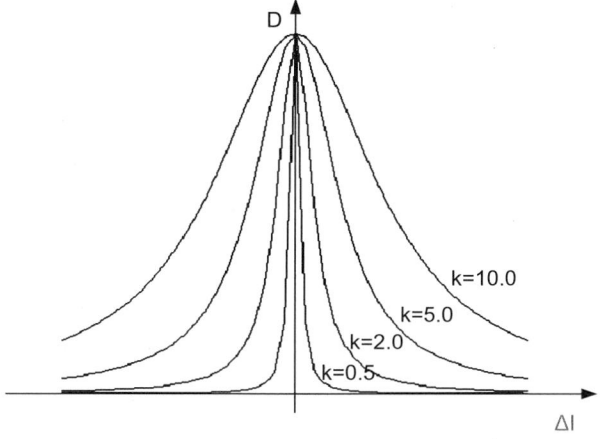

2.3.1 Improved Coefficient of Diffusion

While the formulation for the coefficient of diffusion (3) seems to be a good choice
to preserve the location of edges, as stated in [28], it does not specifically address
our need to preserve the variation of intensity across the edge and features of the
image within the tissue, which might be improved following the lines of [6].

By definition, edges are located in between two areas of perceived distinct intensity levels within the image. Additionally, the OCT background is characterized
by a low average intensity level. Conversely, the tissue due to the differences in the
refractive index, presents a higher average level in the image.

We intend to manipulate (3) to take advantage of these facts. In this way, we aim
to facilitate diffusion at lower intensity level areas (e.g., vitreous, cysts, fluid-filled
regions) and to be conservative within the retinal tissue areas (preserving important
details for analysis). As an advantageous byproduct, edges are better preserved as
diffusion is decreased at the higher level side of the edge.

To this end, we need to locally modify k according to data, increasing k at low
level areas and making it smaller at higher level areas. This is a clear distinction to
the formulation using (3) where k is made constant for the entire image and over
iterations. We proposed to adapt k locally by the use of the function

$$k = k_{Max} + (k_{Min} - k_{Max}) \frac{g - \min(g)}{\max(g) - \min(g)}, \qquad (10)$$

where $\min(g)$ and $\max(g)$ stand for the minimum and maximum of g, respectively,
with g being defined as

$$g = G_{N,\sigma} * \mathrm{Re}(I), \qquad (11)$$

where $*$ is the convolution operator and $G_{N,\sigma}$ is a local average (gaussian) kernel of
size $N \times N$ or $N \times N \times N$ (depending on whether the approach is 2D or 3D) and
standard deviation σ.

Fig. 4 Typical evolution of
the step in time (Δt) for the
proposed adaptive process
in 2D

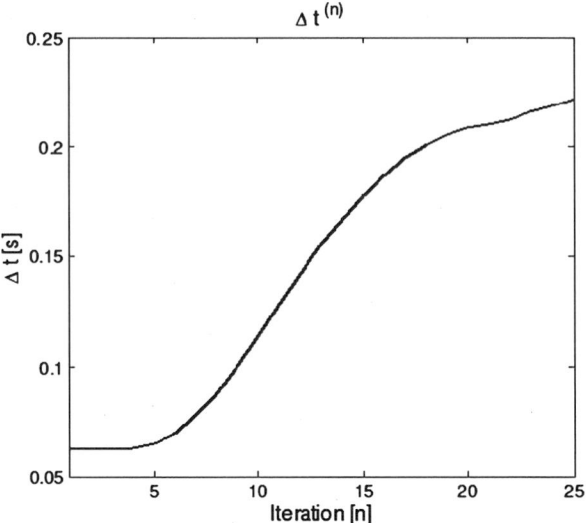

Additionally, using a gaussian filter for D is beneficial to increase speckle removal. While in edges, filtering D does not change D significantly as long as σ is small since Im(I) is smooth [13]. However, at isolated spiky D points, filtering D turns diffusion less conservative and therefore increases speckle reduction without compromising edge preservation.

2.3.2   Adaptive Time Step

As opposed to the majority of nonlinear complex diffusion processes that adopt a constant time step (Δt) close to the time step limit of the convergence of the iterative update process, we opted for an adaptive time step (12). The rational behind this decision is based on the fact that the coefficient of diffusion depends on the gradient of the image (3) and, due to noise, this gradient is much higher in the initial steps of the diffusion process. Therefore we choose iteratively

$$\Delta t^{(n)} = \frac{1}{\alpha} \left[a + b \, e^{-\max(|\mathrm{Re}(\partial I^{(n)}/\partial t)/\mathrm{Re}(I^{(n)})|)} \right], \tag{12}$$

where $\left(\left|\mathrm{Re}\left(\partial I^{(n)}/\partial t\right)/\mathrm{Re}(I^{(n)})\right|\right)$ is the fraction of change of the image/volume at iteration n, α as in (7) and parameters a and b control the time step (with $a + b \leq 1$). The typical evolution of $\Delta t^{(n)}$ over the iterative process in 2D is shown in Fig. 4.

As expected, a small step size is used at the initial iterations in which higher values of D can be found due to the speckle noise. This is, at steady conditions in which changes over time are small (fraction-wise), the time step can be made larger, while at fast changes in time the time step can be made smaller.

2.4 Quality Metrics

For the quantitative evaluation of filters' performance, two quality metrics used in [23, 26] and [28] were applied. The metrics used are the mean squared error (MSE) and the edge preservation parameter (χ).

The MSE is given by:

$$\text{MSE} = \frac{1}{LJ} \sum_{l=1}^{L} \sum_{j=1}^{J} \left(I(l, j) - I_f(l, j) \right)^2, \tag{13}$$

where $I(l, j)$ denotes the original image, $I_f(l, j)$ denotes the filtered image, L and J are the number of pixels in row and column directions, respectively.

To evaluate the edge preservation we use the correlation coefficient χ (14) as in [26, 28], where ΔI and ΔI_f are the laplacian of the original and filtered image, respectively, and the $\Delta \bar{I}$ and $\Delta \bar{I}_f$ the respective mean values.

$$\chi = \frac{\sum_{(l,j)} \left(\Delta I - \Delta \bar{I} \right) \left(\Delta I_f - \Delta \bar{I}_f \right)}{\sqrt{\sum_{(l,j)} \left(\Delta I - \Delta \bar{I} \right) \left(\Delta I - \Delta \bar{I} \right) \sum_{(l,j)} \left(\Delta I_f - \Delta \bar{I}_f \right) \left(\Delta I_f - \Delta \bar{I}_f \right)}}. \tag{14}$$

In order to quantify the smoothness of homogeneous regions (H) the equivalent number of looks (ENL) is computed according to (15).

$$ENL = \frac{1}{H} \sum_{h=1}^{H} \frac{\mu_h^2}{\sigma_h^2}, \tag{15}$$

where μ_h and σ_h^2 are the mean and variance, respectively, of the regions H.

3 Results

In order to evaluate the performance of the filter herewith presented, eyes of 30 healthy volunteers and eyes of patients with age-related macular degeneration (20), diabetic retinopathy (23), cystoid macular edema (2) and choroidal neo-vascularization (13) underwent the high-definition spectral domain Cirrus OCT using both the 200 × 200 × 1,024 and the 512 × 128 × 1,024 Macular Cube protocols.

The volumetric scans were filtered using the here proposed 3D nonlinear complex diffusion filter (3D-NCDF), as well as using its 2D version [28], the Perona-Malik filter (PM) with the diffusion coefficient $d(|\nabla I|) = \exp(-(|\nabla I|/k)^2)$, where $k = 50$ [24], and the adaptive Lee filter with a window of 3 × 3 pixels [22].

The 2D-and 3D-NCDF filters were applied using $k = 10$ and $\theta = \pi/30$, as in [28]. The exact same diffusion time (2.4 s) was used which correspond to 10 and 20 iterations with a step in time of 0.24 and 0.124 s to the 2D and 3D traditional NCDF cases, respectively. For the improve adaptive version we considered the time step as in (12) with $a = 0.25$ and $b = 0.75$. However, to guarantee the stability of the method one needs to consider the stability condition $\Delta t \leq \cos\theta/6 \approx 0.1660$. As remarked in [2], it is advisable to consider more a conservative step in time than the maximum theoretical limit, so we allowed only a maximum step in time of 0.125.

To perform the quantitative measurement of the filter performance the MSE and the χ metrics were computed for each of the 88 volumetric scans. The results from the quantitative analysis are shown in Table 1.

The average computing time for each volume of $200 \times 200 \times 1,024$ voxels OCT data is of 97 min for the Lee filter, 2 min for the Perona-Malik (PM) (2D) filter, 3 min for the 2D-NCDF [28] filter and 11 min for the 3D-NCDF here proposed. The total diffusion time for PM, 2D-NCDF and the 3D filter is of 2.4 s.

These tests were performed using a 2.4 GHz Intel Core 2 Quad Q6600 CPU, 3 GB of RAM to run Matlab on the Ubuntu 10.04 operating system.

Figures 5–7 show the result of the application of the 2D-NCDF to a particular B-scan and the same B-scan after the respective 3D-NCDF filtered data. In Fig. 5 it is shown an healthy volunteer's retina example where is possible to note the good performance of the 3D-NCDF filter in reducing speckle while preserving retinal layers. Figures 6 and 7 show results from a CNV and an AMD cases, respectively. For easy of comparison a region is zoomed in and shown in insets using a pseudo-color (Fig. 7). Please note the good preservation and better visualization of a retinal membrane after the 3D-NCDF application and the increased homogeneity of the vitreous.

To quantify the filters performance in homogeneous areas, one B-scan of each volumetric data was selected and the ENL was computed on a vitreous region. The results are presented in Table 2.

Moreover, we also compared the 3D traditional NCDF with the improved version described in Sect. 2.3, which is illustrated in Fig. 8.

Performance metrics for the comparison of the traditional and improved 3D-NCDF were also performed for three subjects, as a proof-of-concept, for a short diffusion time of $T = 0.75$ s. We obtained a higher ENL for the improved method (ENL_{Impr}) in comparison with the traditional (ENL_{Trad}) one, both in high intensity areas as the nerve fiber layer and the retinal pigment epithelium ($ENL_{Impr} = 176.26 \pm 83.49$ and $ENL_{Trad} = 42.59 \pm 5.54$) and in low intensity areas as the vitreous ($ENL_{Impr} = 106.55 \pm 3.02$ and $ENL_{Trad} = 10.71 \pm 0.78$). This shows that in high intensity areas the improved method quadruplicates the smoothness (measured by the ENL), while for low intensity areas it becomes ten times smoother. As expected the improved method is more conservative in tissue regions (high intensities).

Table 1 Filter performance metrics (m $\pm$ SD)

Metric	Filter	Healthy (N=30)	Diseased eyes			
			AMD (N=20)	DR (N=23)	CNV (N=13)	CME (N=2)
MSE	Lee	129.38 ± 11.51	124.69 ± 9.65	125.15 ± 7.99	120.55 ± 4.64	129.53 ± 14.36
	PM	162.16 ± 13.12	156.23 ± 12.04	158.11 ± 12.04	153.08 ± 5.78	162.58 ± 16.16
	2D-NCDF	119.34 ± 7.35	116.71 ± 6.10	117.95 ± 5.05	115.23 ± 2.91	120.10 ± 8.64
	3D-NCDF	135.62 ± 8.00	132.59 ± 6.96	134.26 ± 5.72	136.40 ± 9.47	131.89 ± 3.69
χ	Lee	0.27 ± 0.00	0.26 ± 0.01	0.27 ± 0.01	0.28 ± 0.01	0.27 ± 0.01
	PM	0.24 ± 0.04	0.19 ± 0.03	0.19 ± 0.03	0.20 ± 0.02	0.20 ± 0.03
	2D-NCDF	0.61 ± 0.03	0.58 ± 0.04	0.57 ± 0.04	0.55 ± 0.01	0.59 ± 0.04
	3D-NCDF	0.70 ± 0.03	0.68 ± 0.03	0.67 ± 0.03	0.69 ± 0.03	0.66 ± 0.02

MSE mean square error, χ edge preservation metric, *PM* Perona-Malik, *NCDF* nonlinear complex diffusion filter, *AMD* age-related macular degeneration, *DR* diabetic retinopathy, *CME* cystoid macular edema, *CNV* choroidal neo-vascularization

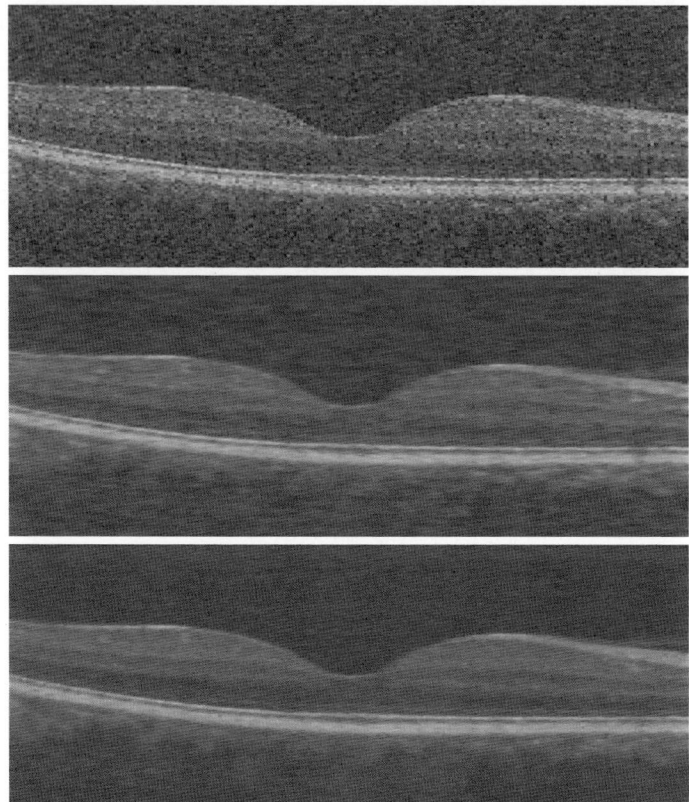

Fig. 5 Original B-scan (*top*) and the respective 2D-NCDF (*middle*) and 3D-NCDF (*bottom*) filtered versions of an healthy volunteer's retina

4   Conclusions

In the work herewith presented we propose to extend the application of a nonlinear complex diffusion filters from 2- to 3-dimensions and quantitatively and qualitatively demonstrate its advantages.

The natural drawback is the required computing time. On the other hand, we should note the increased edge preservation while simultaneously achieving much smoother areas as demonstrated by the χ and ENL parameters, respectively. Moreover the improved version of the NCDF shows better smoothing results than the traditional approach, taking the same roughly the same amount of computational time.

Additionally, the visual inspection allows to see the increased definition of the several retinal layers.

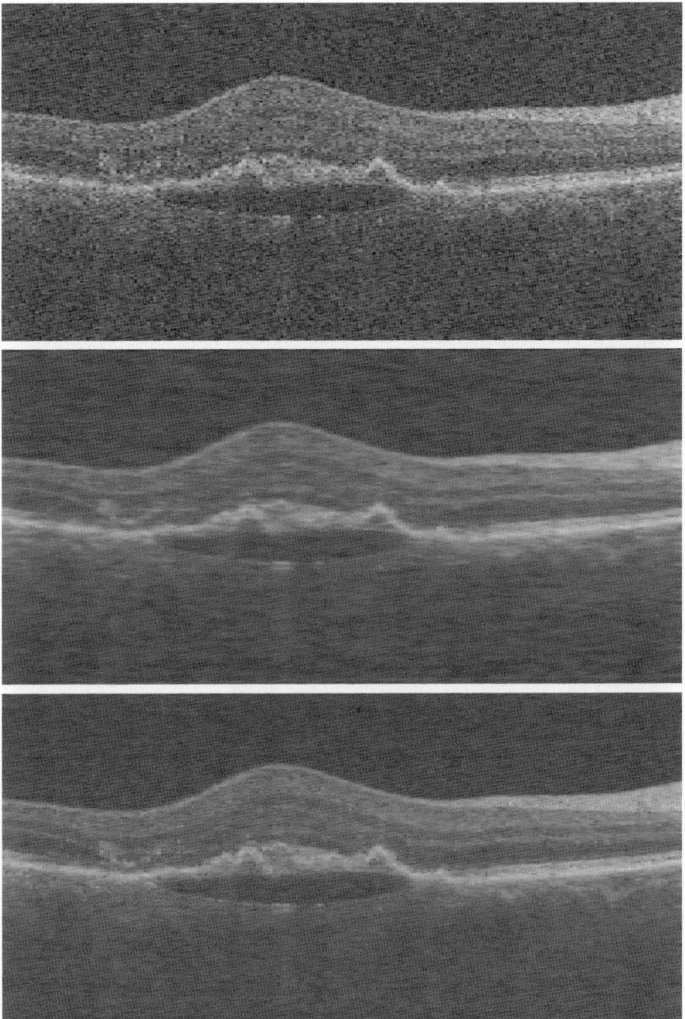

Fig. 6 Original B-scan (*top*) and the respective 2D-NCDF (*middle*) and 3D-NCDF (*bottom*) filtered versions of a CNV diseased eye

These facts allow us to speculate that the 3D filtering presented may represent an important preprocessing towards a better image segmentation process, both manually and by automatic algorithms.

Acknowledgements This study is supported in part by the *Fundação para a Ciência e a Tecnologia* (FCT) under the research project PTDC/SAU-BEB/103151/2008 and program COMPETE (FCOMP-01-0124-FEDER-010930). The authors would like to thanks Dr. Melissa Horne and Carl Zeiss Meditec (Dublic, CA, USA) for their support on getting access to OCT data and AIBILI Clinical Trial Center technicians for their support in managing data, working with patients and performing scans. This study is registered at ClinicalTrials.org (ID: NCT00797524).

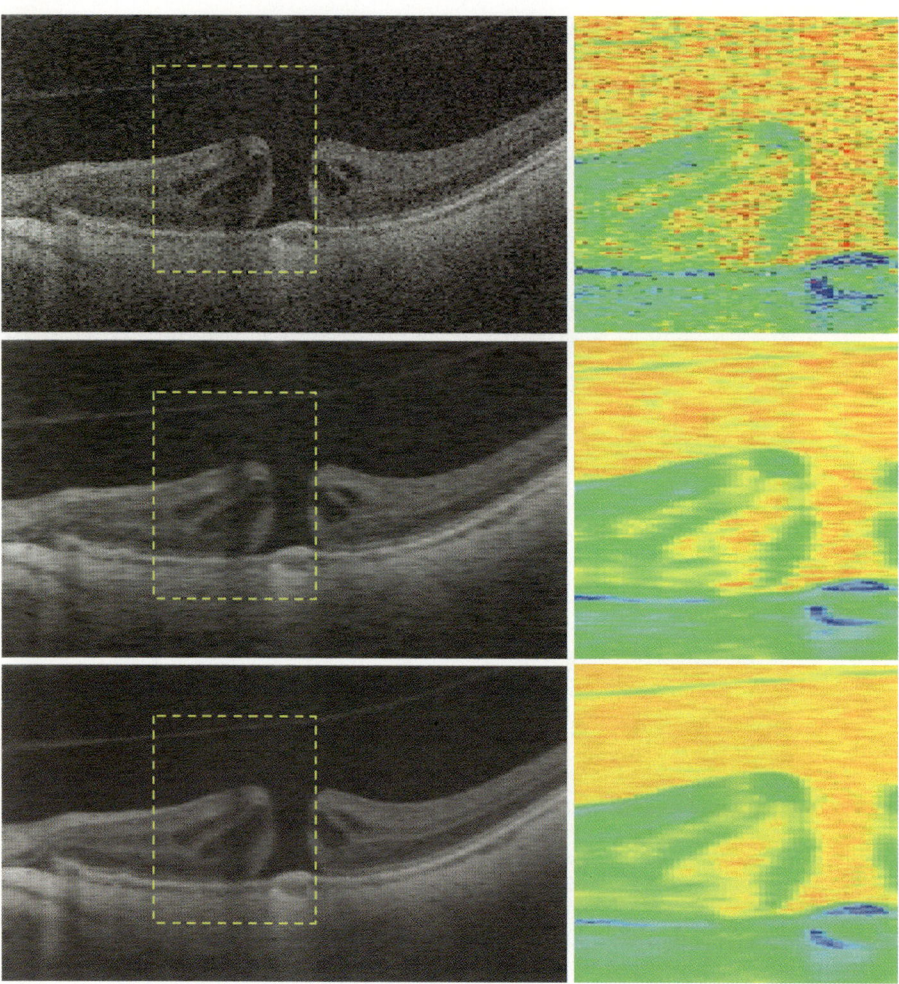

Fig. 7 An original B-scan (*top–left*). *Top–right* color-coded inset from the *dashed area* on the *left*. Filter results for the 2D-NCDF (*middle*) and the 3D-NCDF (*bottom*), with the corresponding color-coded insets on the *right*. All color-coded figures use the same color map and color limits for ease of comparison. Note the well-defined membrane in the vitreous region

Table 2 Equivalent number of looks (ENL) comparison for the original B-scans and the corresponding filters' results ($m \pm SD$)

Filter	Healthy (N=10)	Diseased eyes			
		AMD (N=10)	DR (N=10)	CNV (N=10)	CME (N=2)
Original	5.84 ± 0.77	5.57 ± 0.69	5.53 ± 0.83	5.60 ± 0.99	6.17 ± 0.41
Lee	18.39 ± 2.39	17.13 ± 1.53	16.70 ± 2.60	16.83 ± 4.69	19.25 ± 2.56
PM	71.28 ± 11.45	66.90 ± 10.41	61.45 ± 15.87	69.46 ± 25.73	75.33 ± 9.66
2D-NCDF	39.50 ± 5.79	37.57 ± 3.85	34.73 ± 7.58	37.06 ± 12.23	41.47 ± 5.69
3D-NCDF	111.03 ± 11.99	107.58 ± 8.91	102.74 ± 29.42	99.85 ± 33.54	112.67 ± 2.10

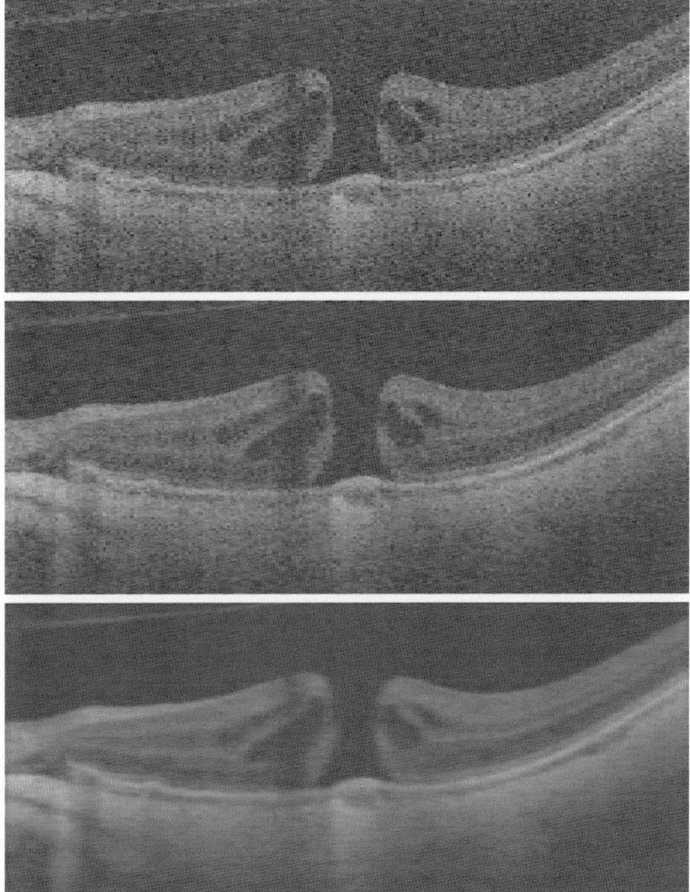

Fig. 8 Original B-scan (*top*) and the respective traditional 3D-NCDF (*middle*) and the improved 3D-NCDF (*bottom*) filtered versions with the same diffusion time of $T = 0.75$ s

References

1. Abbott J, Thurstone F (1979) Acoustic speckle: theory and experimental analysis. Ultrason Imaging 1:303–324
2. Araújo A, Barbeiro S, Serranho P (2010) Stability of finite difference schemes for complex diffusion processes. DMUC report, Estudo Geral, Universidade de Coimbra, pp 10–23
3. Bagci A, Shahidi M, Ansari R, Blair M, Blair N, Zelkha R (2008) Thickness profiles of retinal layers by optical coherence tomography image segmentation. Am J Ophthalmol 146(5): 679–687
4. Baroni M, Fortunato P, Torre AL (2007) Towards quantitative analysis of retinal features in optical coherence tomography. Med Eng Phys 29:432–441
5. Bashkansky M, Reintjes J (2000) Statistics and reduction of speckle in optical coherence tomography. Opt Lett 25(8):545–547

6. Bernardes R, Maduro C, Serranho P, Araújo A, Barbeiro S, Cunha-Vaz J (2010) Improved adaptive complex diffusion despeckling filter. Opt Express 18(23):24,048–24,059. http://www.opticsexpress.org/abstract.cfm?URI=oe-18-23-24048

7. Bernstein R (1987) Adaptive nonlinear filters for simultaneous removal of different kinds of noise in images. IEEE Trans Circuit Syst 34(11):1275–1291

8. Burckhardt C (1978) Speckle in ultrasound b-mode scans. IEEE Trans Sonic Ultrason 25(1): 1–6

9. Drexler W, Morgner U, Ghanta R, Kärtner F, Schuman J, Fujimoto J (2001) Ultrahigh-resolution ophthalmic optical coherence tomography. Nat Med 7(4):502–507

10. Fercher A (2008) Optical coherence tomography: technology and applications, illustrated edn., Chap. 4. Springer, New York, pp 119–146

11. Fernández D, Salinas H, Puliafito C (2005) Automated detection of retinal layer structures on optical coherence tomography images. Opt Express 13(25):10,200–10,216

12. Franceschetti G, Pascazio V, Schirinzi G (1995) Iterative homomorphic technique for speckle reduction in synthetic-aperture radar imaging. J Opt Soc Am A 12(4):686–694

13. Gilboa G, Sochen N, Zeevi Y (2004) Image enhancement and denoising by complex diffusion processes. IEEE Trans Pattern Anal Mach Intell 26(8):1020–1036

14. Goodman J (1976) Some fundamental properties of speckle. J Opt Soc Am 66(11):1145–1150

15. Healey A, Leeman S, Forsberg F (1992) Turning off speckle. Acoust Imaging 19:433–437

16. Iftimia N, Bouma B, Tearney G (2003) Speckle reduction in optical coherence tomography by "path length encoded" angular compounding. J Biomed Opt 8(2):260–263. doi:10.1117/1.1559060

17. Ishikawa H, Stein D, Wollstein G, Beaton S, Fujimoto J, Schuman J (2005) Macular segmentation with optical coherence tomography. Invest Ophthalmol Vis Sci 46(6):2012–2017

18. Kim J, Miller D, Kim E, Oh S, Oh J, Milner T (2005) Optical coherence tomography speckle reduction by a partially spatially coherent source. J Biomed Opt 10(6):064034. doi:10.1117/1.2138031

19. Koozekanani D, Boyer K, Roberts C (2000) Retinal thickness measurements in optical coherence tomography using a markov boundary model. In: Proceedings of IEEE computer society conference on computer vision and pattern recognition (CVPR), vol. 2. Hilton Head Island

20. Kuan D, Sawchuk A, Strand T, Chavel P (1985) Adaptive noise smoothing filter for images with signal-dependent noise. IEEE Trans Pattern Anal Mach Intell 7(2):165–177

21. Kuwahara M, Hachimura K, Eiho S, Kinoshita M (1976) Processing of riangiocardiographic images. In: Preston K, Onoe M (eds) Digital processing of biomedical images. Plenum Publishing, New York, pp 187–203

22. Lee J (1981) Speckle analysis and smoothing of synthetic aperture radar images. Comput Graph Image Process 17(1):24–32

23. Ozcan A, Bilenca A, Desjardins A, Bouma B, Tearney G (2007) Speckle reduction in optical coherence tomography images using digital filtering. J Opt Soc Am A 24(7):1901–1910

24. Perona P, Malik J (1990) Scale-space and edge detection using anisotropic diffusion. IEEE Trans Pattern Anal Mach Intell 12(7):629–639. http://dx.doi.org/10.1109/34.56205

25. Pircher M, Gotzinger E, Leitgeb R, Fercher A, Hitzenberger C (2003) Speckle reduction in optical coherence tomography by frequency compounding. J Biomed Opt 8(3):565–569. doi:10.1117/1.1578087

26. Puvanathasan P, Bizheva K (2007) Speckle noise reduction algorithm for optical coherence tomography based on interval type ii fuzzy set. Opt Express 15(24):15,747–15,758

27. Rogowska J, Brezinski M (2000) Evaluation of the adaptive speckle suppression filter for coronary optical coherence tomography imaging. IEEE Trans Med Imaging 19(12):1261–1266

28. Salinas H, Fernández D (2007) Comparison of pde-based nonlinear diffusion approaches for image enhancement and denoising in optical coherence tomography. IEEE Trans Med Imaging 26(6):761–771. doi:10.1109/TMI.2006.887375

29. Schmitt J (1997) Array detection for speckle reduction in optical coherence microscopy. Phys Med Biol 42(7):1427–1439

30. Schmitt J (1998) Restoration of optical coherence images of living tissue using the clean algorithm. J Biomed Opt 3(1):66–75. doi:10.1117/1.429863
31. Schmitt J, Xiang S, Yung K (1999) Speckle in optical coherence tomography. J Biomed Opt 4(1):95–105. doi:10.1117/1.429925
32. Shahidi M, Wang Z, Zelkha R (2005) Quantitative thickness measurement of retinal layers imaged by optical coherence tomography. Am J Ophthalmol 139(6):1056–1061
33. Shankar P, Newhouse V (1985) Speckle reduction with improved resolution in ultrasound images. IEEE Trans Sonic Ultrason 32(4):537–543
34. Tan O, Li G, Lu A, Varma R, Huang D (2008) Mapping of macular substructures with optical coherence tomography for glaucoma diagnosis. Ophthalmol 115(6):949–956. doi:10.1016/j.ophtha.2007.08.011
35. Wagner R, Smith S, Sandrik J, Lopez H (1983) Statistics of speckle in ultrasound b-scans. IEEE Trans Sonic Ultrason 30(3):156–163
36. Weickert J (1997) A review of nonlinear diffusion filtering. In: Proceedings of the first international conference on scale-space theory in computer vision, Springer, London, pp 3–28
37. Xiang S, Zhou L, Schmitt J (1998) Speckle noise reduction for optical coherence tomography. Opt Imaging Tech Biomonit III Proc SPIE 3196(1):79–88. doi:10.1117/12.297921
38. Yung K, Lee S, Schmitt J (1999) Phase-domain processing of optical coherence tomography images. J Biomed Opt 4(1):125–136. doi:10.1117/1.429942

Using an Infra-red Sensor to Measure the Dynamic Behaviour of N$_2$O Gas Escaping Through Different Sized Holes

Alan Slade, Jan Vorstius, Daniel Gonçalves, and Gareth Thomson

Abstract An anastomosis is a surgical procedure that consists of the re-connection of two parts of an organ and is commonly required in cases of colorectal cancer. Approximately 80% of the patients diagnosed with this problem require surgery. The malignant tissue located on the gastrointestinal track must be resected and the most common procedure adopted is the anastomosis. Studies made with 2,980 patients that had this procedure, show that the leakage through the anastomosis was 5.1%. This paper discusses the dynamic behavior of N$_2$O gas through different sized leakages as detected by an Infra-Red gas sensor and how the sensors response time changes depending on the leakage size. Different sized holes were made in the rigid tube to simulate an anastomostic leakage. N$_2$O gas was injected into the tube through a pipe and the leakage rate measured by the infra-red gas sensor. Tests were also made experimentally also using a CFD (Computational Fluid Dynamics) package called FloWorks. The results will be compared and discussed in this paper.

1 Introduction

An anastomosis is a surgical procedure that consists of the re-connection of two parts of an organ, and is commonly required in cases of colorectal cancer. Approximately 80% of the patients diagnosed with colorectal cancer require surgery [1]. The malignant tissue located on the gastrointestinal track must be resected and the most common procedure adopted is the anastomosis [2]. Unfortunately,

A. Slade (✉) • J. Vorstius • D. Gonçalves
Medical Engineering Research Institute, University of Dundee, Dundee DD1 4HN, UK
e-mail: A.P.Slade@dunde.ac.uk; J.B.Vorstius@dundee.ac.uk; danielsg007@yahoo.com.br

G. Thomson
School of Engineering and Applied Science, Aston University, Aston Triangle,
Birmingham B4 7ET, UK
e-mail: G.A.Thomson@aston.ac.uk

R.M.N. Jorge et al. (eds.), *Technologies for Medical Sciences*, Lecture Notes
in Computational Vision and Biomechanics 1, DOI 10.1007/978-94-007-4068-6_8,
© Springer Science+Business Media B.V. 2012

this procedure is not 100% effective. Studies made with 2,980 patients that has this procedure, show that the leakage through the anastomosis was 5.1% [3]. A gastroesophageal anastomotic leak after cancer resection, for example, has a mortality rate of up to 60% and significant morbidity, no matter what type of treatment is applied after it [4]. A perfect anastomosis depends to a high degree on the surgeon's skill [5], whereas some robot-assisted surgeries, as they do not need direct contact between patient and surgeon, are shown to be more accurate [6]. Therefore, an anastomotic leak has the potential of representing a problem for surgeons [7] and will increase the duration of hospital stay, which is associated with remedial treatment and recovery, causing, as a result, a negative financial impact [2, 8].

Normally leakages can be identified during surgery just after the surgeon finishes the construction of the anastomosis. A number of research techniques to detect, treat, and even prevent an anastomotic leakage are under investigation. However, studies show that these techniques are not always able to prevent an anastomotic leak from occurring [2]. Applying saline through the rectum is a technique widely discussed in previous studies. Gilbert and Trapnell [9] developed this technique and reported it in 1988 in the Annals of the Royal College of Surgeons. However, despite the fact that this technique demonstrated simplicity in its execution, further studies showed that it is not 100% guaranteed that there will be no occurrence of an anastomotic leakage in the future. Instead of applying saline there is also a method that applies air through the rectum. This technique is widely known as "The bubble test". This test is performed by filling the pelvis with saline and the next step is to insufflate air through the rectum. If air bubbles appear, that is an indication that the anastomosis is compromised and further strengthening is required. It was concluded that an air-tight anastomosis is unlikely to leak, but it was recognized that the test is not 100% reliable.

An alternative approach to the problem is presented in this paper and uses a gas sensor and a trace gas to evaluate the leakage rate through the anastomosis. This paper discusses the dynamic behavior of N_2O gas through different sized leakages as detected by an Infra-Red gas sensor and how the sensors response time changes depending on the leakage size. Tests were made experimentally and also using a Computational Fluid Dynamics (CFD) package called FloWorks. The results will be compared and discussed in this paper.

2   The SUSIE Method

The problem with previous techniques is that it was not possible to estimate or calculate the maximum pressure that can be applied safely to the bowel. By distending the bowel by increasing the pressure in the area of the anastomosis might bring about a leakage of bowel faecal contents into the cavity of the abdomen. An alternative method to previous research is discussed in this paper which, instead of using a distension system approach, works by using a sensing system through the colon anastomic join. This new approach presents a safer and more accurate method of detecting leakage as it does not rely on distending the colon wall and thereby having the potential of tearing the suturing, thus creating a leak which might not otherwise have occurred. It uses a gas sensor and a small quantity of trace gas to evaluate leakage through the anastomosis.

The selection of the trace gas and associated sensor required careful study as most gas sensors are usually made to detect dangerous gases, for example there are several sensors readily available to detect poisonous or flammable gases, such as hydrogen sulphide, ammonia, hydrogen and hydrocarbons. However, only a few are built for gases such as helium and nitrous oxide which are classified as safe gases. A problem with helium is that as a noble gas, it is very difficult to detect, as noble gases react to very little. Gases such as carbon dioxide and nitrous oxide are already used in surgical procedures. Carbon dioxide is used to inflate the abdominal cavity during laparoscopic surgery, and that would make any leakage difficult to detect, while nitrous oxide is used in anesthesia, making this gas more suitable for this study. There are two types of sensor available for detecting nitrous oxide: electrochemical or optical. Because a quick and accurate response from the sensor is necessary, optical sensors are better suited to this application than electrochemical sensors.

The procedure starts when the surgeon is about to finish stapling or suturing the colon after a cancer resection or any other surgery that will require an anastomosis at the end. A small opening would be left in the suturing by the surgeon in order to insert a gelatine based, pharmaceutical capsule, into the colon, Fig. 1. Clamps, which are already part of the standard procedure as they are used by the surgeons to manipulate the organs involved, would be used on either side of the join to isolate the area, the capsule placed in the colon and the opening would then be closed.

In order to let the gas in the capsule escape from the capsule, the surgeons will have two choices. The first of them is to wait about 2 min so that the capsule can dissolve and the gas be released. This time can be increased or decreased by altering the thickness of the wall of the gelatine capsule. The other technique would be to compress the colon in the area where the capsule is located, crashing it and releasing the gas, but taking care to not squeeze the anastomosis area, otherwise its integrity could be compromised. Then, after the gas is released, any quantity of it that passes through the anastomosis, indicating a leak, will be detected by the sensing system located outside the colon around the anastomosis.

For laparoscopic procedures, a sensor pipe would be introduced into the abdominal lumen through one of the instrument ports. The abdomen would act then as a sample volume where the gas would effuse. For an open surgery procedure it is envisaged that the sensing system would be a ring with a controlled volume in order to sample any leaking gas, Fig. 1, this would be fitted around the anastomosis and connected to pipes that would act as a link between this sample volume and a gas sensor situated outside the abdominal lumen. If any gas escapes from the colon through the anastomosis, the sensor would then detect it.

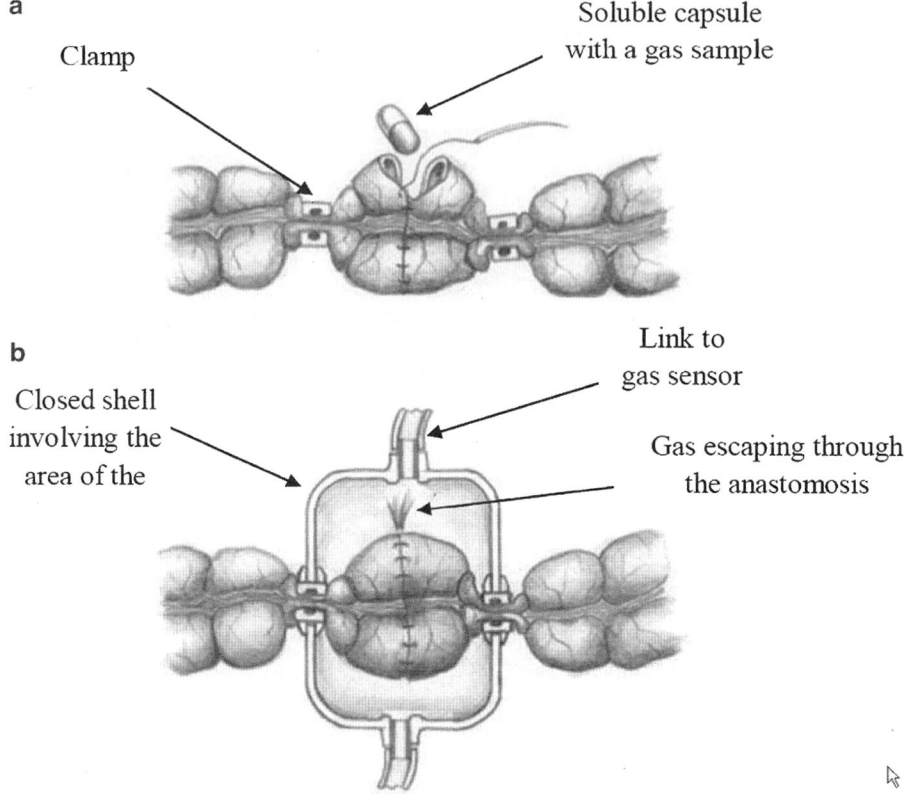

a

Clamp

Soluble capsule
with a gas sample

b

Closed shell
involving the
area of the

Link to
gas sensor

Gas escaping through
the anastomosis

Fig. 1 Proposed colon leak detection system for open surgeries

3   Materials and Methods

For the experimental a box with dimensions of 115 × 115 × 57 mm was used to simulate the interior part of the abdomen. The colon was represented by a sealed rigid pipe placed inside the box. A flexible tube from the box goes to the inlet of the N_2O infra-red sensor and gas is pulled through the sensor by a pump with a flow rate of 1 L/min. An injection pipe goes through the box into the rigid tube to allow gas to be injected into the rigid pipe. The nature of the experimental procedure meant that the methods for releasing the trace gas such as dissolving the gelatine capsule or crushing it through a bowel compression, were not possible. Instead a capsule was placed within a syringe and by compressing the syringe the capsule would be fractured and the released gas would then be injected, via the flexible tube into the rigid pipe (Fig. 2).

To simulate a diversity of anastomotic leak conditions, a series of rigid tubes were produced with holes varying from 1 to 3 mm drilled in them to simulate

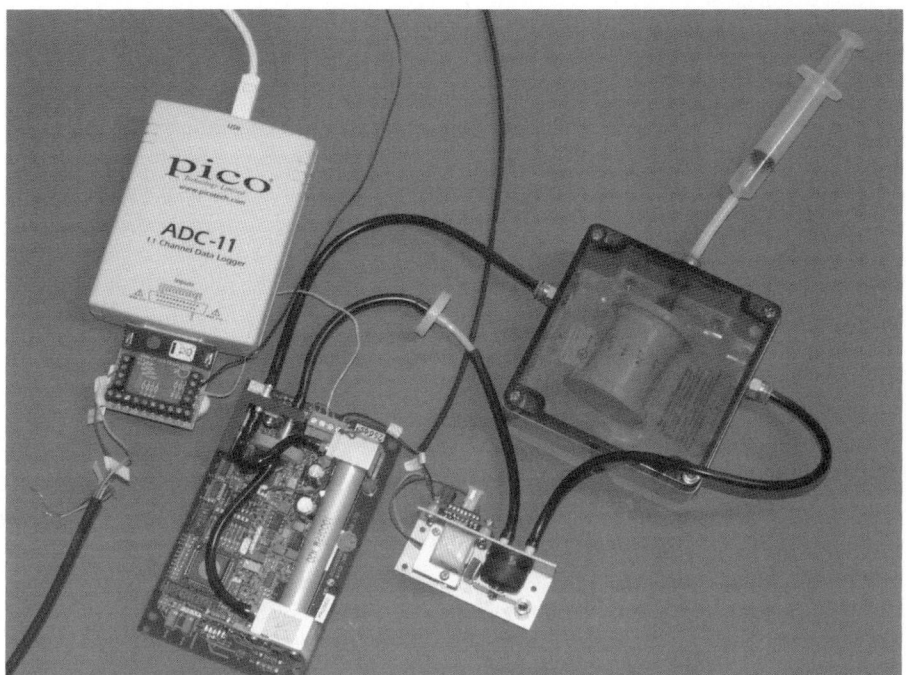

Fig. 2 The experimental apparatus

a leakage. A 0.68 ml gelatine capsule was filled with N_2O gas at a pressure of 2 bar, and placed into a syringe and this was compressed to release the trace gas into the system. The pump was then activated, draining samples of the gas from the abdominal lumen analogue box and transporting it into the gas sensor. Sampling of the gas continued for up to 5 min following initial release of the gas. For each of the tubes the experiment was repeated a number of times and the average values recorded. In order to acquire all the data from the experiments a Pico Data logger system was used. The output signals from the data logger were then converted to ppm (concentration of gas in parts per million) in order to measure the increase of N_2O gas over the time sample for each experiment.

A closed system was used in all experiments, with the gas which was sampled subsequently being returned via another flexible pipe into the abdominal lumen analogue box. With a fixed volume of air in the system at the start of the tests and a fixed quantity of trace gas injected, the aim with a closed system was to check whether a common gas concentration equilibrium would be achieved given enough time, say 2–3 min, regardless of the leak hole size or position used. In a practical clinical setting such a closed system would not be used and instead it is more likely that the inlet vent to the system would be drawn from either the surrounding environment or a supply of medical grade CO_2.

4 Open Surgery Experiments

A second set of experiments were carried out to simulate an open surgical procedure using a sensing ring around the tube. This simulates a closed shell as it is envisaged would be used and is shown in Fig. 3. This model was first created in Solid Works and then built with on rapid prototype machine. It contains one outlet for the N_2O sensor and one inlet for air. The hole made just below the sensor inlet was used to separate the groove in the centre of the ring in two parts, and to create a "directional flow" between this groove and the tube that goes into the testing ring. The separator was introduced to make the air flow in a clockwise direction around the ring pushing the gas in the direction of the sensor outlet and would help to avoid a vacuum in the experiment.

Referring to Figs. 4 and 5, the N_2O gas is injected through the injection tube into the rigid pipe and it would escape through one of the leak holes indicated by the small red circles, shown in Fig. 4 and marked with an angle in order to identify the location of the leak. The gas then circulates in the groove between the testing ring and the colon, and exits through the pipe to the N_2O sensor inlet shown in Fig. 5. It then, passes through the pump, reaches the sensor, which reads the amount in ppm increase over the time of the gas and transmits the information to the computer through the Pico system. The gas is then pumped into the testing ring again through the outlet of the N_2O sensor.

However, some issues were found during the testing phase. One of them was that there was a leakage between the groove and the pipe probably caused by the separator, which was a piece of rubber from an O-Ring, or by an imperfect attachment of the colon analogue into the testing ring leaving it slightly loose

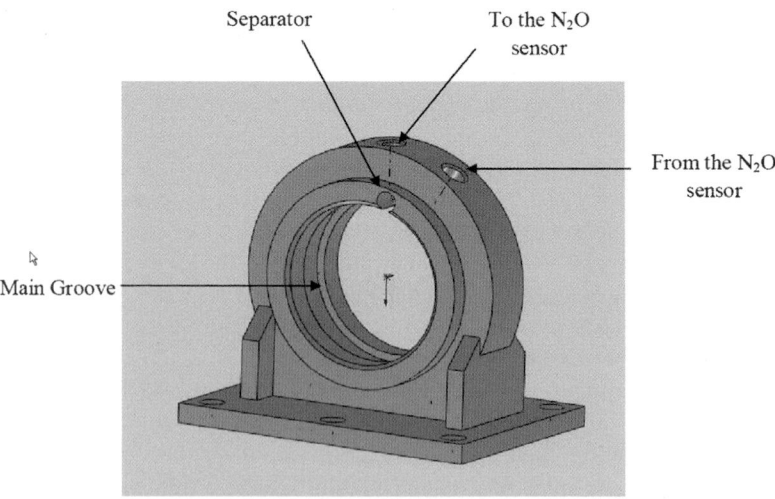

Fig. 3 CAD model of testing ring for one sensor

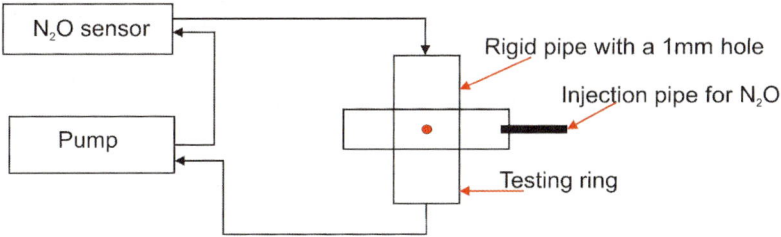

Fig. 4 Arrangement for the experiments using the first model of testing ring

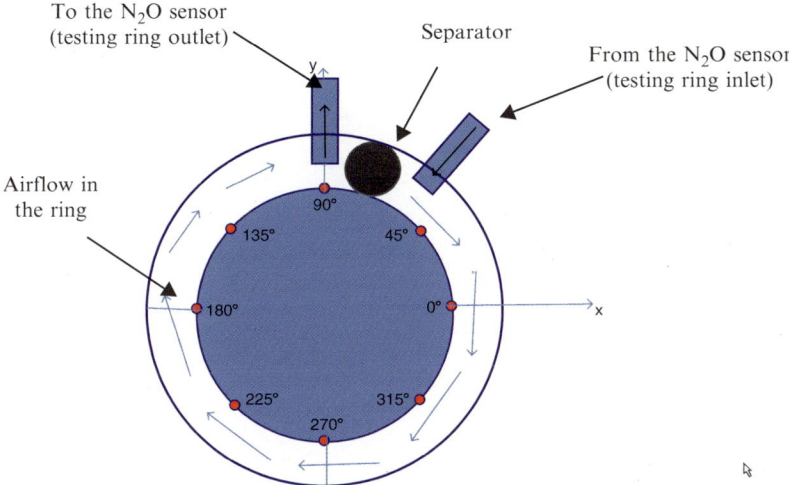

Fig. 5 Front view of the testing ring and orientation used to locate the leak holes

and therefore difficult to maintain the same location for the leak hole for further experiments. The other issue was the correct detection of the leakage spot in order to acquire accurate results. For example, using the reference angles shown in Fig. 5, the values for the ppm curves for different angles should be different for the same interval of time. This is because the further the leakage hole is from the sensor, it will take longer to detect the gas, resulting in different response times.

When the results are compared for the angles of 0° and 90°, it can be seen from Fig. 6 that the green curve (the different colours only represent different experiments for a leakage positioned at the same angle) for the 0° plot is similar to the blue curve for the 90° one. The red curves for both tests look similar, giving a final a concentration close to 500 ppm. A possible reason for these results was that the separator was not blocking the path in the groove properly. The gas was passing through it and going straight to the sensor giving to the 0° position higher readings for the gas concentration.

The same outcome is seen for the comparison between the angles of 180° and 270°. The green and blue curves of ppm increase for the plot of 180° gives a final

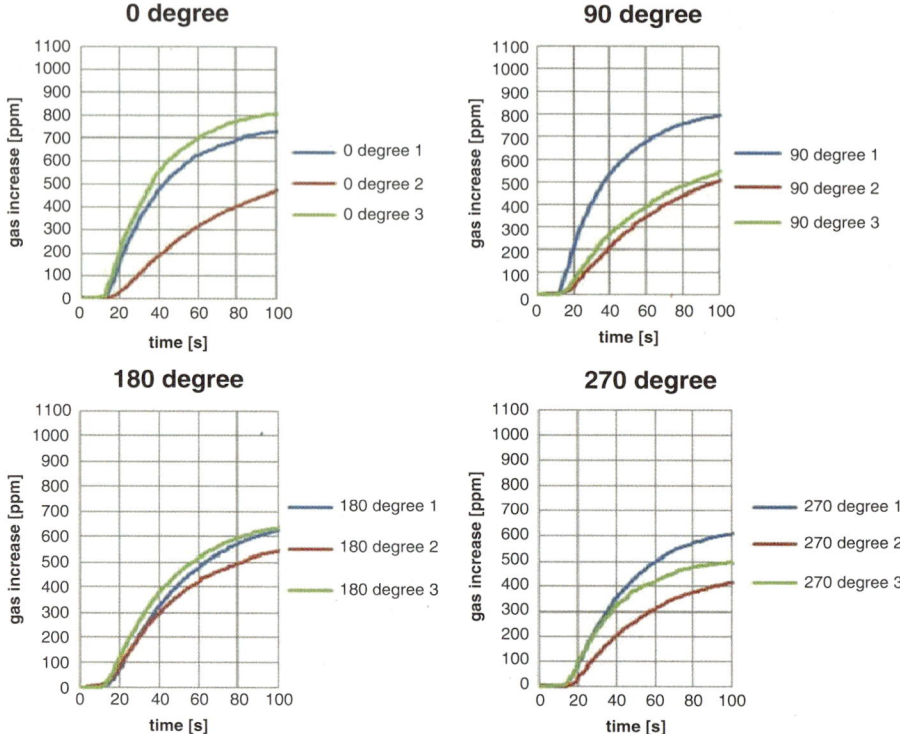

Fig. 6 An effect of the inaccurate positioning of the leak hole and the bad sealing is shown by the high variation of the results

result of 640 ppm close to the result for the blue curve in the 270° plot, 620 ppm whilst they should be giving higher reading of gas concentration than the 0° position because they are closer to the testing ring outlet. Again, a plausible reason is the irregular sealing of the system occasioning these readings of ppm increase over the time.

Because of these problems it became obvious that the testing ring needed to be modified. The first idea was to find a different way of blocking the path in the groove, but no successful design could be found. Then, the idea of modelling another testing ring using two sensors was investigated. Using two sensors would eliminate the need for a separator and also enhance the accuracy of the detection of the leakage spot. This second prototype of testing ring was modelled in Solid Works and then rapid prototyped as before. The second model is shown in Fig. 7.

The small holes around the circumference of the sensing ring are used to fix it to the stand to avoid any changes in its position while the rigid tube is inserted into it. They are also used as a reference for the different angles of rotation. These holes are at 10° intervals to allow for repeatable repositioning of the sensor ring with respect to the "colon".

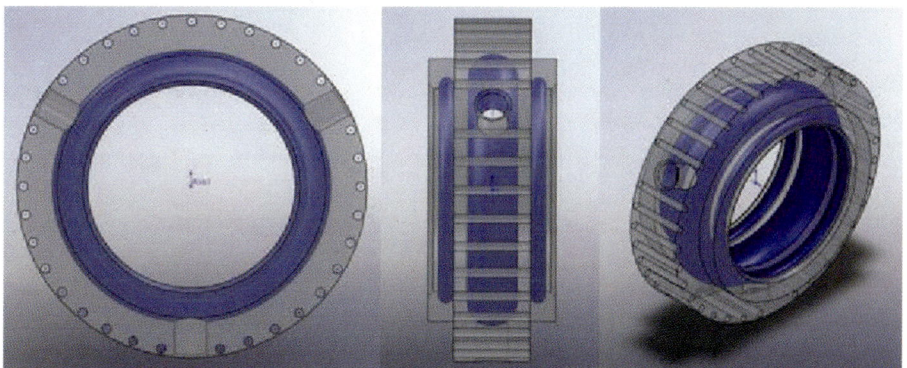

Fig. 7 Model for the second sensing ring built using Solid Works

The bigger holes on the outside of the ring are 120° away from each other. These holes are used to connect two N_2O sensors and an air inlet to avoid creating a vacuum in the system. Also, the main groove, coloured in blue, is bigger and now round in section, instead of rectangular, as in the first model. This new format of groove increases the volume were the gas will be circulating. On each side of it there is a smaller and thinner groove where 'O' Rings can be fitted to seal the device, in case there is a need to perform experiments with a completely sealed environment.

With the sensors connections placed 120° apart it does not matter which connector is attached to which hole as the relative angle between them will be maintained. This would make the device much easier to use in a surgical situation and also makes it easier to develop a control/recording measuring system.

The two thinner outer grooves in the testing ring were considered inappropriate for further measurements due to the fact that, in the real situation there will always be some gaps between the ring device and the real colon. This is because the colon is a flexible surface, making it very difficult for a perfect attachment with a rigid surface. In order words, it would be very difficult to avoid any leakage between the device and colon during an actual surgical procedure. Therefore, a third model of testing ring was created and a change was also made to the colon analogue. Figure 8 shows the third design in Solid Works (Fig. 9).

The other change with this sensor ring is that the locating holes are now at 45° intervals. This corresponds to the angles that it was decided should be studied. Because the O-rings helped locate the "colon" centrally in the sensor ring, changes were also made to the tube to ensure that the tube was centrally located. Some small pads were fitted around the tube with gaps between them. The reason for the gaps is due to the fact that in real life the sensing ring would not be perfectly attached to the colon, and there would be always a certain amount of leakage between both (Fig. 10).

Lastly and one of the most important changes, was the introduction of two flow control valves in the sensing inlet pipes. They are used to balance the volume of gas

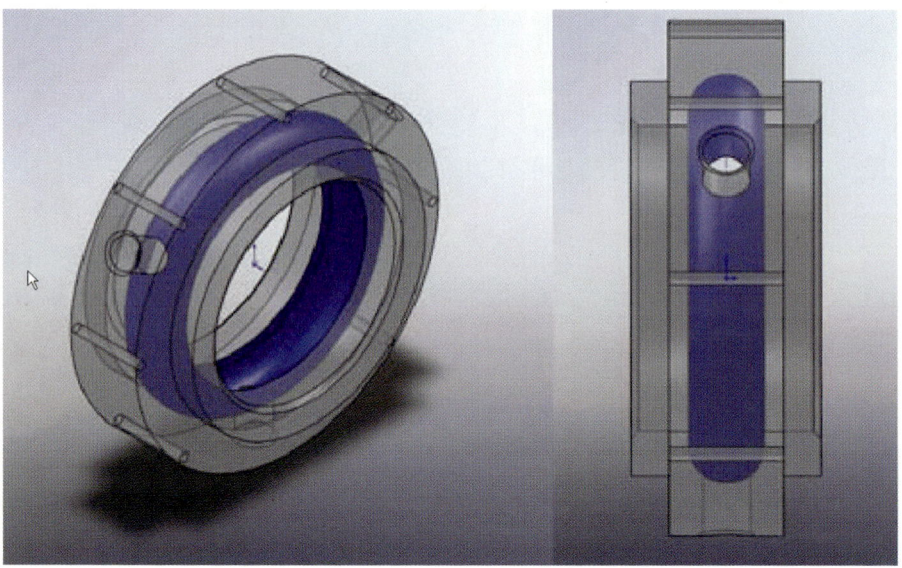

Fig. 8 Final model for the testing ring represented in Solid Works

Fig. 9 Front view of the testing ring showing the possible leakage spots and the arrangement for the inlets

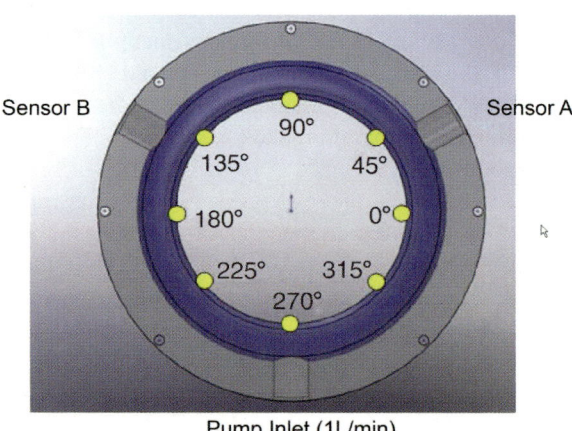

that goes into the inlets of both sensors. Without them, one sensor could be pulling more gas through it than the other one, which could result in an incorrect detection of the leakage spot (Fig. 11).

The sensing ring features two sensing outlets and a balancing inlet connected to a pump. Flows from the sensing outlets pass through control valves to ensure equality of flow rate to each sensing branch. The test arrangement was such that the colon analogue and its leak hole could be rotated relative to the sensing ring. By measuring the relative response of the two sensors in relation to the different hole positions it was hoped that not only could the presence of a leak be detected but an indication of its position around the colon could be estimated.

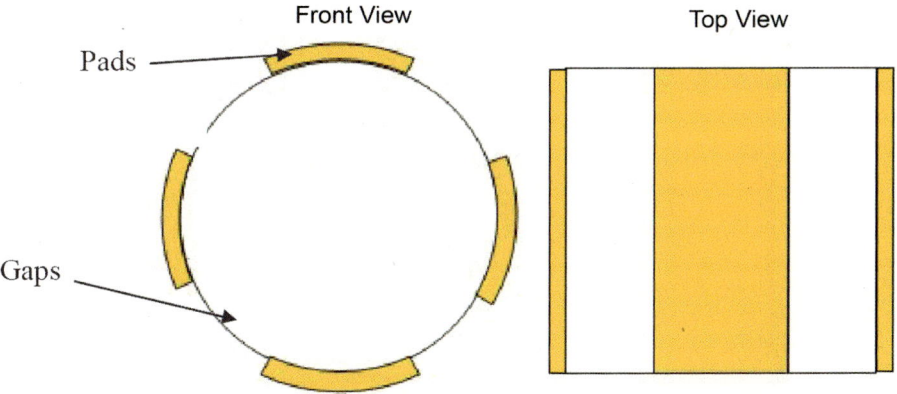

Fig. 10 The addition of a cushion on the colon analogue, in order to fix it in the testing ring

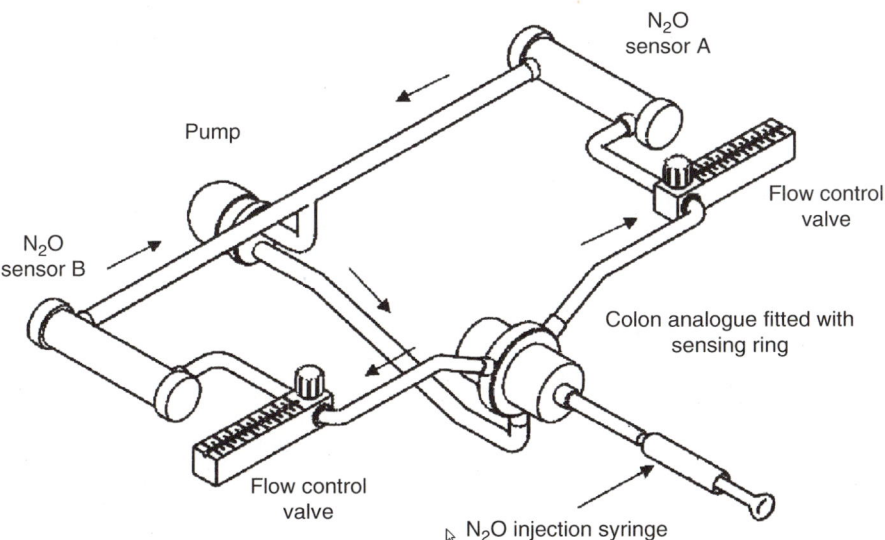

Fig. 11 The new arrangement showing the changes that were implemented and discussed in the text

After these changes, further experiments were undertaken, Fig. 12 shows plots with the results for the positions of 0°, 90°, 180° and 270°, which previously were difficult to separate from the collected data.

From these two plots, it can be seen that the values for the gas concentration [ppm] increase over the time became lower compared to the previous tests. This is because the volume of the groove and the total volume of the sensor ring has increased. As can be seen from the graphs there is also a marked difference in the two curves, which means that now it is possible to differentiate between the two locations.

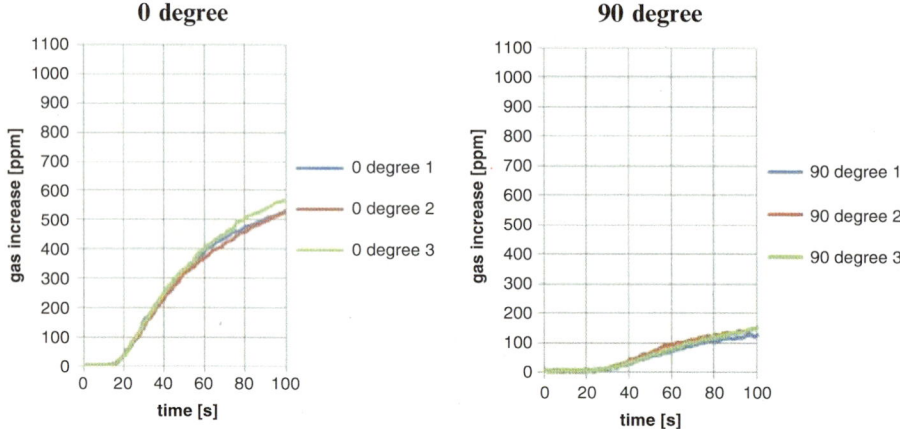

Fig. 12 Comparison between the plots of 0° and 90° with the hew test arrangement

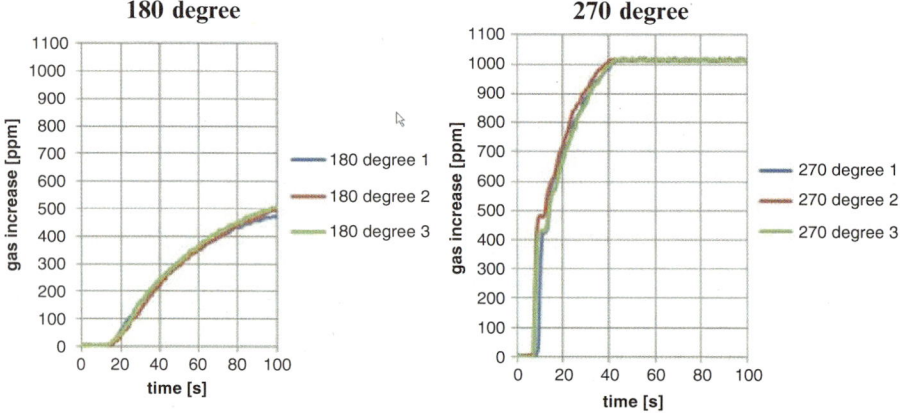

Fig. 13 Comparison between the plots of 180° and 270° with the new test arrangement

From Fig. 13, it can be seen that the results have also changed considerably when compared to the previous ones. Now there is a big difference between the curves of 180° and 270° (Fig. 13).

Figure 14 shows a new reference system that was adopted in order to create an easier and simpler code for a proposed measuring/recording programme that would be used to indicate the possible position and probable size of leak in the "colon". It maintains the same previous functions for each inlet and outlet presented in the testing ring, but with a difference in the angles. Instead of counting from 0° to 270°, it will be divided in positive side and negative side, going from 0° to +180° and from 0° to −180°.

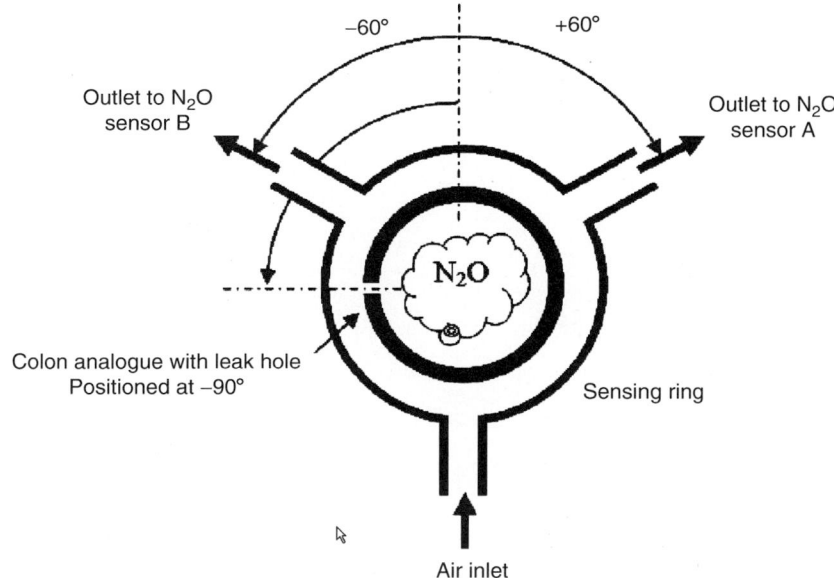

Fig. 14 Sensing ring and colon analogue details showing the relative positions of the leak and the sensing system inlets and outlets

5　Computer Simulation

For the computational analysis, Solid Works was used to generate a model of the actual physical experiment. To detect a ppm increase over the time FloWorks (included in Solid Works) was used. FloWorks uses conservation laws (Navier–Stokes equations). To replicate the same conditions presented as used in the experimental tests, the same conditions as used in the actual experiments were used. Because pumps are not included in the software toolbox the pump used was represented by a fan with a volume flow rate of 1 l/min. This fan will pump out the same amount of gas that was used in the experimental arrange from the test box. The box is filled with air at atmospheric pressure, 101,325 Pa, at a temperature of 293.2 K. The CAD model used for the computer simulations is shown in Fig. 15.

Analyses were performed for three different sized holes (1, 2 and 3 mm) on the pipe's top position for both physical and computational experiments as shown in Figs. 13 and 14 respectively. An average of results from the physical experiments for each size of hole was compared to its computer simulation and are shown in the figures below. For all the computational experiments the injection of N_2O gas started after 5 s.

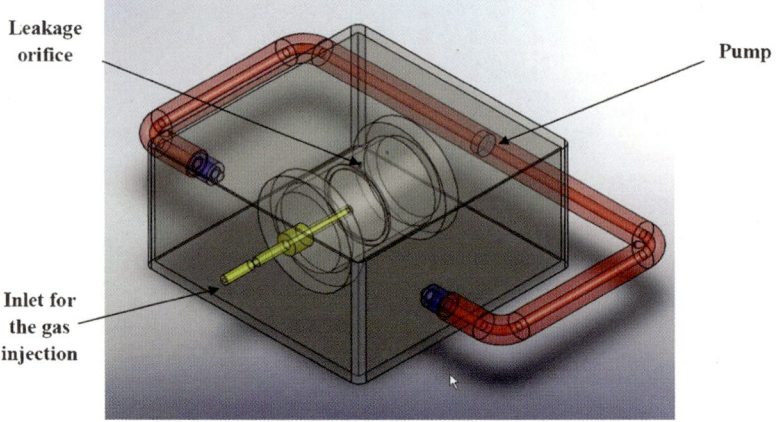

Fig. 15 Computer model used for the CFD analysis

5.1 Case 1: a 1 mm Hole

The analysis of the response time took in consideration the time that each curve would take to start increasing in a constant angle. Figure 16 shows that the physical experiment takes 5 s more to start increasing than the computational one. At the beginning of the experiment the curves would differ by around 12% and after 180 s the values are differing by around 4%. There is a similarity between the slopes of the curves for the first 55 s but after this period there is considerable variation in the curve up to approximately 140 s. Simulations with different meshes and step times were performed to identify the reason for this result, but all of them would show a similar behaviour very close to this same interval. One of the possible explanations for this result is that the simulation in FloWorks does not appear to break up the period of simulation evenly [10]. It appears that FloWorks uses different step sizes for the iterations to calculate the results, and as these step sizes cannot be fixed, this was leading to the unexpected results.

5.2 Case 2: a 2 mm Hole

The response time in this case is faster than case 1 for the physical experiment due to the fact that the area of the hole now is bigger allowing more gas to exit the hole in a shorter time. Figure 17 shows a similar behaviour to that of the previous experiment. Again simulations with different meshes and step times were performed to see if any changes would result, but all of them would show a similar behaviour very close to this same interval (Fig. 18).

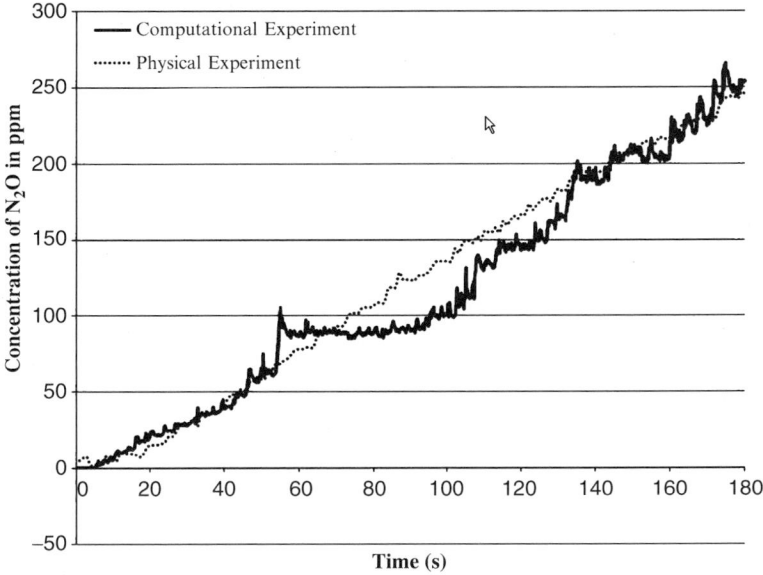

Fig. 16 Comparison of results for a leakage through a 1 mm hole

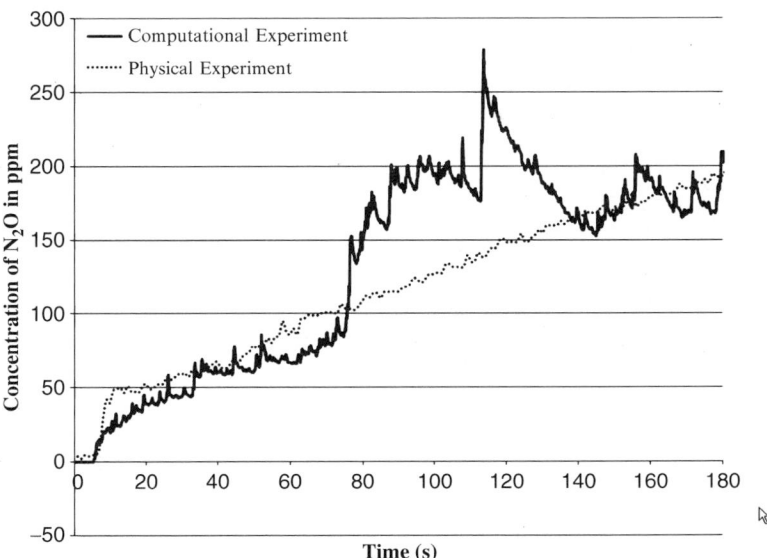

Fig. 17 Comparison of results for a leakage through a 2 mm hole

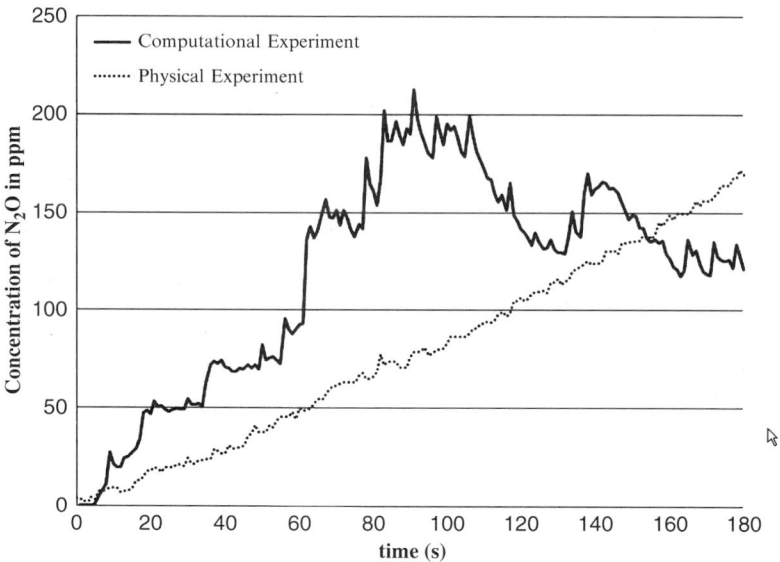

Fig. 18 Comparison of results for a leakage through a 3 mm hole

5.3 Case 3: a 3 mm Hole

Again there is a large discrepancy between the curves which would suggest that FloWorks is not a suitable tool for conducting this type of analysis. At this point all further simulations were stopped.

6 Software Development

The aim of this project was a fully automated system that could be used by surgeons to detect anastomotic leaks. This required the development of a software programme to compare recorded data from a current test a "look up table" and output a "best guess" based on those comparisons.

A programme which is interacting between sensors, obtained data and users was developed. The program currently only exists as a development version. Because of this, the main screen, shown in Fig. 19, is subdivided into an end-user part "Leak detection" on the left and another part "Only for Development" on the right-hand side that is used only for development purposes.

The left part visualises the result of a leakage detecting test. It shows the probable size of a leak on a scale from 0 to 2 mm and gives information about the location of the leak through a symbolized intestine profile. It is possible to detect four different

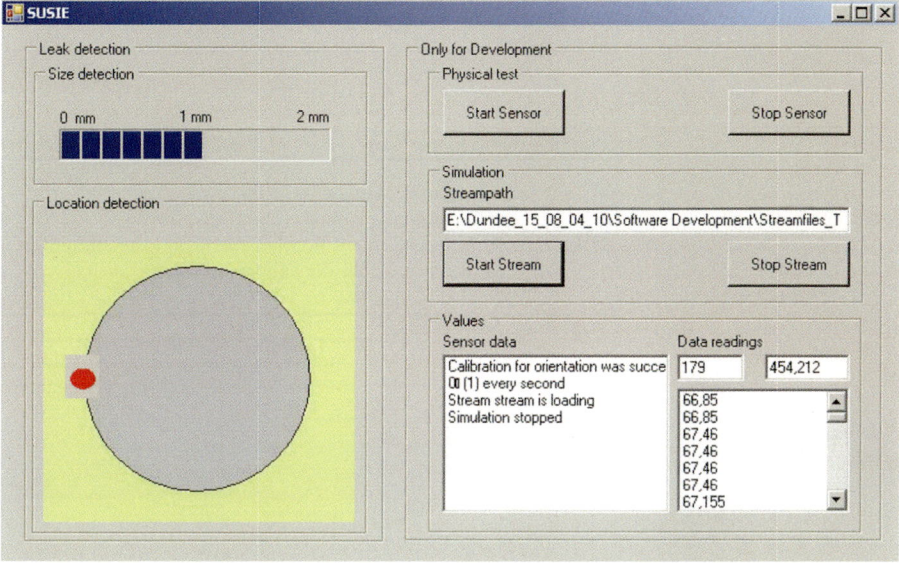

Fig. 19 Main screen of the SUSIE programme interface

leak orientations (0° – dorsal, 90° – dextral, 180° – ventral, 270° – sinistral). Based on this a surgeon will be able to make a decision regarding the severity of the anastomosis.

The right part was programmed to verify the calibration of the system. It is always important to calibrate a system correctly before it is used as a standalone measurement system. A calibration file is stored in the programme directory. It was decided to use the output at a measuring time from 20s to 80s as experience had shown that the data was stable and sufficiently separated to make a judgement on the data at that point.

The first frame "Physical test" is to start and stop a new reading from the sensor. All results are shown under "Leak Detection" and based on the stored calibration file. The measurement data is stored as a .txt file for later evaluation. The middle frame "Simulation" is used to test the programme and the calibration under well-known conditions. Instead of a real-time reading from the sensor a stream file is loadable. The advantage of this stream is that the leak size as well as the orientation of the leak is known through measurements obtained from physical experiments, therefore the programme result is verifiable. The frame "Value" gives information for the programme developer about the programme status and the data the programme has to work with and it is used to detect errors.

The program uses a calibration file to calculate the leak size and orientation. The calibration data is stored as a .txt file that is loadable through the program. Every line of this table is a dataset and must be compared to the sensor reading or the stream reading (Fig. 20). The workflow of this is as follows:

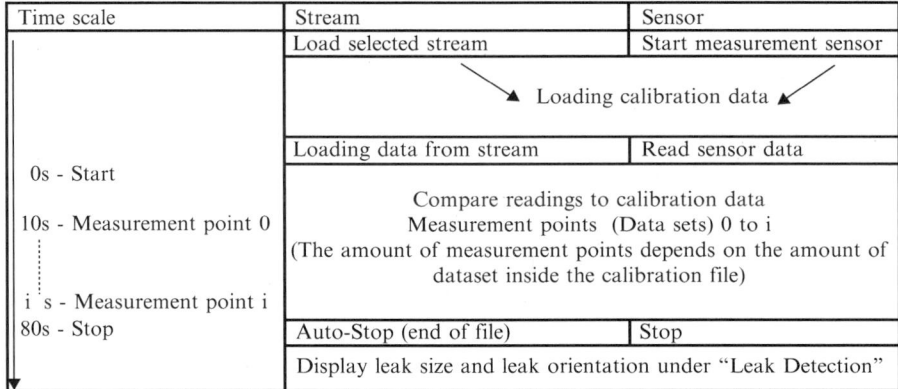

Time scale	Stream	Sensor
	Load selected stream	Start measurement sensor
	Loading calibration data	
	Loading data from stream	Read sensor data
0s - Start	Compare readings to calibration data	
10s - Measurement point 0	Measurement points (Data sets) 0 to i	
i s - Measurement point i	(The amount of measurement points depends on the amount of dataset inside the calibration file)	
80s - Stop	Auto-Stop (end of file)	Stop
	Display leak size and leak orientation under "Leak Detection"	

Fig. 20 The SUSIE workflow diagram

7 Conclusions

The consequences of a failure in the Anastomosis of the colon are serious and any steps that can be taken to reduce the likelihood of such failure must be welcomed. The computer simulations were abandoned after demonstrating weaknesses in the results, also because the simulations were taking close to 48 h for a simulation to finish due to the complexity of the computational arrangement. The main reason for running the simulations was to verify if there was any difference between different sized holes regarding the increase of concentration of nitrous oxide over the time.

For the physical simulations the results presented are very positive because of the stability that was achieved in the results. The curves for the different places where the leakage was spotted around the colon analogue presented similar behaviour over a time of 120 s. It is also possible to see a difference in the increase of nitrous oxide for these different locations, which allows identifying the place of the leakage. However, the objective of this project was to allow the surgeon to identify any anastomosis dehiscence intraoperatively. Such an objective can be achieved with the method proposed in this paper in a short time (60–120 s).

These tests have shown that it is possible to develop a system to detect the presence and location of a small hole in a colon analogue. The use of small quantities of a trace gas coupled to sensing technology should offer more dignified and safer methods to intraoperatively test the integrity of anastomosis than are available at present. The advantages of a gas sensing based approach are also currently being explored by other groups for slightly different procedures though in this case dilute H_2 is used and the work is primarily associated with a pass/fail type test rather than one attempting to evaluate the nature of any leak.

Summarizing the whole process, a N_2O infra-red sensor and gelatin capsules, which would be introduced into the colon during surgery filled with N_2O gas, would then dissolve and release the gas. A leakage containing nitrous oxide could be quickly detected by any sniff system. Therefore, the surgeon would be able to correct the problem in time to avoid further infections caused by bacteria growth at the leakage area.

Acknowledgements The authors wish to acknowledge the support given by the Engineering & Physical Sciences Research Council to this work, under Grant ref. EP/D003040/1.

References

1. Scholefield JH, Steele RJ (2002) Guidelines for follow up after resection of colorectal cancer. Gut 51(V):3–5
2. Fernandez V, Thomson G, Slade A, Vorstius J (2008) Integrity of colorectal anastomosis: a review of technological assets. Biomed Eng. BioMed 2008, 283–287
3. Walker KG, Bell SW, Rickard MJFX, Mehanna D, Dent OF, Chapuis PH, Bokey EL (2004) Anastomotic leakage is predictive of diminished survival after potentially curative resection for colorectal cancer. Ann Surg 240(2):255–259
4. Roy-Choudhury SH, Nicholson AA, Wedgwood KR, Mannion RAJ, Sedman PC, Royston CMS, Breen DJ (2001) Symptomatic malignant gastroesophageal anastomotic leak: management with covered metallic esophageal stents. AJR 176:161–165
5. Fielding LP, Stewart-Brown S, Blesovsky L, Kearney G (1980) Anastomotic integrity after operations for large bowel cancer: a multicentre study. Br Med J 2(1980):411–414
6. Stádler P, Dvorácek L, Vitásek P, Matous P (2008) Is robotic surgery appropriate for vascular procedures? Report of 100 aortoiliac cases. J Vasc Surg 48(4):1065
7. Zurab T, Emanuel S, Geiger TM, Cleveland D, Frazier S, Rawlings A, Bachman SL, Miedema BW, Thaler K (2008) Placement of a covered polyester stent prevents complications from a colorectal anastomotic leak and supports healing: randomized controlled trial in a large animal model. Surgery 144(5):786–792
8. Thomson GA (2007) An investigation of leakage tracts along stressed suture lines in phantom tissue. Med Eng Phys 29:1030–1034
9. Gilbert JM, Trapnell JE (1998) Intraoperative testing of the integrity of left-sided colorectal anastomoses: a technique of value to the surgeon in training. Ann R Coll Surg Engl 70:158–160
10. Ovrebo GK (2005) Simulation of silicon carbide diode heating and natural convection. Army Res Lab

Plantar Pressure Assessment: A New Tool for Postural Instability Diagnosis in Multiple Sclerosis

João M.C.S. Abrantes and Luis F.F. Santos

Abstract Multiple sclerosis (MS) is a chronic inflammatory, demyelinating disease of the central nervous system (CNS), and is the most common progressive neuro-logical disease in young adults. Debilitating motor and sensory function are the major features of the disease. Balance disorders are associated with ambulation difficulties such sustaining an upright posture and performing functional activities such as turning. Those skills predispose people with MS to loss the balance control and fall. An adequate evaluation of postural degree of stability is essential for monitoring the various stages of disease. Sometimes clinical balance tests may not detect subtle deficits in adults with MS who are not yet experiencing functional limitations or disability. It's important to develop new instruments that could identify subtle impairments before they lead to functional decline. The purpose of this study was to determine if centre of pressure (COP) displacement assessed by plantar pressure could be a useful performance-based evaluative measure for adults with MS comparing with a clinical examination using the Berg Balance Scale (BBS). Subjects with MS (n = 29) were compared with healthy adults (n = 28). The subjects with MS were subjected to three tests: (1) Plantar pressure in upright standing position ($\Delta t = 10s$); (2) Right and Left gait stance phase (1-step protocol); and, (3) BBS test. Control subjects performed (1) and (2) tests. COP measures show clear differences when comparing healthy adults with adults with MS and this group had kinematics alterations of COP characteristics. The plantar pressure plate is a

J.M.C.S. Abrantes (✉)
MovLab, Universidade Lusófona de Humanidades e Tecnologias, Lisbon, Portugal
e-mail: joao.mcs.abrantes@ulusofona.pt

L.F.F. Santos
Department of Physical and Medicine Rehabilitation of SAMS, Lisbon, Portugal

ADFisio – Rehabilitation Center, Lisbon, Portugal
e-mail: luis.fernafer.santos@gmail.com

R.M.N. Jorge et al. (eds.), *Technologies for Medical Sciences*, Lecture Notes in Computational Vision and Biomechanics 1, DOI 10.1007/978-94-007-4068-6_9, © Springer Science+Business Media B.V. 2012

useful tool to detect the no visual data. Comparing the results of the present work there is evidence that the exclusive use of the BBS is test is ineffective in small postural disorders.

1 Introduction

Multiple Sclerosis (MS) affects about 2.5 million people in all world and is the most common neurological disorder, with major incapacity in young adults, especially in Europe and North America [1]. We know today that beyond the environmental component, genetic factors have a large influence on the acquisition of the disease, thus, susceptibility to the different responsibilities and racial heterogeneity of ethnic groups, play an important role in the geographical distribution of the disease [2]. Globally, the median estimated prevalence of MS is 30 per 100,000 (with a range of 5–80). Regionally, the median estimated prevalence of MS is greatest in Europe (80 per 100,000), followed by the Eastern Mediterranean (14.9), the Americas (8.3), the Western Pacific (5), South-East Asia (2.8) and Africa (0.3) [3].

The symptoms of MS are very diverse as the disease course. Some patients, throughout their life, just have a small disability, although about 60% can no longer walk in the next 20 years, after the diagnosis [4]. In the disease course, the life expectancy is slightly changed, but the quality of life is seriously affected in recent years. Patients with MS learn to live with the difficulties inherent to the disease progression, but there is a big change in their plans, also in employment and hope for the future. Many of these patients are young adults, in the beginning of their careers and family building [5]. Another stressful aspect is the uncertainty about the future. Many times after adjustment to disability from the last relapse of the disease, a new relapse that causes more disability and limitation, requiring a new period of adjustment and changes in daily life. MS is an inflammatory disease of the central nervous system (CNS) associated with loss of motor and sensory function. These symptoms results from white matter lesions, that causes destruction of axons and myelin sheaths, with a consequent decrease in nerve impulses [6].

A major problem associated with this disease, is the alteration of postural stability [7]. This change of stability puts individuals at risk of falling and serious injury, complicating the handling of these patients, increasing their disability and causing changes in the quality of life [8].

The responsible mechanisms for altering the postural stability in these patients still not very clear. The cause of this instability may be due to an isolated lesion in a single system or neuronal pathway, or often, due to multiple injuries affecting two or more sensor motor systems [7]. If only one system is damaged, the the compensation can be reasonably effective. In the case of many systems affected compensation is more complex and it becomes increasingly difficult as the disease progresses and becomes more severe. The postural stability and joint stability in particular is essential to the success of human movements [4]. In an unstable system, a small variation in initial condition, or a small external perturbation, may lead to an unexpected and inconsistent motor task. On the other hand in a stable system, the same motor command leads to similar moves by controlling small disturbances [9]. This means that the resulting motion can be predicted and planned.

1.1 General Framework

One way of studying the stability, in particular de joint stability is through Biomechanics. In Biomechanics the study objective is the motor production of living beings, constituted and based in knowledge of morphology, cybernetics and mechanics, but it marks autonomy in relation to their biological and mechanical sources [10]. Also according to this author, the biomechanic study of motor behaviour is the non determinist production of the locomotor system, resulting from the mechanical and biological external responses organized by the Kinematics and dynamic point of view. So, the biomechanic, studies the movements and forces that are the consequence of mechanical relationship established and controlled by the performer. Biomechanics can be considered as a complementary method of diagnosis, using in the experimental setups their direct data (obtained from the records of the external forces acting in center of pressure (COP)), or indirect data, that are obtained from the records of the images [11].

One method to access the postural stability is studying the behaviour of the COP, and it can be obtained by Posturography. In this method, the determination of COP is done using one or two force plates [12]. A disadvantage of this method is the lack of parameters that have confidence to be used in evaluation of pathological changes [13]. On the other hand, there is a large gap between the methods of research-based laboratories and those used in the clinical field. Particularly in the biomechanic field, the equipment used to study the gait and postural stability, is fixed to the ground and are very expensive [14]. It is necessary to develop equipment that has portability characteristics, with the ability to perform valid, reliable and safe tests for use in a clinical setting. Taking this into account, as an alternative to the use of one or two force plates, we propose in this study the use of plantar pressure plate to access de COP characteristics.

The plantar pressure has been applied to access the study of COP behavior. A recent study [15] investigated the influence of loading and positioning of school supplies, on the distribution of plantar forces and COP trajectory in students with Baropodometric data, obtained from a plantar pressure plate (Matscan Research, Teckscan). In 2004, another study [16] attempted to verify the risk factors for ankle sprain in students, through the study of the COP, also using a plantar pressure plate (Footscan Pressure Plate RSSCAN International, 2.0 m × 0.4 m, 16,384 sensors, 480 Hz). In 2002, to compare the plantar pressure distribution between hemiplegic children and a healthy control group, some authors [17] used a system of pressure insoles (Parotec, Paromed GmbH, D-8201, Neubeuern Markt, Germany). Another study conducted in 2006 [18] used a system of insoles (F-scan system) to identify characteristics in the distribution of plantar pressure foot deformities and to identify changes in these parameters after corrective surgery in children with spastic cerebral palsy. Robain and his colleagues [18] conducted a study with the aim of analyzing the path of the COP during gait using hemiplegic patients, also using an F-Scan system (Teckscan, Inc., South Boston MA).

Another method to access postural stability is often made by clinical tests such as the Berg Balance Scale (BBS) [19], however these instruments often fail to detect minimal changes in postural stability in patients without visible changes, or functional abnormalities. An evaluation that detect small disturbances before the functional changes, allowing early intervention, preventing deterioration and functional limitation. In this work, we perform a characterization of the center of pressure in the standing position, and as much as possible a characterization during the gait in individuals with multiple sclerosis. It is intended in addition, to relate the characteristics of the COP with the results obtained by applying the Berg Balance Scale. To date, few studies have been published on the application of plantar pressure in the assessment of postural stability in individuals with MS.

2   Bibliographic Review

2.1   Multiple Sclerosis

Multiple Sclerosis (MS) is a chronic disease of the central nervous system (CNS) characterized by: immuno-inflammatory response, astrocytic gliosis and focal demyelination of axons [7]. It is the most common neurological disease in young adults between 18 and 50 years of age, and the peak of the first relapse occurs in the third decade of life. It affects about two or three times more women than men, being the major source of economic losses [20]. His prognosis is well known, 15 years after diagnosis 50% of patients using walking aids (crutches and walkers) and 29% a wheelchair [21, 22]. During the first 10 years of evolution, from 50% to 80% of patients stop working, however life expectancy is only slightly reduced [23]. The exact etiology of MS remains unknown, but it is believed that neuro-degeneration is secondary to an auto-immune mediation, however there is no precise explanation on the induction of abnormal immune response towards the CNS [24]. Some authors [25] consider that there is an agent associated with the onset of the disease. The Epstein-Barr virus is a biologically plausible candidate, but this assumption is not fully proven.

This disease also shows a latitudinal discrepancy, because it occurs more frequently in temperate regions far from the equator [2]. The lesions can occur anywhere in the CNS, but there are certain areas of predilection, such as the optic nerve, the cerebellum and spinal cord [26].

2.1.1 Symptomatology

The symptoms or disorders associated with MS can be from various types such as motor, sensory, cognitive [27] and psychosocial [28]. Vary widely from individual to individual and also with the evolutionary stage of the disease [29]. The motor symptoms include impaired speech and swallowing, bladder dysfunction, bowel and sexual [30, 31], fatigue [32], spasticity [33], tremor [34], muscle weakness, paresis, clonus, impaired postural stability [35] and gait abnormalities, being a major factor the ataxia [36]. Ataxic patients give priority to the maintenance of postural stability by a propulsive movement, with increased proximal muscle activity, step towards extending the medio-lateral and extended period of double support (which corresponds to the time that both feet are in contact with support).

This type of gait ataxia identifies a incoordination in the lower limbs, in which the angular displacements of joints are getting smaller with a consequent decrease in gait speed [37]. Fatigue is another symptom that patients identify as one of the most adverse factors for the activities of daily living, followed by bladder problems and changes in postural stability. New evidence suggests that fatigue may be related to dysfunction of the regulation of body temperature [38]. The bladder disorders are highly disabling in daily life and spinal cord injuries appear to be the cause of pelvic dysfunction. These disorders are characterized by urinary urgency as a result of the Detrusor hyper-reflex or by decreasing the storage capacity of the bladder. In sensory symptoms is identified the changes in vision, dizziness, paresthesia and sexual dysfunction.

2.1.2 Types of Multiple Sclerosis

We consider that there are three major types of Multiple Sclerosis [20]: Relapsing-Remitting, Secondary Progressive and Primary Progressive.

- The Relapsing-Remitting type accounts for 25% of total cases and is characterized by an exacerbation of neurological symptoms lasting more than 24 h [39]. Typically occurs between several days to 2 weeks, followed by a complete or nearly complete remission of symptoms. The frequency of relapses varies greatly, but on average one case per year [40]. Especially with more severe relapses, there may be long periods of recovery and the persistence of residual symptoms. Some authors [41, 42] consider that there must be at least a period of 30 days between two exacerbations, to be considered two distinct relapses. The most frequent symptoms in this type of MS are the visual and sensory disturbances. The patient often resorts to an evaluation by a neurologist in the second or third relapse, with the disease already installed in the progressive phase.
- Secondary progressive type accounts for 60% of total cases and is a continuation of relapsing-remitting [43]. It is characterized by a progression of relapses, with worsening of symptoms with a minimum period of 6 months, in which may occur another severe relapses [44]. In this type of MS disorders are frequently associated with gait and motor abnormalities, such as paresthesia.

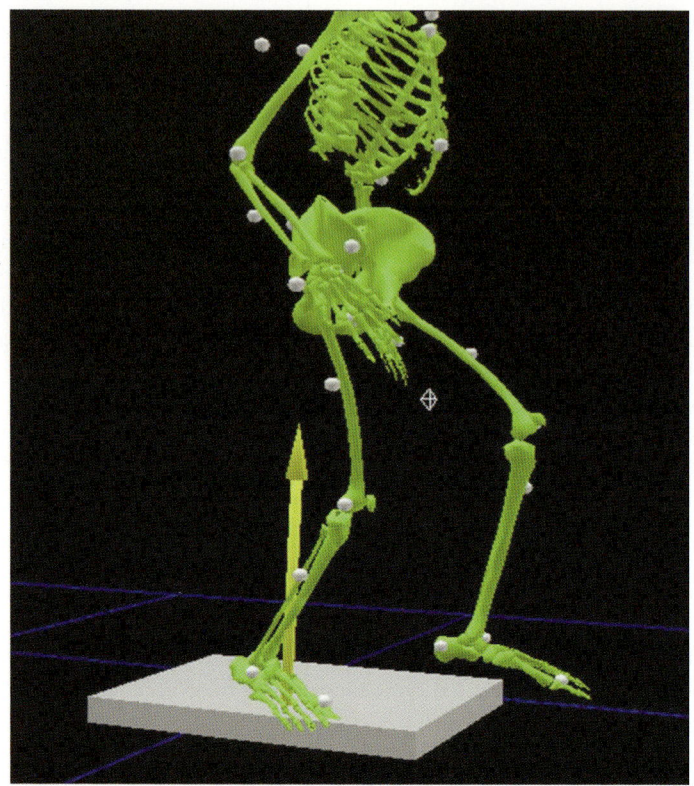

Fig. 1 Ground Reaction Force (GRF) identified by *Yellow* vector

- Primary progressive MS represents the minority of cases with 15%. Characterized by a progression from the beginning of the disease, without existence of any
  relapse, more characteristic in older men and often associated in elderly [45]. In
  this form of MS, the lesions are usually located in the spinal cord and develop
  less cognitive problems compared with other forms.

2.2 Dynamometry and Center of Pressure (COP)

A device developed to measure forces and moments of forces is called a dynamome-
ter [46]. The moment of a force is the tendency of this force to produce torsion or
rotation around an axis [10]. During the gait or simply in the standing position, the
contact of foot with the support develops a force called the ground reaction force
(GRF) (Fig. 1).

The human plantar support dynamometry allows graduate the deformation on
the surfaces of the plates (force and pressure) and thus obtains the value of GRF.

The evaluation of this GRF, permit to calculate the moments of force by inverse dynamics (mechanic of rigid body methodology), and study the behavior of the system in relation to a motor task [47]. Winter defined the COP [48] as the point of application of the vertical ground reaction force. Represents the weighted average of the pressures on the surface and is considered a major kinetic variable in the study of postural stability. The COP determination using a single force plate, results in a two-dimensional diagram (spatial and temporal), which results from the vector sum of the anterior-posterior and medial-lateral components of force [49]. The center of mass (COM) is considered the major kinematic variable in the study of postural stability, and is defined as the point representing the total body mass in a global reference system. In the human body, the COM coincides with the center of gravity (COG), but is independent of any gravitational field [50]. The COM is determined by the weighted average COM of each body segment, in a space defined by a three dimensional referential.

The standing position is not a static position, presents oscillations that allow in indirect way describing the stiffness and postural control [11]. In standing position, humans have a postural sway with an average frequency of 0.27–0.45 Hz [51], which is related to the constant change of neural inputs, primarily originated from the spinal cord level [48, 52]. These small oscillations are associated with angular changes of about $1.0°$–$1.5°$ of the ankle, knee and hip [53], which causes horizontal displacement of COM nearly about 4–28 mm [54]. To ensure that the COM remains in the ideal position, the COP has to suffer larger displacements than COM. Considering the COP behaviour a consequence from the individual control of postural stability, accessing the variability of this variable during the standing position or in gait, we can access the strategies used in postural control in both planes (sagittal and frontal) [55], with the advantage of being immediately, non invasive and easily acquired. When assessing the standing position we obtained the "stabilograms", which is the projection of the COP trajectory in a two-dimensional space [56]. It was demonstrated in multiple sclerosis patients, at an early stage disease, when there are no major functional changes, the static tests are less sensitive [57]. Moreover the dynamic tests, usually through balance tasks to achieve, do not reproduce the postural changes during walking, so it is essential to perform an evaluation based on this functional activity.

2.3 Plantar Pressure

One method to study the COP in standing position or during gait is using the plantar pressure plate [58]. The information obtained from this system is very important because it allows to verify the relationship between plantar pressure and body posture, as well as defining the COP variability [59]. This evaluation was recognized as an important factor to access gait disturbances in neurological diseases. The multidimensional and complex nature of postural stability, prevents this type of information to be obtained with a single test [16]. The matrix of plantar pressure

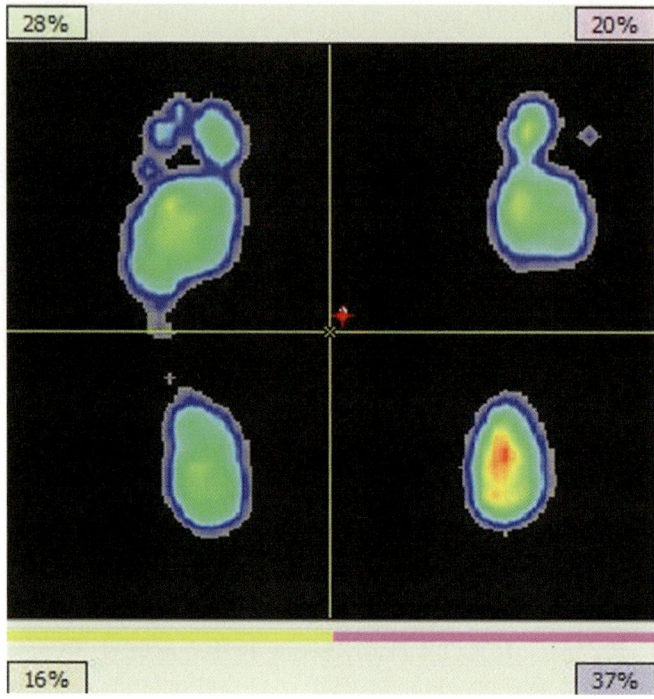

Fig. 2 Plantar pressure distribution in standing position. Image obtained by RSSCAN software – footscan 7.7 balance 2nd generation

plates includes many sensors that allow the different pressures by colour (Fig. 2). The red and orange colours represent areas of higher pressure while the green and blue colours, representing areas of lower pressure [47].

Plantar pressure plates allow us to examine all plantar pressure support, allowing changes evaluation since the initial contact until the final contact (Fig. 3). During the support we can also observe the COP trajectory, by analyzing the medial-lateral and anterior-posterior component [16].

Laboratory tests should be included in the diagnostic of postural stability changes, as a complement to the clinical test usually used. The evaluation of plantar pressure must be included in a gait analysis laboratory, in association with other laboratory tests [60]. The data obtained with these systems, help the health professionals to anticipate the intervention or changes in treatment programs, in order to increase the effectiveness of rehabilitation.

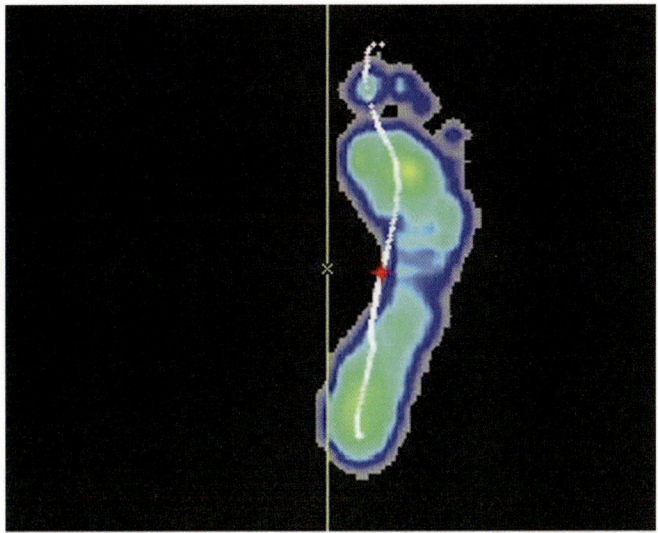

Fig. 3 Plantar pressure distribution in right foot contact

2.3.1 Foot Contact Phases and COP Trajectory

The foot performs several functions during ground contact, and may be divided into several phases. In the beginning of contact, the foot acts as a shock-absorbing structure, followed by a total support phase, when behaves as a stable object [61]. In the final phase, foot acts as a catalyst, by moving the body structure in the direction of progression. Winter defined five stages in foot ground contact [62] (Fig. 4):

- Initial contact, or foot contact with ground support, normally by Hell (Fig. 4a).
- Contact of the fifth Metatarsal (Fig. 4b).
- Total contact, or contact of all Metatarsals (Fig. 4c).
- Heel elevation, or heel is no longer in contact with the ground support (Fig. 4d).
- Final contact, or last anatomical structure in ground contact, normally the first toe (Fig. 4e).

The COP trajectory begins with the heel contact (assuming that the initial contact begins in this area) and moves towards to the final contact in first toe [47]. However, in the literature, there are no descriptions about this normal COP trajectory. In the normality, there is a tendency to an external COP trajectory between phase 1 and phase 2. To determine the tendency of COP trajectory (internal or external), is important to define the longitudinal axis of the foot. This axis is the imaginary line passing through the heel and the space between the head of the 2nd and 3rd metatarsal [63]. If the trajectory of the COP is located outside this line, it occurred on the outer edge of the foot. If the trajectory of the COP is more internal in respect to this line, it was in the inner edge.

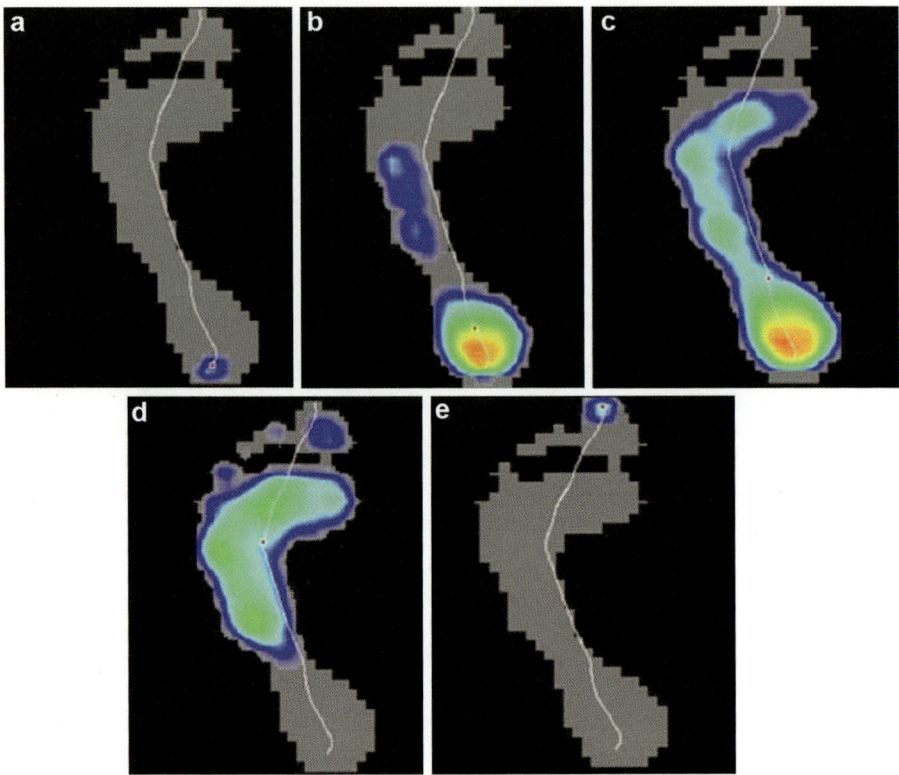

Fig. 4 Foot contact phases. (**a**) Initial contact. (**b**) Contact of the fifth metatarsal. (**c**) Total contact (all metatarsal). (**d**) Heel elevation. (**e**) Final contact (toe off). (Adapted from [61] with permission)

2.4 Postural Stability

For a long time it was implicitly assumed that the postural sway was a stationary process. However, this assumption is not true in most cases, which led some authors [64] to applied the stochastic theory in analysis of postural control mechanism. They hypothesized that the COP profile, reflects the Fractional Brownian Motion (also known as the Analysis of Diffusion Stabilograms [65]), which consists of two processes: a process of short duration, approximately one second (1 s) called "open-loop", in which displacement of COP and COM are virtually simultaneous, and another long process, longer than one second (>1 s), called "close-loop", in which displacement of COP has a considerable delay comparing to COM. However, a deeper analysis of postural control [66] suggested that these two processes were insufficient to characterize this mechanism and the stochastic properties of COP trajectory in the standing position were yet to be elucidated. Some authors tried to characterize the mechanism of postural control from the nonlinear dynamics perspective and chaos theory, bringing new concepts and tools for detecting chaos in physiological systems [67]. The characterization in the linear view is correct and applicable only to simple systems, which in fact is not applicable to living organisms due to its extraordinary complexity, with large numbers of structures and processes [68].

In the postural system there are large nonlinearities, due to the elastic property and the shortening of the muscles and the nonlinear control of the nervous system [69]. Thus, the displacements of COM and its relation with the oscillation of COP are good candidates to assess inter-segmental movements in the standing position. Initially it was established that the existence of reflex mechanisms in the spinal cord and brainstem, were responsible for maintaining the standing position, adjusting the configuration and reflexes of postural control by disruption of rectification [70]. Recently an alternative hypothesis was developed, taking into account an argument originally proposed by Morasso [71]. This argument suggests that the standing position is no different from other forms of movement, because it requires planning anticipation and monitoring of internal models, such as the movement of a human limb in a controlled manner. However, these control mechanisms are not obvious in the standing position because the body movements and muscle movements has reduced amplitude.

The control of postural stability is usually associated with the process control of a inverted pendulum [72]. Modelling postural stability as an inverted pendulum, it is assumed that there is a rigid structure on top of both ankles and this structure fluctuate around these rigid structures. However, the human body is a multi-segmented structure capable of motion in all joints above the ankles [53]. This model relates a variable that is controlled (COM) and a variable that controls (COP), predicting that the difference between COP and COM is proportional to the horizontal acceleration of COM but with a negative correlation, i.e., in the anterior-posterior plane, when COP is ahead of the COM, the acceleration is posterior, when the COP is behind the COM acceleration is anterior [72]. The same correlation was observed when the COP and COM are in the medial-lateral plane. These findings were validated experimentally by Winter and colleagues [54]. In standing position when the feet are placed side by side, maintaining the COP in the limits of stability depends of two different strategies [73]:

• Ankle Strategy – in small perturbations, posture control is maintained through the dorsal and plantar flexors of the foot, acting alone to maintain postural control in the anterior-posterior plane.
• Hip Strategy – in large postural disturbances, when the ankle strategy can not be sufficient to maintain postural stability, the central nervous system acts with hip strategy. In this case a hip flexion displaces the COM in the posterior direction and a hip extension moves the COM in anterior direction [74].

With these strategies, it's intended to maintain the COM position within the limits of the base support [75]. Clearly, the COP follows the COM displacement and oscillates at his side to keep the COM in the desired position between the 2 ft. Therefore and because the COP oscillates from either side of the COM, its displacement is always slightly larger than the COM [54]. On the other hand, during an intermediate position of the feet 45° (when in double support phase, during walking), the control strategy appears to be mixed, and both mechanisms act in opposite ways to maintain the postural control. During the standing position, the generated moments at the various body kinetic chains are transmitted to the base of support, seeing as a signal of the COP component.

Considering the COP behaviour as a measure of body dynamics, there is access to a greater representation of the various neuromuscular components that act on different joints. These neuromuscular components and their characteristics are strongly dependent on the stimuli that control the postural stability [76]. Disorders in stimuli processing, such as occurs in neurological disorders, lead to changes in COP characteristics [77]. The standing posture is defined by mutual relations between the body segments and the vertical orientation of the body in the gravitational field, thus, this guidance (in conjunction with the small airfoil and body architecture) determines the potential for postural instability [78].

2.4.1 Joint Stability

The joint stability results from motor control over the elements acting on each joint. Thus, the effect of control over the active elements (neuromuscular) is associated with the effect of passive elements (mechanical properties of joint materials) [10] act simultaneously to produce an adequate stability. Joint stability should provide adequate stiffness and resistance to external forces, when the objective is maintain postural stability [10]. One of the key components of joint stability is related to muscle stiffness. The concept of stiffness as an important factor in the stability control was introduced in 1998 [54]. The key point of these arguments (based on experimental evidence) was that the controlled variable (COM) was virtually in phase with the controlling variable (COP) [79].

The role of the CNS in this postural control is to maintain a steady supply of muscle tone, capable to support the gravitational load and shift the COP faster than the COM, to maintain this position. In anterior-posterior direction, when a subject is in the standing position, usually presents the COM about 5 cm below the ankle. When an oscillation occurs, is necessary that the ankle muscles generate a tone with sufficient stiffness to move the COP faster than COM. If the reactive control is normal, the afferent and efferent latencies combined with biomechanical delays of muscle recruitment, resulting in a delay of COP about 100 ms after the initial COM movement [80]. In standing position the amount of gravitational COM movement, increases linearly with the increase in ankle dorsal-flexion, but the frontal body collapse is controlled by the ankle joint moment, produced by the activity of triceps and soleus muscle [81]. The activation of this muscle generates an intrinsic joint stiffness, causing a force moment in response to the instantaneous change in the joint angle, without any intervention from the CNS. If the stiffness is less than the gravitational movement, the COM is mechanically unstable, with need for neural modulation of joint moment to produce stability [71].

It has been postulated that the CNS performs the modulation of joint stiffness to control postural sway [54, 82]. However the experimental results of another study

[83] revealed that the intrinsic stiffness has a little change when compared to the ankle moment, despite a large change in muscle activation. It is unlikely that the muscle stiffness is the source of joint stiffness, but the aponeurosis, tendon and bone architecture of the foot. So in the standing position the stiffness is not on neural control, but is a biomechanic constant. Thus, increased the idea that the stiffness increases when the ankle movements are smaller and slower [83]. However, when there is an angular displacement during walking, we noticed a stiffness in the joint, which was called dynamic stiffness [84].

As expressed in the introduction, the postural stability evaluation is often made by clinical tests such as the Berg Balance Scale [19]. However, these instruments often fail to detect minimal changes in postural stability in patients who have not shown functional changes. An evaluation that can detect small perturbations before the functional changes, allows early intervention, prevents deterioration and functional limitation.

3 Methodology

3.1 Objectives

The purpose of this study was to characterize the center of pressure behaviour in the standing position and in the stance phase of gait (1-step protocol) in subjects with multiple sclerosis. Based on previous studies [12, 57, 85, 86] the present study used five COP parameters sensitive to postural balance and MS postural changes: Medial-lateral COP displacement (ML); Anterior-posterior COP displacement (AP); Total COP displacement (TD); Ellipse area (EA) and Total Contac Time (CT). Were also tried to establish relations between the results obtained in COP evaluation and scores obtained in Berg Balance Scale

3.2 Subjects

The study was conducted with support from Portuguese Society of Multiple Sclerosis. Inclusion criteria for participation were: (1) clinical diagnosis of MS, conducted by a neurologist; (2) aged between 18 and 65; (3) ability to maintained upright standing position for 60 s; (4) ability to perform the 1-step protocol. Exclusion criteria were: (1) other neurological conditions such stroke or brain trauma; (2) cardiovascular diseases or other causes that interfere with the implementation of the evaluation protocol; (3) cognitive deficits; (4) included in another study of MS. To verify the inclusion criteria, a questionnaire was sent by email, to each subject with MS, who intended to participate. Before test procedures, each subject performed an interview to collect demographic, anthropometric and clinical characteristics including age, gender, foot size, type of MS and disease duration. Twenty-nine subjects with MS, 12 male and 17 female, mean age $43,24 \pm 12,08$, were included in the study. Control subjects were eligible to participate if they met the same inclusion criteria as the subjects with MS, with the exception of having a diagnosis of MS and were recruited from a variety of sources of convenience. The same exclusion criteria also applied to the control group. Twenty-eight control subjects, 9 male; 19 female, mean age $36.79 \pm 8,96$, met the criteria for the study and were tested. All subjects provided written informed consent prior to test procedures and the study was approved by ethic commission of Portuguese Catholic University were the study was presented. All subjects participated in one testing session which included plantar pressure assessment and clinical test. The study was conducted in accordance to recommendations guiding biomedical research involving human subjects (Helsinki Declaration).

3.3   Assessment and Data Collection

In this study, in order to obtain all necessary information to verify the variables, we used two measurement instruments. One technical instrument, the plantar pressure plate (Footscan® – 3D Gait Scientific System from RSSCAN®) kindly supplied by the Laboratory of Physical Therapy, School of Health Alcoitão. The other instrument is the Berg Balance Scale, a clinical instrument to measuring postural stability. We also used video cameras to obtain images, to characterize the clinical status of participants.

3.3.1   Berg Balance Scale

The Berg Balance Scale (BBS) consists of 14 standardized sub-tests (13 tests in the standing position and 1 test in the sitting position), scored on five-point scales (0–4), with a maximum (best) score of 56 [19]. Scores are based on the time that a position can be maintained, the distance that the upper limb is capable of reaching in the front of the body and the time to complete a specific task. Reliability and validity have been demonstrated in elderly people [87], and scores below 45 indicate increased risk of falling for elderly people [88]. Reliability and validity of the BBS have not been established in persons with MS. However, the BBS has been found to change in response to rehabilitation in adults with clinically stable MS [89] and many studies included this scale to evaluate postural stability in MS [8, 90, 91]. A recent systematic review [92] to identify measurement tools of balance activity in people with neurological conditions, concluded that BBS is psychometrically robust and feasible to use in neurological disorders and clinical practice.

3.3.2 Plantar Pressure Assessment

Plantar pressure assessment was performed with Footscan 1 m – 3D Gait Scientific System – RsScan® International – Belgium. The plate consists of two units of 0.5 m × 0.5 m installed in carbon mat and synchronized with each other. Each unit has dimensions: length 578 mm × width 418 mm × height 12 mm, and 4096 sensors (5.08 mm × 7.62 mm).Thus, it is possible to operate as a unit of 1 m to gait analyses, or only using one unit of 0.5 m to balance evaluation. The 1 m plantar pressure plate use resistive technology using 8192 sensors (5.08 mm by 7.62 mm). The dimensions are, 1068 mm, length by 418 mm width and 12 mm height. The actual study used the left unit.

The plate was connected to analog-digital unit – Footscan® Interface 3D Box to synchronize the entire system and convert the signal in digital values to pressure data. The software provided by the manufacturer (Footscan 7.7 Balance 2nd Generation) was installed in one computer system to collect and store pressure data. The 100 Hz sample frequency was used to collect data from upright standing position (10 s) and 250 Hz sample frequency for the stance phase of gait (4 s).

3.4 Protocol

In order to test the whole experimental procedure previously projected, as well as verify its feasibility, before the real study two pilot studies were developed. These studies, allowed determining the adequate space, the necessary equipment and its assembly, the procedures to plate calibration. Also allowed to test the protocols and establish routines for collecting and recording data. Simultaneously with this process, we carried out a detailed study of the software (Footscan 7.7 Balance2nd Generation), to check if the proposed variables for study were possible to achieve with his instrument. The plate was placed on the ground at a distance of 1.5 m from front wall and calibrated by manufacturer's specifications. Each upright standing position test data was collect for 10 s. Each subject performed three trials. The subjects stood on plate, barefoot, in her/his free selection usual natural position more stable self considered. They were instructed to stay as quiet as possible during the trial. To avoid disturbing effects due to eye movements over postural control, the subjects were required, during the trial, to stare at a target. This target consisted in a blue circle (diameter = 0.16 m) drawn on a white sheet, positioned in the front wall at 1.6 m of the ground. During the trials, an assistance stay close to subjects to prevent instability and fall risk. Trial, in which the feet were not contacted with the whole plate, was not saved for data analysis and was repeated. Some authors [59] identified that fatigue affects the process of muscle excitation, and the efficiency of the muscular mechanism, affecting the gait pattern.

In order to prevent possible cases of fatigue and its possible effects on biomechanical parameters, the plantar pressure assessment was performed first. If necessary, between trials, subjects with greater postural instability were allowed to sit for 2 min. For gait stance phase, the study used the 1-step protocol [93]. Each subject performed three times with right foot and three times with left foot. The subjects stood in upright standing position behind the plate, and were instructed to perform a step moving inside the plate just with one foot, and place the other foot out of plate. If the first test was performed with the right foot, then the other two tests were also conducted with the same foot. After the pressure assessment, subjects were evaluated by a clinical test (Berg Balance Scale – BBS) based on a qualified scale and applied by a specialist. The assessment is done by the visual direct observation of the balance behaviour characteristics.

3.4.1   Phases of the Study

Due to the characteristics of this disease, which leads to difficulties in mobility, and due to constraints associated in mounting of experimental environment, it was not possible to collect the data only on a certain date and at the same place. Thus, the study had to be done in several phases. As the participants were recruited and selected, they were sequentially introduced in to the study. The study was conducted in four phases:

- Phase 1 – Testing in Clinical Center of Medical and Social Services (SAMS) in Lisbon – six participants with MS were tested
- Phase 2 – Tests on the National Headquarters of Portuguese Society of Multiple Sclerosis – 11 participants with MS were tested
- Phase 3 – Testing for control group in Clinical Center of Medical and Social Services (SAMS) in Lisbon – 28 participants without neurological or orthopaedic surgery were tested
- Phase 4 – Testing in the Sea Clinic (Matosinhos) – 12 participants with MS were tested

3.4.2   Protocol for Plantar Pressure Assessment

In plantar pressure study, data are collected to obtain a representative estimate of the true plantar pressure of each participant. In this sense, they are used several walking tests, ranging from the midgait protocol (3 steps protocol), to the lower protocols, involving just one or two steps before contact with the plate [94]. However, the better protocol choice, as well the number of tests, must be appropriate to the aims of investigation. Collected data shall be valid and reliable when compared to the

Table 1 Demographic, anthropometric and clinical characteristics of study population

Variable	Mean ± S.D. (Range)	
	MS Subjects N = 29	Healthy Subjects N = 28
Age (years)	43,2 ± 12,1 (20–63)	36,8 ± 8,96 (19–62)
Gender	17 females; 12 males	19 females; 9 males
Ratio	1.4:1	2.1:1
Foot Size[a]	39,2 ± 2,48 (35–43)	38,5 ± 2,57 (35–44)
Berg balance scale	46,6 ± 9,97 (21–56)	55,7 ± 0,47 (55–56)
Disease duration (years)	8,72 ± 6,18 (0,17–22)	–

[a]Foot size in continental European system (adults)

normal gait. The midgait protocol requires higher space and time to perform the tests, due to a larger number of steps and the effect of "target". This "Targeting Effect" is considered the necessary adjustments to perform a accurate contact on the plate surface [95]. According to some authors [96], the 1step protocol and 2 step protocol do not show significant differences in peak pressure and pressure–time integral when compared to 3-step protocol. The same study also concluded that the 1 step protocol provides a higher confidence in the register of plantar pressure when compared with the 3-step protocol. The variability in 1 and 2 steps protocol may be affected, because in these methods, the pressure is evaluated during gait initiation, which is considered a instability phase, defying the control system until the stabilization is acquired [97]. Moreover, the abbreviated protocols are not representative of steady gait, but reduce the number of eliminated trials due to the "target" effect, so they are widely used. There are no comparative studies of these protocols in MS patients. The validity and confidence in the register of plantar pressure in this population, remains unknown. However, there are studies in this population that used the 1 step protocol [98, 99]. In our study, we used the 1 step protocol based on the participant's safety, and to minimize any fatigue effects.

3.5 Statistical Analysis

Statistical analysis was performed using the software Statistical Package for the Social Sciences (SPSS), version 17.0 software for Windows XP SP2 (SPSS, Chicago, IL, USA) and Microsoft® Excel 2003. We calculated Spearman correlation coefficients to evaluate the validity of the postural stabilization parameters for the considered population of MS subjects.

Demographic, anthropometric and clinical characteristics (mean, standard deviation and range) for all subjects are listed in Table 1.

Table 2 Upright standing
position – Results

MS subjects				Healthy subjects			
ML	AP	TD	EA	ML	AP	TD	EA
6,7	11,1	145,0	5,5	2,0	3,3	85,3	0,9

Values are the mean of 3 trials for 29 MS subjects and 28
healthy subjects in millimetres
ML Medio-lateral COP displacement, *AP* Anterior-
posterior COP displacement, *TD* Total COP displacement, *EA* Ellipse area (mm2)

3.6 Berg Balance Scale

Fourteen of 28 MS subjects scored ≥ 51 points in BBS (maximum 56), with higher
scores indicating better performance. However the average BBS score in MS group
is approximately nine points less than the average score in healthy group. Ten MS
subjects scored <44, below the score (45) from which increases the risk of falls
and corresponds to 34.48% of total group. Nine healthy subjects scored 55 points,
remaining subjects reached the maximum score.

3.7 Upright Standing Position

Results for upright standing position are shown in Table 2. In MS group, medio-
lateral and anterior-posterior data demonstrate a substantially displacement than
control group. A similar behavior is observed in total displacement and ellipse area
values. For each trial, an ellipse area is calculated. All the centre of pressure points
within 1 standard deviation is represented in this ellipse, so the ellipse is a representation of the spreading of the centre of pressure line. Lower values correspond
to stable measurements. Medio-lateral COP displacement in MS subjects is the
triple value than verified in healthy subjects. Similarly the anterior-posterior COP
displacement in MS subjects has a triple value too, compared to the other group.
Comparing the results for ellipse area, the results demonstrate that the difference
is even greater, and the result is five times higher in MS subjects. These results
identified impairments in balance and greater postural instability in MS group.
To verify the behavior of the upright standing position stability parameters in
individuals with little impairment, we constitute another MS group, with 12 subjects
who have BBS score ≥ 52 points. Table 3 shows the results of this new group.

Unlike what happened with the initial group of MS, when compared healthy
subjects with this restricted group of 12 MS subjects, there are no statistical
differences between BBS averages scores. However, the upright standing position
stability parameters of this new MS group continue to demonstrate a substantially
displacement than control group. The value for ellipse area is four times higher than
verified in healthy subjects. As expected we found that disease duration positively
correlated with age and impairments. There was a moderately negative correlation

Table 3 Results for MS group with BBS ≥ 52

	Subjects												
	1	2	3	4	5	6	7	8	9	10	11	12	M*
BBS	54	55	52	55	54	56	55	55	56	56	56	54	55
ML	4,0	3,3	2,7	2,7	2,0	6,7	3,0	3,3	1,7	6,3	2,3	3,3	3,4
AP	9,0	9,7	7,0	4,0	5,3	12	8,3	3,0	3,0	13	3,7	4,3	6,9
TD	99	88	114	88	87	108	117	113	84	106	91	94	99
EA	5,5	3,6	3,3	2,4	1,4	14	3,6	1,5	0,7	10	0,7	4,4	4,3

Values are the mean (M*) of 3 trials for 29 MS subjects and 28 healthy subjects in millimetres
ML Medio-lateral COP displacement, *TD* Total COP displacement, *AP* Anterior-posterior COP displacement, *EA* Ellipse area (mm2)

Table 4 Support phase of gait – results

	MS Subjects			
	ML	AP	TD	CT
Right foot	37,73	209,28	369,63	1,35
Left foot	35,45	215,37	370,91	1,35

	Healthy Subjects			
	ML	AP	TD	CT
Right foot	34,12	226,54	334,00	1,03
Left foot	29,08	228,26	342,36	1,01

Values are the mean of three trials for 29 MS subjects and 28 healthy subjects in millimetres
ML Medio-lateral COP displacement, *AP* Anterior-posterior COP displacement, *TD* Total COP displacement, *CT* Contact time (s)

between BBS and ML, AP, TD ($p < 0,05$), indicating that high values of BBS are associated with low values of ML, AP and TD. The ML displacement has strongly positive correlation with the AP displacement ($rs = 0.835$), EA ($rs = 0,763$) and also a positive moderate intensity with TD ($rs = 0,555$).

3.8 Support Phase of Gait

Results for plantar pressure assessments in support phase of gait (1-step protocol) are listed in Table 4. In 1-step protocol, ML, TD and CT values for both feet are higher compared to control group. In both groups (MS and healthy) the ML COP displacement for left foot is inferior than registered in right foot.

We also observed in MS group that the AP COP displacement is lower than they were assessed in the control group. This is because some subjects did not perform the initial contact with the heel but with metatarsal region. This difference in first contact area decreased the AP COP displacement, contrary to what would be expected. In total displacement we assisted to opposite behavior to that seen in ML parameter. For both groups (MS and healthy) the TD value is superior than registered in right foot. Another interesting finding is the result of CT value in MS group, is equal in both foot and superior to healthy group, more 31% in right foot and 33% in left foot. The disease duration has a positive correlation and moderate intensity with CT in both feet (rs = 0.472), indicating that the higher disease duration tend to be associated with higher CT. The BBS has a negative correlation and moderate intensity with the TD (rs = −0.585) indicating that high values of BBS tend to be related to low values of DT.

4 Discussion

The main aim of this study was to study if patients with multiple sclerosis, when in upright standing position and in the stance phase of gait, do have kinematics changes associated to COP when compared with a healthy group. To perform this study we compare plantar pressure assessment with a clinical test. The primary limitation of the investigation is related to the disease itself. Multiple sclerosis is a chronic, inflammatory autoimmune central nervous system, causing motor and sensory changes. The disease course is variable and is related to changes in the inflammatory process, causing changes in symptoms over time [27]. So it's very difficult to recruit subjects with the same characteristics and the same evolutionary stage of the disease. In this sense and in order to achieve the greatest number of subjects, we considered all patients with MS which satisfied the inclusion criteria, regardless the type and stage of MS evolution. Also, the study did not compare balance performance between subcategories of people with MS, such as those with spasticity, ataxia or sensory loss. These factors increased the group variability in the MS sample.

An important factor in data collection of plantar pressure is the test time. Test periods with short time may lead to results that aren't representative of postural stability. On the other hand long periods, in certain clinical situations, might influence the results due to increased fatigue. However it's necessary to establish what the optimum testing time, allowing the collection of data with confidence, without developing factors that may influence the results. A study with MS patients, to obtain the offset AP with eyes open and closed in upright standing position, used three trials with time 10 s [100]. The validity and confidence in gait assessment with plantar pressure in this population is unknown. There are however studies on plantar pressure in subjects with MS, who used a first step protocol [98, 101]. In our study, we used the same protocol based on the subject safety and to minimize any effects of fatigue. The analysis of test results in MS group shows that the variables are higher when compared to control group. In standing position an increase of ML is strongly correlated with increased AP, TD, and EA. In our study the statistical correlation between BBS and data obtained in the plate are not linear, showing large variations. BBS maintains the relationship with ML, AP and TD. A high value on BBS tends to be related to reduce values of ML, AP and TD. In 1-step protocol the correlation shows that a high value of BBS tends to be associated with a reduced value of the CT and TD, but with high value of AP. A major advantage of plantar pressure assessment is the ability to visualize the whole course of COP during foot contact. Thus it is possible to analyze and determine whether or not a stable support, and also visualize areas of the foot contact. This is particularly important when we are dealing with subjects with high scores in BBS. The relation between BBS and COP is more evident in standing position. There are situations in which BBS identifies increased instability, but tests on the plate indicate the maintenance of stability. Moreover, in some situations of maximum score in the BBS, this instrument is unable to detect the real situation of stability, because, as a compensatory response to postural instability, subjects can adopt a position or a more conservative gait pattern, to increasing security, reducing the risk of falls and reducing the variability of position and gait.

5   Conclusion

COP measures show clear differences when comparing healthy adults with adults with MS. The study found kinematics alterations on COP properties in all positions in multiple sclerosis group. As show, a clinical approach that usually tests postural stability (BBS) is ineffective in small postural disturbances. Specific and accurate analysis of postural stability in subjects with MS in upright standing position can be a useful tool to monitorize MS evolution and can be used to advise target oriented rehabilitative management of MS patients. Information obtained from pressure systems is also useful from a research perspective to address many questions regarding the relationship between plantar pressure and lower-extremity posture. The instrumented measures used here may be more sensitive than common clinical tests for objectively documenting both deficits and improvements in balance. With pressure technology becoming more common in physical therapy clinics, these parameters would be easy to capture as part of a physical therapy assessment. Because MS is a progressive disease, tools to measure balance impairments during early stages of the disease may lead to identification of people at risk for future decline. Specific and accurate analysis of postural stability in subjects with MS in upright standing position and support phase of gait can be a useful tool to monitorize MS evolution and can be used to advise target oriented rehabilitative management in these patients.

References

1. WHO (2006) Neurological disorders: public health challenges. World Health Organization, Library Cataloguing-in-Publication Data, Geneva
2. Rosati G (2001) The prevalence of multiple sclerosis in the world: an update. Neurol Sci 22(2):117–139

3. WHO (2008) Atlas multiple sclerosis resources in the world 2008. World Health Organization, Library Cataloguing-in-Publication Data, Geneva
4. Polman C, Thompson A, Murray T, Bowling A, Noseworthy J (2004) Multiple sclerosis: the guide to treatment and management, 6th edn. Demos Medical Publishing, New York
5. Murray J (2005) Multiple sclerosis: the history of a disease. Demos Medical Publishing, New York
6. Waxman S (2005) Multiple sclerosis as a neuronal disease. Elsevier, California
7. Burks J, Johnson K (2000) Multiple sclerosis, diagnosis, medical management and rehabilitation. Demos Medical Publishing, New York
8. Cattaneo D, De Nuzzo C, Teresa Fascia T, Macalli M, Pisoni I, Cardini R (2002) Risks of falls in subjects with multiple sclerosis. Arch Phys Med Rehabil 83:864–867
9. Burdet E, Tee KP, Mareels I, Milner TE, Chew CM, Franklin DW, Osu R, Kawato M (2006) Stability and motor adaptation in human arm movements. Biol Cybern 94(1):20–32
10. Abrantes J (2008) Fundamentos e Elementos de Análise em Biomecânica do Movimento Humano. MOVLAB. http://movlab.ulusofona.pt/cms/templates/movlab/files/publicacoes/2008%20Fundamentos%20e%20Elementos%20de%20An%C3%A1lise%20em%20Biomec%C3%A2nica%20do%20Movimento%20Humano.pdf. Accessed 12 Dec 2010 10h40
11. Abrantes J (2009) Estabilidade Articular na Tibiotársica - Adaptabilidade da rigidez dinâmica associada. Paper presented at the I Simposium Internacional de Biomecânica Y Podologia Deportiva. Sevilla-Spain; 5 e 6 Junio de 2009, Sevilla, Spain, 5 e 6 Junio de 2009
12. Doyle R, Hsiao-Wecksler E, Ragan B, Rosengren K (2007) Generalizability of center of pressure measures of quiet standing. Gait Posture 25(2):166–171
13. Goebel JA, Sataloff RT, Hanson JM, Nashner LM, Hirshout DS, Sokolow CC (1997) Posturographic evidence of nonorganic sway patterns in normal subjects, patients, and suspected malingerers. Otolaryngol Head Neck Surg 117(4):293–302
14. Doyle T, Newton R, Burnett A (2005) Reliability of traditional and fractal dimension measures of quiet stance center of pressure in young, healthy people. Arch Phys Med Rehabil 86:2034–2040
15. Rodrigues S, Montebelo M, Teodori R (2008) Plantar force distribution and pressure center oscillation in relation to the weight and positioning of school supplies and books in student's backpack. Rev Bras Fisioter 12(1):43–48
16. Willems T, Witvrouwa E, Delbaerea K, De Cockb A, De Clercqb D (2004) Relationship between gait biomechanics and inversion sprains: a prospective study of risk factors. Gait Posture 21(4):379–387, in press
17. Femery V, Moretto P, Renaut H, Thevenon A, Lensel G (2002) Measurement of plantar pressure distribution in hemiplegic children: changes to adaptative gait patterns in accordance with deficiency. Clin Biomech (Bristol, Avon) 17(5):406–413
18. Park E, Kim H, Park C, Rha D, e Park C (2006) Dynamic foot pressure measurements for assessing foot deformity in persons with spastic cerebral palsy. Arch Phys Med Rehabil 87(5):703–709
19. Robain G, Valentini F, Renard-Deniel S, Chennevelle JM, Piera JB (2006) A baropodometric parameter to analyze the gait of hemiparetic patients: the path of center of pressure. Ann Readapt Med Phys 49(8):609–613
20. Berg K, Wood-Dauphinee S, Williams J, Maki B (1992) Measuring balance in the elderly: validation of an instrument. Can J Public Health 83(Suppl 2):S7–11
21. McDonald W, Ron M (1999) Multiple sclerosis: the disease and its manifestations. Philos Trans R Soc Lond B Biol Sci 354(1390):1615–1622
22. Banwell B, Ghezzi A, Bar-Or A, Mikaeloff Y, Tardieu M (2007) Multiple sclerosis in children: clinical diagnosis, therapeutic strategies, and future directions. Lancet Neurol 6(10):887–902
23. Confavreux C, Vukusic S (2002) Natural history of multiple sclerosis: implications for counselling and therapy. Curr Opin Neurol 15(3):257–266
24. Finlayson ML, Peterson EW, Cho CC (2006) Risk factors for falling among people aged 45 to 90 years with multiple sclerosis. Arch Phys Med Rehabil 87(9):1274–1279, quiz 1287

25. Hayes CE, Acheson DE (2008) A unifying multiple sclerosis etiology linking virus infection, sunlight, and vitamin D, through viral interleukin-10. Med Hypotheses 71(1):85–90
26. Lunemann JD, Kamradt T, Martin R, Munz C (2007) Epstein-barr virus: environmental trigger of multiple sclerosis? J Virol 81(13):6777–6784
27. Breij EC, Brink BP, Veerhuis R, van den Berg C, Vloet R, Yan R, Dijkstra CD, van der Valk P, Bo L (2008) Homogeneity of active demyelinating lesions in established multiple sclerosis. Ann Neurol 63(1):16–25
28. Kelleher KJ, Spence W, Solomonidis S, Apatsidis D (2009) Ambulatory rehabilitation in multiple sclerosis. Disabil Rehabil 1–8
29. Kalb R (2007) The emotional and psychological impact of multiple sclerosis relapses. J Neurol Sci 256(Suppl 1):S29–33
30. Hirst C, Ingram G, Pearson O, Pickersgill T, Scolding N, Robertson N (2008) Contribution of relapses to disability in multiple sclerosis. J Neurol 255(2):280–287
31. Barak Y, Achiron A, Elizur A, Gabbay U, Noy S, Sarova-Pinhas I (1996) Sexual dysfunction in relapsing-remitting multiple sclerosis: magnetic resonance imaging, clinical, and psychological correlates. J Psychiatry Neurosci 21(4):255–258
32. Zivadinov R, Zorzon M, Locatelli L, Stival B, Monti F, Nasuelli D, Tommasi MA, Bratina A, Cazzato G (2003) Sexual dysfunction in multiple sclerosis: a MRI, neurophysiological and urodynamic study. J Neurol Sci 210(1–2):73–76
33. Johansson S, Ytterberg C, Hillert J, Widen Holmqvist L, von Koch L (2008) A longitudinal study of variations in and predictors of fatigue in multiple sclerosis. J Neurol Neurosurg Psychiatry 79(4):454–457
34. Sadiq SA, Poopatana CA (2007) Intrathecal baclofen and morphine in multiple sclerosis patients with severe pain and spasticity. J Neurol 254(10):1464–1465
35. Alusi SH, Glickman S, Aziz TZ, Bain PG (1999) Tremor in multiple sclerosis. J Neurol Neurosurg Psychiatry 66(2):131–134
36. Thoumie P, Lamotte D, Cantalloube S, Faucher M, Amarenco G (2005) Motor determinants of gait in 100 ambulatory patients with multiple sclerosis. Mult Scler 11:485–491
37. Mills RJ, Yap L, Young CA (2007) Treatment for ataxia in multiple sclerosis. Cochrane Database Syst Rev 2:1–15
38. Ienaga Y, Hiroshi Mitoma H, Kubota K, Morita S, Mizusawa H (2006) Dynamic imbalance in gait ataxia, characteristics of plantar pressure measurements. J Neurol Sci 246:53–57
39. Baker DG (2002) Multiple sclerosis and thermoregulatory dysfunction. J Appl Physiol 92(5):1779–1780
40. Confavreux C, Vukusic S, Moreau T, Adeleine P (2000) Relapses and progression of disability in multiple sclerosis. N Engl J Med 343(20):1430–1438
41. Pender MP (2004) The pathogenesis of primary progressive multiple sclerosis: antibody-mediated attack and no repair? J Clin Neurosci 11(7):689–692
42. McDonald W, Alistair Compston A, Edan G, Goodkin D, Hartung H, Lublin F, McFarland H, Paty D, Polman G, Reingold S, Sandberg-Wollheim M, Sibley W, Thompson A, Van den Noort S, Weinshenker B, Wolinsky J (2001) Recommended diagnostic criteria for multiple sclerosis: guidelines from the international panel on the diagnosis of multiple sclerosis. Ann Neurol 50:121–127
43. Palace J (2001) Making the diagnosis of multiple sclerosis. J Neurol Neurosurg Psychiatry 71(2):ii3–8
44. Chwastiak LA, Gibbons LE, Ehde DM, Sullivan M, Bowen JD, Bombardier CH, Kraft GH (2005) Fatigue and psychiatric illness in a large community sample of persons with multiple sclerosis. J Psychosom Res 59(5):291–298
45. Confavreux C, Vukusic S, Adeleine P (2003) Early clinical predictors and progression of irreversible disability in multiple sclerosis: an amnesic process. Brain 126(Pt 4):770–782
46. Miller DH, Leary SM (2007) Primary-progressive multiple sclerosis. Lancet Neurol 6(10):903–912
47. Dvir Z (2004) Isokinetics: muscle testing, interpretation and clinical applications. Churchill Livingstone, Edinburgh

48. Winter D (2005) Biomechanics and motor control of human movement, 3rd edn. Wiley, New York
49. Winter D (1995) Kinetics: our window into the goals and strategies of the central nervous system. Behav Brain Res 67(2):111–120
50. Winter D, Patla A, Ishac M, Gage W (2003) Motor mechanisms of balance during quiet standing. J Electromyogr Kinesiol 13(1):49–56
51. Abrantes J (2005) BIOMECÂNICA - Apontamentos de apoio às aulas teóricas. http://www.fmh.utl.pt/biomecanica/aponteoricos.pdf. Accessed 03 Dec 2010 18:56
52. Carpenter M, Frank J, Winter D, Peysar G (2001) Sampling duration effects on centre of pressure summary measures. Gait Posture 13(1):35–40
53. Tokuno C (2007) Neural control of standing posture. Karolinska Instituted, Stockholm
54. Gage W, Winter D, Frank J, Adkin A (2004) Kinematic and kinetic validity of the inverted pendulum model in quiet standing. Gait Posture 19(2):124–132
55. Winter D, Patla A, Prince F, Ishac M, Gielo-Perczak K (1998) Stiffness control of balance in quiet standing. J Neurophysiol 80(3):1211–1221
56. Doyle R, Dugan E, Humphries B, Newton R (2004) Discriminating between elderly and young using a fractal dimension analysis of centre of pressure. Int J Med Sci 1:11–20
57. Pascolo P, Barazza F, Carniel R (2006) Considerations on the application of the chaos paradigm to describe the postural sway. Chaos Soliton Fract 27(5):1339–1346
58. Karst GM, Venema DM, Roehrs TG, Tyler AE (2005) Center of pressure measures during standing tasks in minimally impaired persons with multiple sclerosis. J Neurol Phys Ther 29(4):170–180
59. Hallemans A, D'Aout K, De Clercq D, Aerts P (2003) Pressure distribution patterns under the feet of new walkers: the first two months of independent walking. Foot Ankle Int 24(5):444–453
60. Bisiaux M, Moretto P (2008) The effects of fatigue on plantar pressure distribution in walking. Gait & posture Article in press:6 pages
61. Orlin MN, McPoil TG (2000) Plantar pressure assessment. Phys Ther 80(4):399–409
62. Hagman F (2005) Can plantar pressure predict foot motion? Technische Universiteit Eindhoven, Eindhoven
63. Winter D (1991) Biomechanics and motor control of human gait: normal, elderly and pathological, 2nd edn. Wiley, New York
64. Nordin M, Frankel V (2001) Basic biomechanics of the musculoskeletal system, 3rd edn. Lippincott Williams & Wilkins, Baltimore
65. Collins J, De Luca C (1995) The effects of visual input on open-loop and closed-loop postural control mechanisms. Exp Brain Res 103(1):151–163
66. Rougier P (1999) Influence of visual feedback on successive control mechanisms in upright quiet stance in humans assessed by fractional Brownian motion modelling. Neurosci Lett 266(3):157–160
67. Newell KM, Slobounov SM, Slobounova ES, Molenaar PC (1997) Stochastic processes in postural center-of-pressure profiles. Exp Brain Res 113(1):158–164
68. Accardo A, Aìnito M, Carrozzi M, Bouquet F (1997) Use of the fractal dimension for the analysis of electroencephalographic time series. Biol Cybern 77:339–350
69. Recordati G, Bellini TG (2004) A definition of internal constancy and homeostasis in the context of non-equilibrium thermodynamics. Exp Physiol 89(1):27–38
70. Myklebust JB, Prieto T, Myklebust B (1995) Evaluation of nonlinear dynamics in postural steadiness time series. Ann Biomed Eng 23(6):711–719
71. Loram ID, Maganaris CN, Lakie M (2005) Human postural sway results from frequent, ballistic bias impulses by soleus and gastrocnemius. J Physiol 564(Pt 1):295–311
72. Morasso P, Baratto L, Capra R, Spada G (1999) Internal models in the control of posture. Neural Netw 12(7–8):1173–1180
73. Winter D (1995) Human balance and posture control during standing and walking. Gait Posture 3:193–214

74. Karlsson A, Lanshammar H (1997) Analysis of postural sway strategies using an inverted pendulum model and force plate data. Gait Posture 5(3):198–203
75. Winter D, Prince F, Patla A (1996) Interpretation of COM and COP balance control during quiet standing. Gait Posture 4(2):174–175
76. Blaszczyk JW (2008) Sway ratio - a new measure for quantifying postural stability. Acta Neurobiol Exp (Wars) 68(1):51–57
77. Blaszczyk OR, Duda-Klodowska D, Opala G (2007) Assessment of postural instability in patients with Parkinson's disease. Exp Brain Res 183(1):107–114
78. Latash ML, Ferreira SS, Wieczorek SA, Duarte M (2003) Movement sway: changes in postural sway during voluntary shifts of the center of pressure. Exp Brain Res 150(3):314–324
79. Blaszczyk KW (2001) Postural stability and fractal dynamics. Acta Neurobiol Exp (Wars) 61(2):105–112
80. Winter D, Patla A, Rietdyk S, Ishac M (2001) Ankle muscle stiffness in the control of balance during quiet standing. J Neurophysiol 85(6):2630–2633
81. Rietdyk S, Patla AE, Winter DA, Ishac MG, Little CE (1999) Balance recovery from medio-lateral perturbations of the upper body during standing. J Biomech 32(11):1149–1158
82. Morasso P, Schieppati M (1999) Can muscle stiffness alone stabilize upright standing? J Neurophysiol 82(3):1622–1626
83. Gatev P, Thomas S, Kepple T, Hallett M (1999) Feedforward ankle strategy of balance during quiet stance in adults. J Physiol 514(Pt 3):915–928
84. Loram ID, Lakie M (2002) Direct measurement of human ankle stiffness during quiet standing: the intrinsic mechanical stiffness is insufficient for stability. J Physiol 545(Pt 3): 1041–1053
85. Houdijk H, Doets H, Middelkoop M, Veeger H (2008) Joint stiffness of the ankle during walking after successful mobile-bearing total ankle replacement. Gait Posture 27:115–119
86. Chernikova L, Peressedova A, Zavahshin I (2005) Postural disturbances in multiple sclerosis. Gait Posture 21:S128–S129
87. Zabjek K, Hill S, Gage W, Danells C, Closson V, Maki B, McIlroy W (2005) Gait and standing posture in patients with multiple sclerosis. Gait Posture 21(Supplement 1):S136
88. Berg K, Wood-Dauphinee S, Williams J (1995) The balance scale: reliability assessment with elderly residents and patients with an acute stroke. Scand J Rehabil Med 27(1):27
89. Maki BE, Holliday PJ, Topper AK (1994) A prospective study of postural balance and risk of falling in an ambulatory and independent elderly population. J Gerontol 49(2):M72–84
90. Lord S, Wade D, Halligan P (1998) A comparison of two physiotherapy treatment approaches to improve walking in multiple sclerosis: a pilot randomized controlled study. Clin Rehabil 12(6):477
91. Cattaneo D, Jonsdottir J, Zocchi M, Regola A (2007) Effects of balance exercises on people with multiple sclerosis: a pilot study. Clin Rehabil 21(9):771
92. Smedal T, Lygren H, Myhr K, Moe-Nilssen R, Gjelsvik B, Gjelsvik O, Strand L (2006) Balance and gait improved in patients with MS after physiotherapy based on the Bobath concept. Physiother Res Int 11(2):104–116
93. Tyson S, Connell L (2009) How to measure balance activity in clinical practice? A systematic review of the psychometric properties and clinical utility of measurement tools in neurological conditions. Clin Rehabil 23(9):824–840
94. Bus S, Lange A (2005) A comparison of the 1-step, 2-step, and 3-step protocols for obtaining barefoot plantar pressure data in the diabetic neuropathic foot. Clin Biomech 20(9):892–899
95. Bus SA, de Lange A (2005) A comparison of the 1-step, 2-step, and 3-step protocols for obtaining barefoot plantar pressure data in the diabetic neuropathic foot. Clin Biomech (Bristol, Avon) 20(9):892–899
96. Wearing SC, Urry S, Smeathers JE, Battistutta D (1999) A comparison of gait initiation and termination methods for obtaining plantar foot pressures. Gait Posture 10(3):255–263
97. Peters EJ, Urukalo A, Fleischli JG, Lavery LA (2002) Reproducibility of gait analysis variables: one-step versus three-step method of data acquisition. J Foot Ankle Surg 41(4): 206–212

98. Miller CA, Verstraete MC (1996) Determination of the step duration of gait initiation using a mechanical energy analysis. J Biomech 29(9):1195–1199
99. Abdurakhmanov M, Stolyarov I, Il'vesa A, Tsvetkova T, Lebedev V (2006) Measuring the distribution of plantar pressures during walking in patients with multiple sclerosis to evaluate treatment efficiency. Hum Physiol 32(2):154–156
100. Tsvetkova T, Stoliarov I, Ivko O, Ilves A, Abdurahmanov M, Prakhova L, Nikiforova I, Lebedev V (2008) Dynamic plantar pressure distribution in multiple sclerosis patients with different neurological status. Clin Biomech//Abstr 23:662–720
101. Daley M, Swank R (1981) Quantitative posturography: use in multiple sclerosis. IEEE Trans Biomed Eng 28(9):668–671
102. Tsvetkova T, Stoliarov I, Ivko O, Ilves A, Abdurahmanov M, Prakhova L, Nikiforova I, Lebedev V (2008) Dynamic plantar pressure distribution in multiple sclerosis patients with different neurological status. Clin Biomech 23(5):691

Recent Progress in Studying the Human Foot

V.C. Pinto, M.A. Marques, and M.A.P. Vaz

Abstract This chapter has the objective of illustrate some of the work being done on human foot studies in the last years related to its structure and its influence on human locomotion, namely gait, as a mean of detecting physical or pathological problems. One of the aims of this work is to describe the experimental techniques available, some of them developed by the authors, and their fields of application. This description will start with a brief approach to gait characteristics as an introduction to the purpose of using the experimental techniques. First, experimental data acquisition and processing techniques are described, by indicating the type of available systems and then a brief literature review on the research developments on measuring plantar pressures and forces. At last, a section is dedicated to describe numerical techniques and methodologies used today in plantar forces analysis.

1 Introduction

Since primitive times, when Homo Australopithecus locomotion was supported on four limbs, natural evolution and morphological adaptation of the species related to the need for survival by grabbing food from high places for example, led to a gradual

V.C. Pinto (✉)
Institute of Mechanical Engineering and Industrial Management – University of Porto, Campus da FEUP, Rua Dr. Roberto Frias, 4200-432 Porto, Portugal
e-mail: vpinto@inegi.up.pt

M.A. Marques
Physics Department, School of Engineering – Polytechnic of Porto, Rua Dr. Antonio Bernardino de Almeida, 4200-072 Porto, Portugal

M.A.P. Vaz
LABIOMEP – Institute of Mechanical Engineering and Industrial Management – University of Porto, Rua Dr. Roberto Frias, 4200-432 Porto, Portugal

R.M.N. Jorge et al. (eds.), *Technologies for Medical Sciences*, Lecture Notes in Computational Vision and Biomechanics 1, DOI 10.1007/978-94-007-4068-6_10, © Springer Science+Business Media B.V. 2012

change in human locomotion tending to a vertical position supported mainly on two limbs – lower limbs. This transformation led to a derived species known as the "Homo Erectus" which still presented a big head and therefore a curved spine and long upper limbs, in spite of already showing some intelligence.

Nowadays, human species presents morphology very similar to Homo Sapiens Sapiens, where locomotion is definitely supported by lower limbs. It is undeniable that in our species, and since early stages of birth, the foot is the sole support of the human body, being therefore crucial for human balance. When children learn to walk, their balance is critical as the whole body is still adapting and perfecting to the new position according to body weight, height, physiology and bone structure. Therefore, as the body grows and turns into an adult, a good skeletal structure, associated to efficient muscles and good physiological conditions are necessary to prevent injuries resulting from external unforeseen loads or impacts on the human body.

In medicine, it is well known that diseases like peripheral neuropathy, diabetic neuropathy, osteoarthritis or rheumatoid arthritis, poliomyelitis, cerebrovascular accident, among others, or even a prolonged immobilization, can affect human locomotion, either by affecting different parts of the nervous system or the muscular system. Plantar force measurement is an important technique helping the physician or doctor performing a reliable diagnosis.

For example, for patients with peripheral or diabetic neuropathy, lower limbs sensitivity is reduced leading to an higher probability of developing ulcers. Using plantar pressure profile measurement during gait as a prevention method, abnormal high pressures will be detected, allowing for ulcer prevention [3]. This information also plays an important role in cases of musculoskeletal deformities or pathologies, like supination or pronation, flatfoot, since pressure distributions can help designing appropriate shoes or orthosis for normal people or people with impairments [11, 28]. By redistributing loads in the plantar surface, these hyper-pressures are acted upon and therefore an adequate gait profile can be achieved. Also, in cases of severe joint or bones malformations, a surgical procedure can be prepared taking into account this information [7]. On the other hand, not only the absolute values are important, but also the profile itself. In rehabilitation, plantar pressures measurements are used to assess the efficiency and adequacy of lower limbs prostheses or orthoses, or even to evaluate the results of an hip implant, by evaluating the changes in gait [38, 39].

Any abnormal gait profile allows identifying probable causes, instead of acting only on the consequence as stated before. In sports like long or high jumps, during training of high performance athletes, it is important to measure plantar pressures distributions mainly during the last support phase, just before propulsion, which will allow adjusting the athletes' performance to the shoes or pavement conditions, in order to achieve a better jump. Also, in fencing, shoes can affect the athletes' performance, due to fast movements and rapid changes in direction involved in this sport [19].

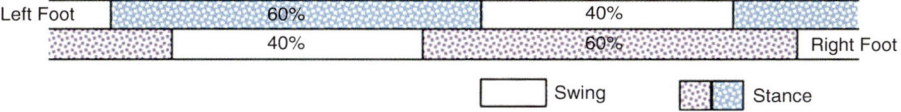

Fig. 1 Gait cycle division according to [47]

1.1 Characterization of Plantar Forces

Since gait is a common movement for all humans, gait analysis is an area of study transversal to several fields of study in the area of Biomechanics. Gait kinetics [42] and kinematics [41] have been extensively studied [37, 46]. Physical quantities like, acceleration, velocity, cadence, gait period, step and stride length, single stance and swing phase durations can be experimentally measured for a kinematical description of the movement. Others, like flexion and dorsiflexion angles, segment angular velocity, plantar pressures and reaction forces provide a more specific characterization related to the way the subject performs the movement. Therefore, temporal and spatial knowledge are two combined aspects of plantar forces characterization describing a certain movement.

A detailed description of the gait cycle can be found in both Winter et al. and Vaughan et al., who are cited extensively and their division of the gait cycle has been widely adopted as a reference. Both consider gait cycle divided in two phases: stance and swing phases as illustrated in Fig. 1. The differences between these two authors are quite small, since Winter considers a division of 60/40 [47] and Vaughan establishes a 62/38 gait phases division [46].

Considering standing position, for a normal foot, forefoot, rear foot (or heel) and lateral area are those in contact with the ground. Due to inter-subject variability, one can find a large variety of foot geometries being common in the forefoot to observe quite different contact areas under the toes. Nevertheless, the intensities of their pressures are very similar exhibiting peak values corresponding to a vertical force of 1.1–1.2 times Body Weight (BW).

During gait, the heel is the first body part to support body weight right after initial contact (IC). This phase occurs during the period of single stance starting with loading response with a maximum peak force occurring at around 25% of the gait cycle, at which the whole foot is in contact to the ground (midstance).

In kinematic terms, during initial contact the center of pressure accelerates until single stance, decreasing afterwards and regaining acceleration after heel rise (HR), corresponding to the terminal stance phase, which determines the beginning of the second double support phase. The period elapsed between these instants, i.e., between IC and HR, is around 50% of the gait cycle. This acceleration evolution is related to the magnitude of the horizontal anterior-posterior component of the ground reaction force (GRF). This description is generally accepted as a typical gait profile, in spite of substantial differences found between every individual pattern, as seen in literature.

In general, gait analysis is performed using force or pressure platforms to acquire kinetic data, namely ground reaction force information, which associated to video capture and inverse dynamic analysis will provide complete kinematical characterization [12]. Also, by introducing the movement recorded in video to a biomechanical model, it is possible to develop further biomechanical studies [33, 47].

2   Measurement of Plantar Forces

2.1   Commercially Available Systems

Every time the primary interest is measuring plantar forces for describing a certain movement, the first experimental technique chosen will be using a force platform. If, in addition, there is a need to characterize plantar pressure distribution, namely, in order to study the contact between the foot and the ground or shoe during stance phase, the common choice will be using pressure platforms or pressure insoles.

On the other hand, when choosing either platforms or insoles, measurement conditions will be the relevant factor. When using platforms, it is common to ask subjects to walk for a few minutes in order to warm-up, and also to adjust their steps and velocity to get the foot right into the middle of the platform. This preparation is considered to have some influence on the subject normal gait. If using insoles, this problem will not exist, since the patient can walk freely without worrying where to step on. The measurements can be taken anytime, and superfluous information can be disregarded. This system is of particular interest in the study of foot-shoe interaction, providing important information for orthoses design. Another advantage is the fact of being a portable system, which can be taken for outside studies or other type of movements, like running and dancing, for example. The negative aspect is that fact that due to in-shoe conditions like, humidity and temperature, these systems have a shorter lifetime.

Either force or pressure platforms or pressure insoles are commercially available. Some examples are Bertec Corporation, Kistler Corporation, AMTI-Advanced Mechanical Technology, Inc. force platforms, pedar®, footscan® and F-scan® pressure insoles and also pressure platforms solutions from novel, RSscan International, Tekscan® and Xsensor® Technology Corporation.

Force platforms provide Ground Reaction Force (GRF) measurement in terms of its components: medial-lateral, anterior-posterior and vertical. The latter represents the pressure exerted during contact in a certain instant. The other two components represent the in-plane force component, which is related to the lateral deviation and the direction or movement progression. The force components values are obtained with the signal from four sensors located at the four corners of the platform, by measuring their local deformations. With these instantaneous signals, the system calculates the three force components F_x, F_y and F_z, and the three torques M_z,

M_x and M_y. Since at every instant, the actual foot plantar area in contact with the platform surface varies, the signal obtained is an overall response of the deformation. These force and torque are averaged values related to the instantaneous area of contact. Even though, force platforms represent the only commercially available system capable of measuring the complete GRF vector

Using pressure insoles or platforms, the type of information obtained is different. These can map the pressure distributed in the whole plantar surface, which is of great relevance when the main purpose is the foot instead of the movement itself. Depending on the model and manufacturer, these systems can have a spatial resolution varying between 1 cm [pedar®] and 1 mm [Xsensor®], which determines the plantar pressure mapping discreteness. Commercially available platforms have always a better resolution than insoles. This mapping provides a more detailed picture on the evolution of the force distribution for each area in contact at every moment, instead of an overall value as with the force platforms. Nevertheless, the drawback is the fact of measuring only the GRF vertical component. This aspect associated to the difficulty of developing a system or sensor capable of measuring the three plantar force components, simultaneously and locally, either inshoe or on the floor surfaces, have been subject of research for several decades.

In his revision work on sensors to measure plantar pressures [45], Stephen Urry refers that, considering the various attempts to measure shear plantar forces and the difficulties and limiting factors encountered by researchers, this task is an even more exigent and time consuming than pressure measurement. One interesting point of view of this author is that the optimum sensor is not the one with the best performance and technological characteristics in the point of view of engineers, but the one adjusting the best to the purpose for which it was developed, i.e., taking into account the application and its limitation is as important as developing a sensor with outstanding technical characteristics. Therefore the optimal solution is a natural commitment between these two aspects.

To measure horizontal or shear plantar force components, sensor measurement range should be chosen to represent between 20% and 26% the body weight, since according to Lebar et al., this is the expected magnitude for these components [25].

2.2 Research Developments

2.2.1 Measuring Plantar Pressures

In research, the first instrumented shoe, identified by the authors as "CyberShoe" [35], was a prototype incorporating a variety of different sensors, allowing the measurement of angular velocities with gyroscopes, accelerations with accelerometers, pressures in pre-determined areas using piezoresistive sensors and contact instants with piezoelectric sensors. This prototype was developed with a broader concept since it was designed to be applied in dancers in order to follow their steps and movements and correlate this information with the music played.

Fig. 2 An example of a
pedobarograph system

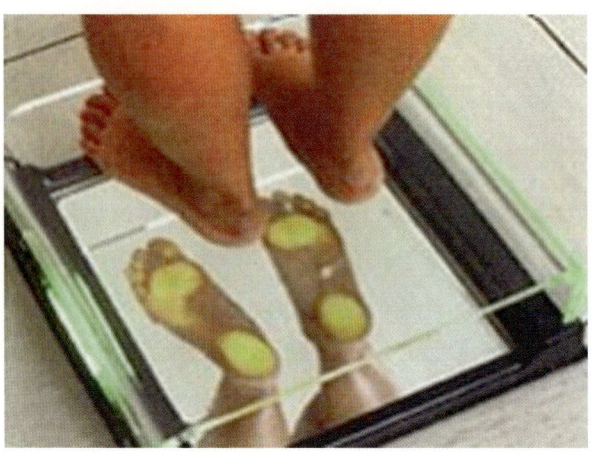

It is interesting to follow the evolution suffered with plantar pressure measurement techniques. According to J. Stott et al., one of the first registered attempts consisted on printing the foot depression in a cast mould. With this technique, the information provided was obviously static and related to the foot profile. The pressures were determined by the depth of the printed foot profile [40]. Since then, several approaches have been developed and systems with different operational principles have been implemented. The podoscope is, what we could considered, a previous and simplified version of the plantar pressures platform, since it provided a qualitative and comparative measure of the pressure distribution in the plantar surface static images projected on a mirror. This technique also evolved, and at present, the dynamic al version of these systems is called pedobarograph (Fig. 2), since being instrumented with load cells, measurement of observed pressures is possible.

A different optical technique proposed by Hughes et al. used optical interferometry by developing a platform composed by a PMMA layer (due to its optical transparency and being a slightly deformable material as a result of applied forces) together with a CCD camera to determine the changes in the interference pattern due to the applied plantar pressure [22]. As stated by the authors, this system presents a good resolution of 70 pixels/cm^2, when compared to novel$^®$ system having 4 sensors/cm^2.

A different approach developed by Zhu et al. [49] uses Force Sensitive Resistors, FSR's as the key element to measure pressure in seven foot areas, chosen previously as those showing higher vertical loads.

Another approach consisted on developing a micro-transducer based on a piezoelectric thin film of PVDF (polivinilidene fluoride) with dimensions from *25 μm^2 to 4 cm^2*. This micro-transducer could be used as the sensing element in the fabrication of force or pressure platforms [17, 50].

The presented approaches aim to illustrate just different operating principles for plantar pressure measurements, since this type of data can be obtained from commercial available solutions as described before.

2.2.2   Measuring Plantar Shear Forces

In an attempt to achieve tridimensional characterization of local plantar surface force distribution, allowing mapping the three plantar force components, as achieved with pressure insoles for the vertical component, several authors developed different approaches.

In 1980, Tappin et al. presented a centre-tapped magneto resistor in a bridge configuration with a magnet placed centrally above it, to measure shear forces under the toe and metatarsals heads. In this solution, any lateral movement of the magnet will unbalance the bridge, thus generating a signal proportional to the magnet movement which, in, is proportional to the shear force responsible for that movement [43]. With this solution they measure these forces in barefoot subjects as well as a variety of footwear to test their effect in modifying and redistributing shear forces.

One symptomatic aspect related to the intrinsic and major difficulty of measuring plantar shear forces is the fact that, more than a decade after this work, in 1992, other authors using also magneto-resistor devices, developed different approaches for the same purpose [24, 29]. When looking for different approaches in plantar shear force measurement, one can find the solution proposed and validated by Lebar et al., using optoelectronic devices consisting on a photodiode and a surface mounted LED of 660 nm emission wavelength, both mounted on a shell mainly composed by an upper and lower component where the light emitter-receiver set is located [26]. The sensor has a diameter of 15 mm by 3.8 mm thick, weighting 0.85 g. Also, in 1998, Davis et al. developed what could be thought of as a small platform consisting on 4×4 sensor matrix measuring the shear component, covering a total area of 10.5×10.5 cm2 [14]. Each sensor is an aluminum cylinder on top of which one can find an S-shaped load cell with strain-gages which measure the deformation suffered by the load cell faces, as a result of the shear force due to foot movement. This may be one of the first well succeeded attempts of designing a 3D plantar force mapping platform. The authors recognized that their solution was not appropriate for inshoe measurements, thus the acquired data will always represent the force between the shoe and the floor surface.

In an overall look at the temporal development published on this subject, it appears that two techniques are popular: optical and magneto-resistive sensor techniques.

Indeed, in 2000, Hosein et al. presented a bi-axial magneto resistive sensor, together with the F-scan® insoles for the vertical component measurement, characterizing completely the three plantar vector force components in five plantar areas: four underneath the metatarsals heads and the fifth under the calcaneous (heel) [21]. As for optical techniques, Koulaxouzidis et al. developed the first optical sensor based on Fiber Bragg Grating (FBG) disposed in three directions constituting a

3-axis referential [23]. Due to the use of Bragg gratings, they could measure the in-plane (or horizontal force component) in the direction of each fiber. Unfortunately, these authors did not present any results related to the application of this sensor on the measurement of plantar forces.

Perhaps the two most well sustained, tested and validated solutions were proposed by Razian et al. and Faivre et al. The first developed what they called "*The Kent in-shoe system*" since it was developed at Kent University. Each sensor consisted on a layer of a piezoelectric copolymer of 500 μm thick, in contact with three layers of double-faced printed circuit boards, constituting the electrode connections necessary to obtain the electrical signal representing the three orthogonal force components. These authors tested and validate their approach, by incorporating four sensors in an insole, which in turn was used introduced in a shoe and used for gait locomotion of a non-pathological individual [36]. The four locations were chosen as those showing an intensity peak in the vertical component [49]. The solution by Faivre et al. used dynamometric rings together with strain-gages in the outer surfaces. The ring deformation is transmitted to the strain-gauge [16]. These authors also validated their sensors by developing a shoe with eight holes to accommodate the sensors. The regions to position the sensors were chosen in accordance to several authors [3, 34] as being those where the information obtained could have more significance.

Finally, in 2008, Marques et al. [30] developed an in-plane sensor based on piezoelectric devices, which is patented [32], whose main purpose was measuring plantar shear force components, even though the vertical component was also measured. This approach represents a novelty, since it's the first approach where all the sensing elements are distributed in the same plane. The sensor consisted on three piezoelectric ceramic elements, with in-plane polarization, distributed around a central point, with an angular separation of 120°. In the central point, a small piezoelectric film was placed to measure the vertical force component. The complete assembly was about 25 mm diameter and 4 mm thickness, with an average weight of 2.5 gf. The combination of the three ceramic elements electrical signals will provide information about F_x and F_y components, these being the medio-lateral and the anterior-posterior components, respectively. Another output alternative was to combine the signals to get the intensity and direction of the in-plane horizontal force. Its resolution is about 0.3 N for the force and 10° for the angular direction. Also, it showed 10% linearity for the force and 3% for the direction angle. This sensor was also characterized in terms of frequency and temperature, since piezoelectric materials are also pyroelectric (i.e., output electrical signal depends on temperature), showing a negligible dependence in both parameters. To validate this sensor, authors designed a shoe (Fig. 3) to accommodate the sensor in three different locations: underneath the 1st-2nd metatarsal heads, the 3rd-5th metatarsal heads and under the hallux. These regions are known to be those presenting higher intensities with the exception of the heel [50].

The proposed integration solution presented one disadvantage. As the sensor's main purpose was measuring the in-plane force, and since the geometry has to allow for this type of measurement, these two factors resulted in the need of a previous

Fig. 3 Shoe design to integrate the sensors for in-plane plantar vector force measurement [30]

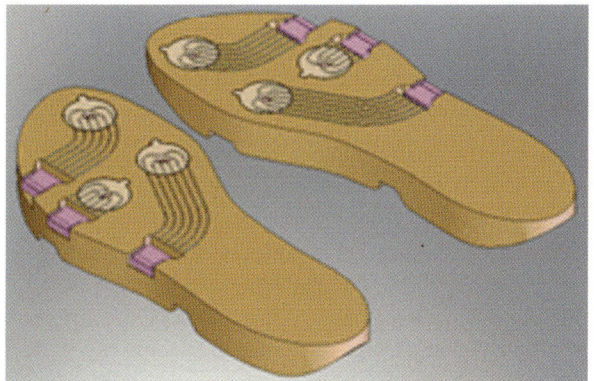

in-place calibration. The calibration was achieved using an indirect methodology, with the help of a force platform. Comparing the results from these two techniques, one gets a procedure where the sensor is previously calibrated. Only after this step, the system is ready for any kind of plantar force measurements. In the gait analyses conducted, obtained results were in agreement with those published by Hosein et al., showing a peak value in the anterior-posterior component, happening about 22%- of the gait cycle (e.g. 40% single contact phase) with a forward direction and another at about 50%–55% of gait cycle in the backward direction [21].

Therefore, during normal gait, these results show that when the foot contacts the ground, apart from the well-known plantar pressure profile, one can state that anterior-posterior component first increases in the forward direction at about 60° towards lateral direction (or left for the right foot), while decreasing during total contact and increasing afterwards until reaching a peak in the posterior direction, at about 240°.

One interesting application of the GRF information obtained with force platforms is the work developed by Burnfield et al. With the vertical and in-plane (or shear) components, these authors defined a coefficient CoF_u – "utilized" Coefficient of Friction – calculated as a ratio between the shear and vertical components, which is used to determine a risk factor to classify the friction coefficient in order to define a probability of falling by losing adherence [5]. This type of study can also be used in the choice of materials for pavement design namely in public or exterior areas [8].

If the sensing elements or matrix are positioned inside the shoe, the knowledge can be used to study the insole or shoe sole materials causing a better force distribution and hence giving the sensation of best comfort. This approach will be very interesting for shoe industry. At present, this aspect is overcome by introducing orthoses in the shoe, which results in an effective way of reducing abnormal pressures [6, 15, 28], although, as shown by Hennig et al., the design and the fabrication process are the major factors responsible for the pressures observed in the foot. Even though, only a medical study on the occurrence of injuries related to the use of sportive shoes will enable a better understanding of the relevant factors [20]. From an opposite side of view of comfort shoes, there are the high heel shoes, which were confirmed by Yung et al., as being those which would profit a lot from orthoses, since due to their design, they shift the center of pressure during gait to the forefoot, apart from showing hyper pressures [48].

3 Techniques for Plantar Forces Analysis

As explained before, when analyzing gait, a variety of factors have to be accounted for due to alteration on gait pattern or plantar forces, like body weight and height, gait characteristics, foot geometry and deformities, patient tissues physiological conditions, pathologies and others. In the case of diabetic patients, one can predict the areas where ulcers will most probably be developed. It is known that shear forces act as enablers in the weakening of plantar surface tissues, being more critical during heel contact and during stance final phase, namely right before toe-off, than during mid stance. Since GRF horizontal in-plane component is greater in these time instants, the corresponding contact areas, namely under the calcanous and under the metatarsal heads, are regions of major ulceration for a patient with diabetes. To reduce the ulceration risk it is to use orthoses that allows redistributing plantar forces into superior areas, since better foot accommodation reduces relative movement between the two contact surfaces, decreasing shear stress.

With availability of new tools and technologies, it has become recent practice to use CT images to obtain 3D computer body models. These models lead to realistic simulation results and by associating them with experimental values is possible to determine body internal stress and strains and predict their influence in the individual comfort, namely by designing foot orthoses [27]. Geometry is a key factor when studying strain, stress and plantar shear forces therefore any simulation has to be well controlled and defined process. With geometrically well defined anatomical structures, namely for the foot, it is possible to simulate all types of situations affecting gait and stability of an obese patient, for example.

Nowadays there are many tools to create 3D anatomical model, some of them will be explain in the next sections of this chapter. Nevertheless and in what concerns the foot, the major difficulty is to obtain CT scans where the foot is in positions usable for certain simulation studies, since the majority of CT scans are done with the person lying down, leading to foot relative position being quite different from adequate positioning for gait studies, for example.

3.1 Scanning 3D Objects

With a 3D scanner is possible to obtain and analyze a real object, in respect to its shape and appearance, in a static or dynamic way. This collects data that can be used to construct three dimensional models useful for several applications like industrial design and inspection, orthotics and prosthetics, reverse engineering and prototyping (Fig. 4), structures quality control and documentation of cultural artifacts [2].

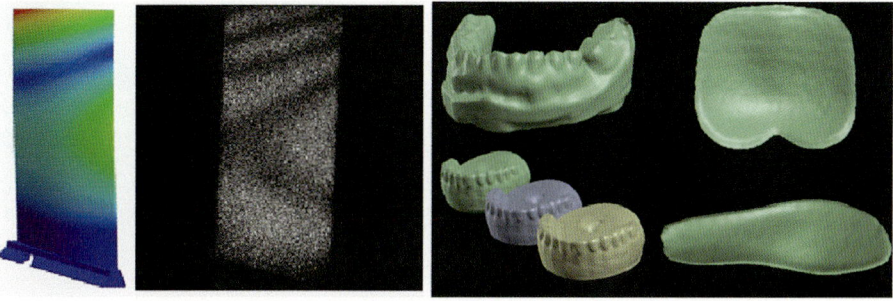

Fig. 4 Experimental techniques at LOME/INEGI (*left*) reverse engineering with 3D scanning [44]; (*right*) 3D scans

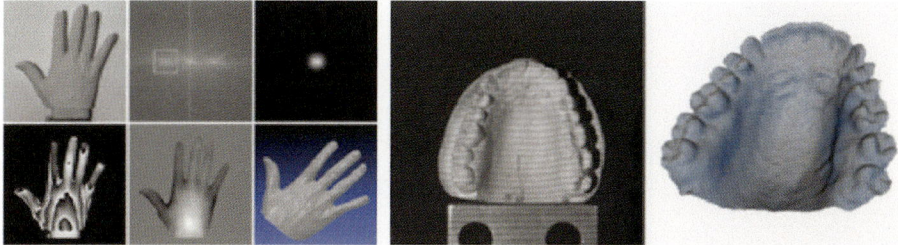

Fig. 5 Objects, models and techniques available at LOME/INEGI

3D scanner methodology is used to create a point cloud of geometric samples on the object surface, resulting in a very dense and accurate point set [13]. These points will be used in the reconstruction of the object (Fig. 4), by extrapolating its shape and the result can be several types of models depending on how reconstruction occurs and for which application it is. Point cloud files are used in CAD models (Solidworks®, CATIA®), polygon mesh models are used for visualization with reconstruction software (MeshLab®, Photomodeler®, Rapidform®), surface models, which are editable, have the advantage of being lighter and more adaptable when exported to CAD (Rapidform®, Geomagic®, Rhino®), solid CAD models, also editable, are used in industry and engineering applications, with special relevance on part design, allowing modelers to create not only the CAD model but also shape and design of the 3D object (Geomagic®, Imageware®, Rhino®).

At Optics and Experimental Mechanics Laboratory (LOME)/Institute of Mechanical Engineering and Industrial Management (INEGI) at Porto, 3D scanning techniques, like photogrammetry and digital videogrammetry, based on different optical techniques, such as coherent light, Moiré pattern, laser stripes, holography and others, are been used (Fig. 5). Two of these techniques are illustrated in Fig. 6. The first, Coherent Fringe Projector, consists on a camera and a projector accommodated in a flexible cart-like structure which can move around and enables 3D acquisition of rather large objects based on phase measurement profilometry

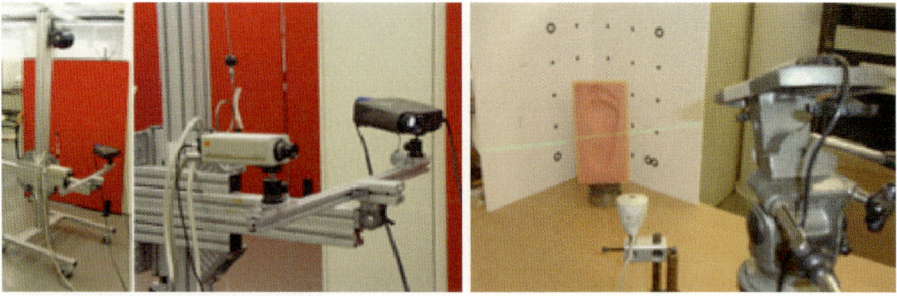

Fig. 6 (*left*) Coherent fringe projector and (*right*) simple set up for 3D scanning of plantar impression

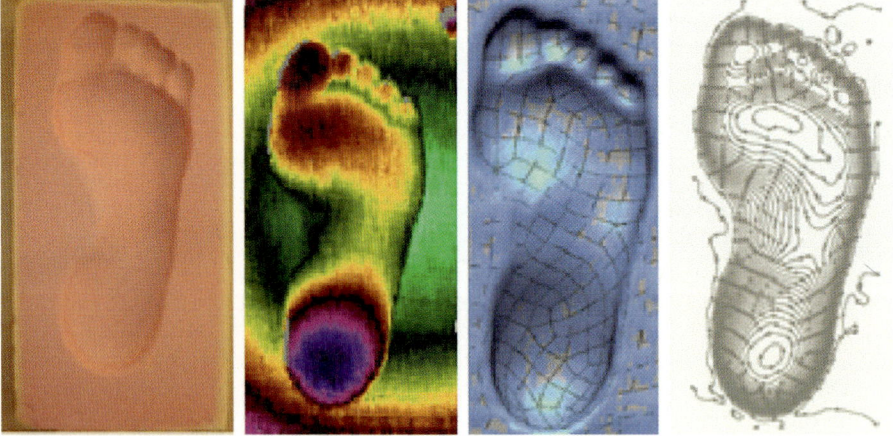

Fig. 7 Results from methodology used to study plantar topography population: (from *left* to *right*) sponge with plantar impression, 3D scanning that leads to 3D models and 3D models analysis

[44]. The second (right), also shows a set-up including a camera, a laser and the target. This system has appropriate modeling reconstruction software to obtain plantar impression geometry with laser stripes.

By creating a point cloud taken from foot impression, it is possible to have a functional plantar impression 3D model, which was used, for example, to characterize plantar topography with the purpose of creating a database of obese population in Portugal, during 2009 and 2010. With the help of reverse engineering, having 3D foot CAD models, one can analyze strain and stress with finite element methodologies (Fig. 7) and determine simple prototype solutions to improve comfort for each population subject [4].

It is also possible to have real-time 3D scanning with some of the same optical techniques, but for now, the hard work in real-time it is to fuse images from different sides of the object to reconstruct the 3D model.

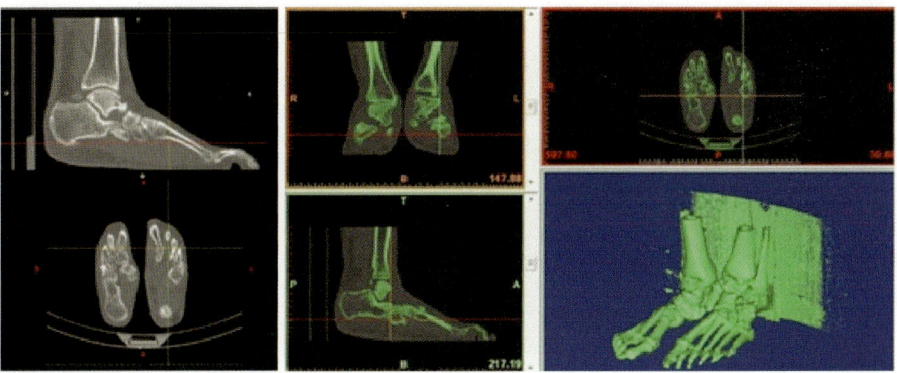

Fig. 8 CT from an individual feet and software Mimics®

3.2 3D Foot Models

In the attempt to find and develop a reliable and efficient method to build 3D anatomical structures for reverse engineering, a methodology including the use of different interconnected software, was validated. It consists on using medical imaging files to develop the 3D model, using design software, for Finite Element Method (FEM) simulation, making possible to obtain a 3D foot model of each individual. There are similar methodology studies, starting from CT scans and using CAD software (CATIA®) to develop a model ready to be tested on FEM simulation (Abaqus®) in order to find either, strain and stress on the foot, or to see stress differences considering specific tendons and muscles or even stress for different foot positioning for 2D and 3D foot models [1, 9, 10, 18, 31].

These studies showed it is possible to take a file from medical images, CT, MRI or even Micro-CT scanner, even though the latter aren't point clouds but rather a set of 2D slices which are unified to produce a 3D representation. During a subject CT or MRI exam, it is important that each foot is in the position adequate for the study objective, allowing for original tissue assembly and avoiding wrong 3D objects manipulation. For example, to study the foot evolution during gait, which is obviously done in the standing-up position, when doing a CT scan, and because this medical exam is done lying-down in a table, it is important to have the patient feet vertically aligned as they would be in the focused movement. As a curiosity, for high heels studies subject's feet must have the calcaneous slightly raised.

Using software like Mimics®, and taking patient feet medical images (DICOM files) it is possible to get a single file with the corresponding point clouds, according to tissue density (Fig. 8). Therefore, one can get 3D objects corresponding to bones, with or without cartilage, and soft tissues, with or without differentiating muscles tissue, fat tissue, skin tissue, using density segmentation techniques related to the different masks provided by the software (Fig. 9).

For our study mesh clouds were divided into two groups: bone structure (that includes bones and cartilage) and soft tissue. They were then exported as STL files,

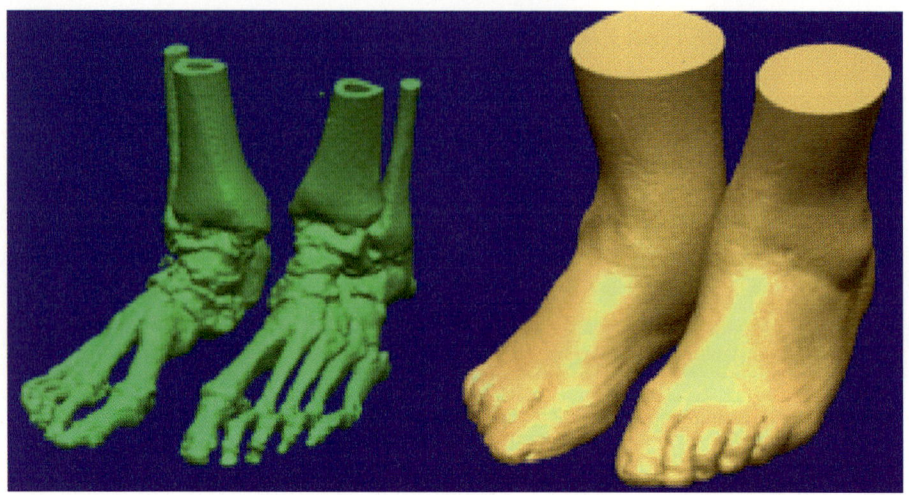

Fig. 9 Bone structure and soft tissues from CT by Mimics® for obese individual

to a CAD software, like Solidworks®,CATIA® or Rapidform®, being afterwards edited and improved, resulting in a solid part for each 3D object. Since foot bone structure is complex, being difficult for the software to generate surfaces along all the structure, it is necessary to divide anatomically the bone structure into five pieces: tibia and fibula; calcaneous and talus; cuboid, cuneiforms and navicular; metatarsals and phalanges, separately. A solid part for all these individual objects is generated (Fig. 10). Finally, by combining them, results in a unified bone structure, which was assembled together with the soft tissue and a rigid support under the foot whose purpose was to simulate the ground (Fig. 11).

3.3 Numerical Simulation: Finite Element Method Analysis

Some experimental methods already described in this chapter for pressure, stress and strain foot analysis, acquire these values using different sensing systems or matrices. FEM processes and calculates these parameters, or other mechanical material characteristic, by solving mathematical equations applied to a model. Therefore, this method works better when every dependent factor is defined the most realistic possible. Geometry is the key factor for a better performance, so it is necessary to have a 3D foot model most approximated to the real model, attending to foot-ground positioning, foot position during CT, geometry adjustments during foot assembly, human tissue properties and others.

After constructing the 3D foot model, reverse engineering is possible, enabling biomechanical analysis in every anatomic structure defined: strain, internal stress,

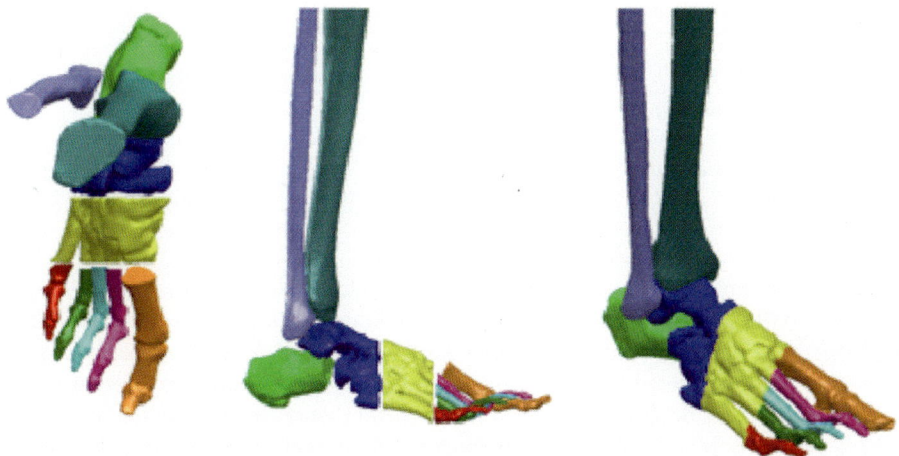

Fig. 10 Solid parts of bone structure and soft tissue part

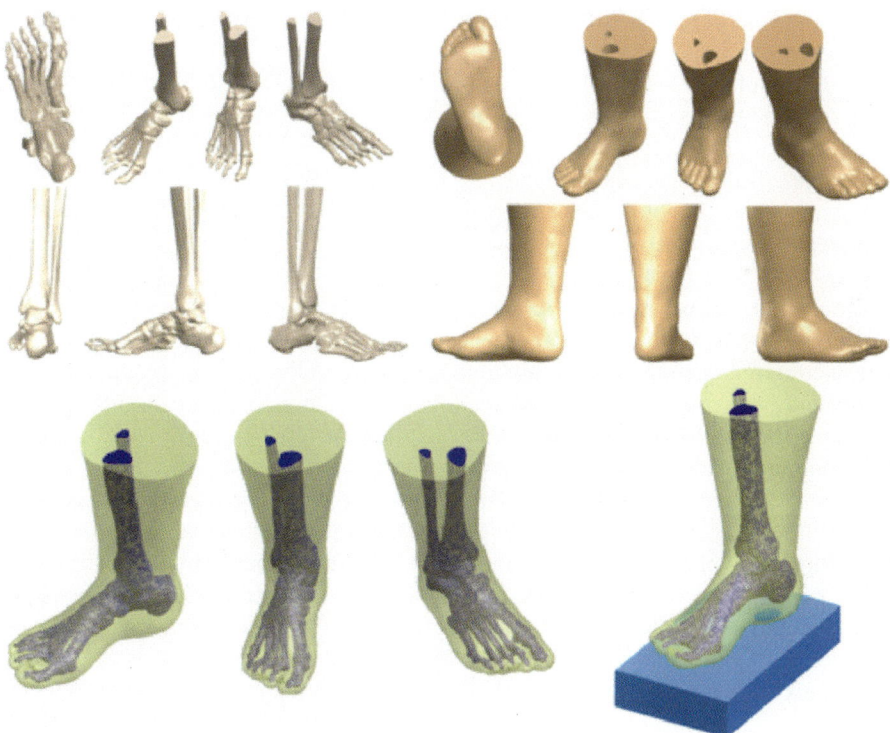

Fig. 11 Bone structure and soft tissue parts in solidworks® and final assembly

Table 1 Mechanical properties of human tissue

	Young's modulus (MPa)	Poisson coeficient	Elements
Bone structure	7,300	0.3	3D tetrahedrics
Soft tissue	0.15	0.45	3D tetrahedrics
Plantar fascia tendons	350	–	3D tetrahedrics
Ground	2.10×10^5	0.3	quadrilaterals

plantar shear stress, plantar pressure, displacement, etc. In order to achieve it, 3D foot model file is exported to FEM analysis software, like Ansys® or Abaqus®, for example. The next step before simulating is to choose static or flexible dynamics simulation, either related to static or non-static conditions, enabling different kinds of foot movements or activities. It is possible to simulate just standing foot position, where feet are in pure compression (balanced standing position), or one can analyse different gait phases instances separately, knowing which foot parts are in contact with ground. The results obtained in each simulation must be looked at, in order to search for foot areas most affected during gait or run, i.e., search for plantar pressure maximum peaks or shear stress maximum peaks, which are aspects of most concern in this context.

FEM simulation starts with the definition of initial conditions, bonding conditions, applied forces or loads and supports. In the case of the foot, it was defined that bone structure and soft tissues were bonded in the corresponding contact surfaces and edges. Soft tissue and ground can have three types of bonding conditions: frictional, bonded or no contact, depending on the simulation goal. Also, there is the need to apply different initial contact conditions according to the chosen contact areas.

The FEM software allows completing the 3D foot model with tendons or ligaments, by adding springs to the bone structure in the plantar fascia or in calcaneous, representing Achilles tendon, extensor tendons, flexor tendon, peroneus tertius and longus, plantar fascia tendons and others. As human tissues have nonlinear behaviour and variable mechanical characteristics, in order to simplify this computational procedure tissue extrapolation was done. Muscles, fat tissue, and skin were consider soft tissue, and also no bone constitutes distinction was done for trabecular and cortical bone, therefore estimating their mechanical properties, such as Young's modulus and Possion's ratio [31]. In addition, bone structure, soft tissue and tendons were considered to be linearly elastic, isotropic and homogeneous [9]. These values are shown in Table 1. Soft tissue can also be defined as having an hyperelastic behaviour which is closer to reality [1].

For each 3D model a mesh is built, dividing the model into elements, depending on model complexity, enabling mechanical study. These elements are also defined in Table 1. As an example, Fig. 12 shows a model which, due to its complexity, the generated mesh has more than 173,300 nodes and 97,700 elements, using 3D tetrahedral elements.

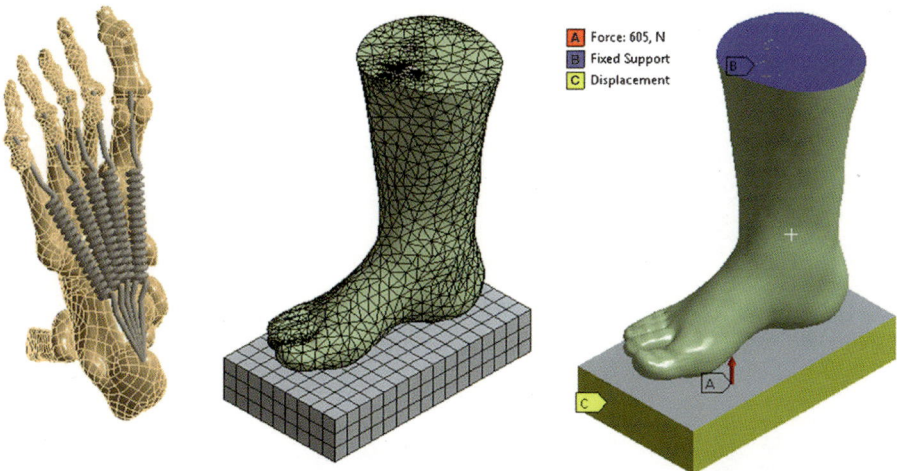

Fig. 12 Mesh of the assembly: springs simulating tendons on the plantar fascia, mesh model and set up model in Ansys®

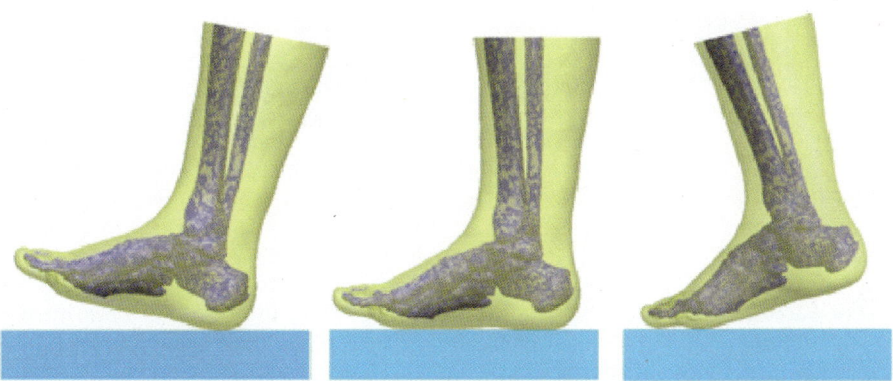

Fig. 13 3D foot model for three gait stages

When setting-up the simulation, the objective pursued determines the movement restrictions. For instance, when studying effects of ground reaction force in order to evaluate plantar foot damage related to body weight, a vertical restrain is imposed to the ground body which is considered rigid with no longitudinal expansion, tibia and fibula are fixated and force is applied vertically on the ground surface, perpendicularly to the foot (Fig. 12).

For different movements, assemblies, mesh and set up for simulations are different. Figure 13 shows an example of a FEM static simulation for different gait stance phase stages.

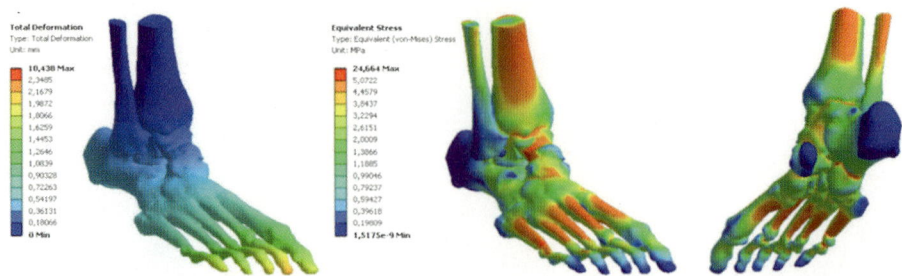

Fig. 14 Bone structure stress distribution and displacement for an healthy foot in the standing position

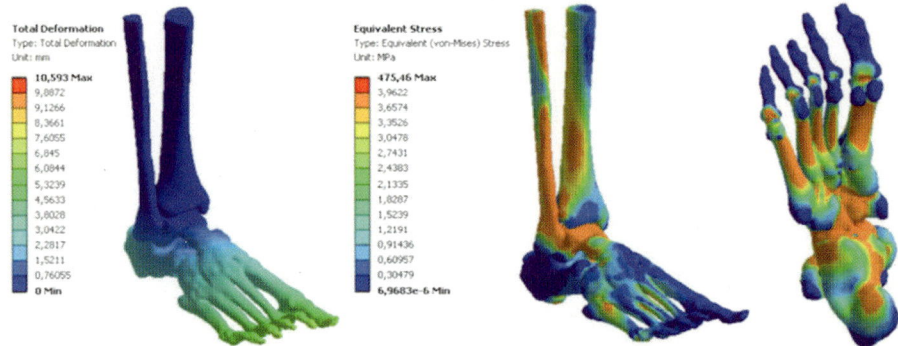

Fig. 15 Bone structure stress distribution (equivalent von Mises stress) for an obese foot for standing position

For each gait stage, contacts will change according to how foot areas hit the ground. Three gait cycle stance phase stages were simulated: heel contact (HC), midstance (MS) and toe off (TO). For this, it is necessary to build either three 3D models, one for each foot-ground contact position and corresponding three FEM simulations if a static structural simulation is conducted, or only one model if flexible dynamic simulation is chosen. In the situation illustrated in Fig. 13, the choice was a static structural simulation by analysing each gait stage chosen. For midstance stage, it is possible to assume the foot is in pure compression just like in standing position. Simulation results can be foot displacements, internal stress distributions in bone structure, which are most interesting indicators to search for healthy feet solutions (Fig. 14).

These results were compared with similar simulation for an obese foot. In this case, apart from bone structure internal stresses, plantar pressure and soft tissues displacements were studied (Figs. 15–18).

The knowledge and data obtained from these techniques are very important in identifying critical foot areas, which will be relevant in the design and construction of an orthosis in order to minimize plantar pressure, decreasing discomfort.

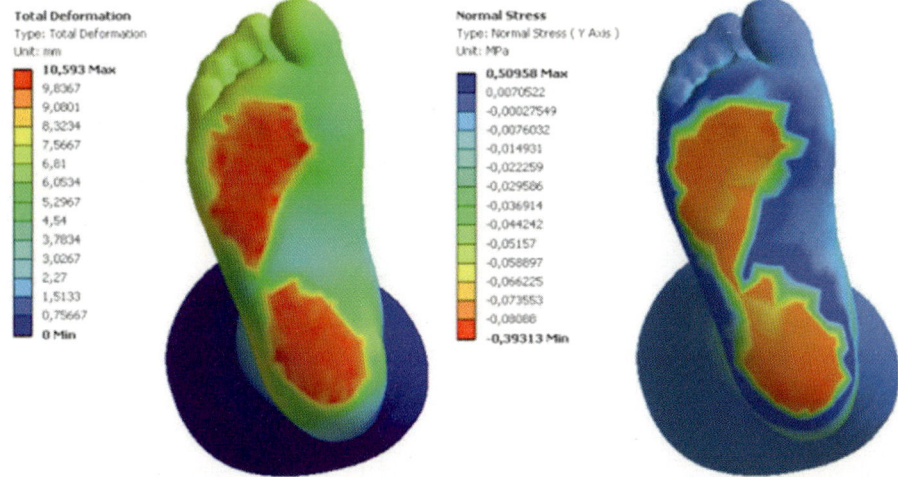

Fig. 16 Displacement and plantar pressure for an obese foot for midstance position

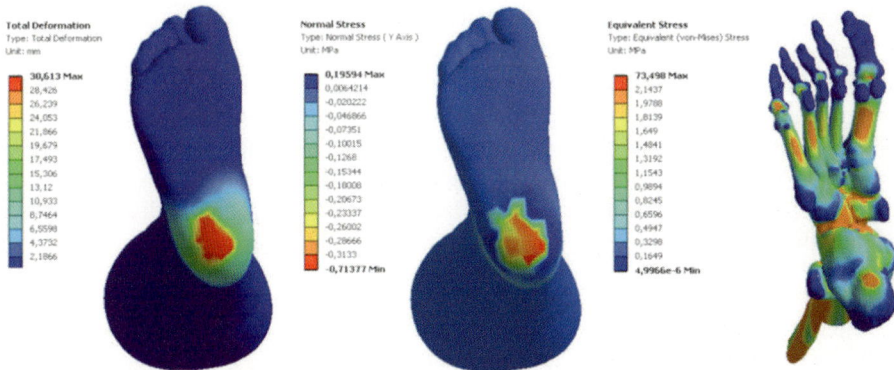

Fig. 17 Displacement, internal stress and plantar pressure for an obese foot for heel contact position

4   Conclusion

Human foot is a complex structure with 26 bones like metatarsals and calcaneous, tendons, such as well known Achilles tendon, which rupture can cause pain and locomotion difficulties. There are also muscles and ligaments that are essential to gait like ligaments from plantar fascia and fat tissue, which is a matter issue on today's fat pad discussion.

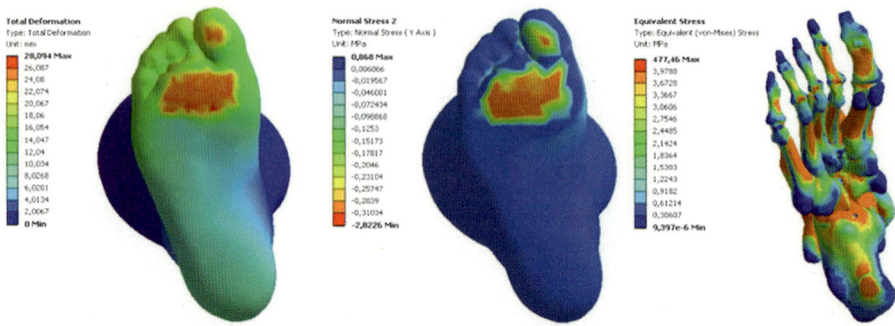

Fig. 18 Displacement, internal stress and plantar pressure for an obese foot for toe-off position

Locomotion and support are feet primarily functions, being important their analysis and study. This can be accomplished by studying data obtained from force and pressure platforms, pressure insoles, computational processes associated with mechanical methods, revealing information on pressure, strain, stress, ground reaction force and other important parameters allowing a complete study of foot dynamics. Some of aspects were illustrated in the previous sections.

Nowadays Sports, Orthopedics, Rehabilitation Medicine, Podology and Biomechanics, amongst others, are foot interventional areas looking to improve measurement, methods and systems. As shown, experimental data taken from force platforms can be integrated as load forces in a FEM foot simulation, after obtaining the 3D foot model from CT images. The results will enable the development of personalized orthoses, in order to optimize gait, relieving pain and discomfort, by minimizing stress and pressure.

References

1. Antunes PJ, Dias GR et al (2007) Non-linear finite element modelling of anatomically detailed 3D foot model. Mimmics Innovation Awards 2007
2. Bernardini F, Rushmeier HE (2002) The 3D model acquisition pipeline. Comput Graph Forum 21(2):149–172
3. Bhatia MM, Patil KM (1999) New on-line parameters for analysis of dynamic foot pressures in neuropathic feet of Hansen's disease subjects. J Rehabil Res Dev 36(3)
4. Birtane M, Tuna H (2004) The evaluation of plantar pressure distribution in obese and non-obese adults. Clin Biomech 19:1055–1059
5. Burnfield JM, Tsai Y-J et al (2005) Comparison of utilized coefficient of friction during different walking tasks in persons with and without a disability. Gait Posture 22:82–88
6. Bus SA, Ulbrecht JS et al (2004) Pressure relief and load redistribution by custom-made insoles in diabetic patients with neuropathy and foot deformity. Clin Biomech 19(6):629–638
7. Cavanagh PR, Ulbrecht JS et al (2000) New developments in the biomechanics of the diabetic foot. Diabetes Metab Res Rev 16(S1):S6–S10
8. Cham R, Redfern MS (2002) Changes in gait when anticipating slippery floors. Gait Posture 15:159–171

9. Cheung JT, Zhang M et al (2004) Effects of plantar fascia stiffness on the biomechanical responses of the ankle-foot complex. Clin Biomech 19:839–846

10. Cheung JT, Zhang M et al (2005) Three-dimensional finite element analysis of the foot during standing – a material sensitivity study. J Biomech 38:1045–1054

11. Colagiuri S, Marsden LL et al (1995) The use of orthotic devices to correct plantar callus in people with diabetes. Diabetes Res Clin Pract 28:29–34

12. Cordero AF, Koopman HJFM et al (2004) Use of pressure insoles to calculate the complete ground reaction forces. J Biomech 37(9):1427–1433

13. Curless B et al (2000) Surface light fields for 3D photography SIGGRAPH 2000, New Orleans, LA, pp 24–28

14. Davis BL, Perry JE et al (1998) A device for simultaneous measurement of pressure and shear force distribution on the plantar surface of the foot. J Appl Biomech 14:93–104

15. Erdemir A, Saucerman JJ et al (2005) Local plantar pressure relief in therapeutic footwear: design guidelines from finite element models. J Biomech 38:1798–1806

16. Faivre A, Dahan M et al (2004) Instrumented shoes for pathological gait assessment. Mech Res Commun 31(5):627–632

17. Gallagher M, Abboud RJ et al (1999) The role of microengineering in pedobarography. Foot 9:79–83

18. Gefen A (2003) Plantar soft tissue loading under the medial metatarsals in the standing diabetic foot. Med Eng Phys 25:491–499

19. Geil MD (2002) The role of footwear on kinematics and plantar foot pressure in fencing. J Appl Biomech 18:155–162

20. Hennig EM, Milani TL (1995) In-shoe pressure distribution for running in various types of footwear. J Appl Biomech 11(3):299–310

21. Hosein R, Lord M (2000) A study of in-shoe plantar shear in normals. Clin Biomech 15:46–53

22. Hughes R, Rowlands H et al (2000) A laser plantar pressure sensor for the diabetic foot. Med Eng Phys 22:149–154

23. Koulaxouzidis AV, Holmes MJ et al (2000) A shear and vertical stress sensor for physiological measurements using fibre Bragg gratings. In: 22nd annual international conference of the IEEE engineering in medicine and biology society, Chicago

24. Laing P, Deogan H et al (1992) The development of the low profile liverpool shear transducer. Clin Phys Physiol Meas 13(2):115–124

25. Lebar AM, Harris GF et al (1993) Development of a miniature plantar shear force sensing transducer. In: Proc IEEE EMBS, San Diego, CA, 15:989–990, Oct. 28–31, 1993

26. Lebar AM, Harris GF et al (1996) An optoelectric plantar "shear" sensing transducer: design, validation and preliminary subject tests. IEEE Trans Rehabil Eng 4(4):310–319

27. Lemmon D, Shiang TY et al (1997) The effect of insoles in therapeutic footwear - a finite element approach. J Biomech 30(6):615–620

28. Lobmann R, Kayser R et al (2001) Effects of preventative footwear on foot pressure as determined by pedobarography in diabetic patients: a prospective study. Diabet Med 18:314–319

29. Lord M, Hosein R et al (1992) Method for in-shoe shear stress measurement. J Biomed Eng 14(3):181–186

30. Marques A (2008) Desenvolvimento de Estruturas Planas com Caracterização Dinâmica de Forças em 3D - Aplicação ao Pé. Engineering Sciences. Porto, Universidade do Porto. PhD: 321. (in portuguese)

31. Marques MA, Nabais C et al (2008) Modelação do pé para o estudo de tensões internas localizadas. 7º Congresso de Mecânica Experimental Vila Real. (in portuguese)

32. Marques MA, Ribeiro R et al (2010) Sensor Portátil para Medição de Forças Plantares em 3D. INPI. Portugal, Universidade do Porto e Instituto Politécnico do Porto. (in portuguese)

33. Nagano A, Yoshioka S et al (2005) A three-dimensional linked segment model of the whole human body. Int J Sport Health Sci 3:311–325

34. Orlin MN, McPoil TG (2000) Plantar pressure assessment. Phys Ther 80:399–409

35. Paradiso J, Hu E et al (1999) The cyberShoe: a wireless multisensor interface for a dancer's feet. International Dance and Technology, Tempe, p 99

36. Razian MA, Pepper MG (2003) Design, development, and characteristics of an in-shoe triaxial pressure measurement transducer utilizing a single element of piezoelectric copolymer film. IEEE Trans Neural Syst Rehabil Eng 11(3):288–293
37. Schmidt MW, Lopez-Ortiz C et al (2003) Foot force direction in an isometric pushing task: prediction by kinematic and musculoskeletal models. Exp Brain Res 150:245–254
38. Sousa D, Tavares J et al (2006) A gait analysis laboratory for rehabilitation of patients with musculoskeletal impairments. CompIMAGE - C Computational Modelling of Objects Represented in Images: Fundamentals, Methods and Applications, Coimbra
39. Sousa D, Tavares J et al (2007) Análise Clínica da Marcha Exemplo de Aplicação em Laboratório de Movimento. 2º Encontro Nacional de Biomecânica, Évora, Portugal. (in portuguese)
40. Stott JRR, Hutton WC et al (1973) Forces under the foot. J Bone Joint Surg 55B(2):335–344
41. Sutherland DH (2002) The evolution of clinical gait analysis: part II kinematics. Gait Posture 16(2):159–179
42. Sutherland DH (2005) The evolution of clinical gait analysis part III - kinetics and energy assessment. Gait Posture 21(4):447–461
43. Tappin JW, Pollard J et al (1980) Method of measuring 'shearing' forces on the sole of the foot. Clin Phys Physiol Meas 1:83–85
44. Tavares P (2010) Three dimensional geometry characterization using structured light fields. Faculdade de Engenharia, Universidade do Porto. PhD
45. Urry S (1999) Plantar pressure-measurement sensors. Meas Sci Technol 10:R16–R32
46. Vaughan CL, Davis BL et al (1999) Dynamics of human gait, Kiboho Publishers, Cape Town
47. Winter DA (2005) Biomechanics and motor control of human movement. Wiley, Hoboken, ISBN-0-471-44989-X-90000
48. Yung-Hui L, Wei-Hsien H (2005) Effects of shoe inserts and heel height on foot pressure, impact force, and perceived comfort during walking. Appl Ergon 36:355–362
49. Zhu H, Hams GF et al (1991) A microprocessor-based data-acquisition system for measuring plantar pressures from ambulatory subjects. IEEE Trans Biomed Eng 38(7):710–714
50. Zhu HS, Maalej N et al (1990) An umbilical data-acquisition system for measuring pressures between the foot and shoe. IEEE Trans Biomed Eng 37(9):908–911

The Scapular Contribution to the Amplitude of Shoulder External Rotation on Throwing Athletes

Andrea Ribeiro, Augusto Gil Pascoal, and Nuno Morais

Abstract Traditional clinical testing of the shoulder ER imposes a fixed scapula in order to assess the glenohumeral joint, despite the recognized importance of the scapular mobility and stability on shoulder function. Here the scapular contribution to the amplitude of humeral axial rotation (internal and external) was tested on the dominant shoulder of two groups of 12 subjects, the thrower athletes and the non-athletes group. The scapular 3D position recorded at the end-range of GH and TH IR and ER rotations was compared across groups using a mixed-model two-way ANOVA. At the end-range of humeral ER, throwers showed less GH and TH amplitude and a scapula more in retraction. A positive correlation was found between scapular spinal tilt and TH and GH angles at the end-range of ER. The throwers group showed a scapula more in retraction in maximal external rotation of the humerus, and less external rotation in active motion. On volleyball players, the scapula assumed a position of posterior spinal tilt when the humerus was positioned more in external rotation. No such correlation was found in the control group or the handball players group, possibly due to sports adaptation.

1 Introduction

Overhead throwers are a population at risk of developing shoulder injuries. The mechanics of the throwing action, where a ball is released or stroked at maximum speed when the hand is placed over the head, puts an enormous stress on

A. Ribeiro (✉) • A.G. Pascoal
CIPER - Neuromechanics of Human Movement Research Group,
Technical University of Lisbon, Lisbon, Portugal
e-mail: andrear77@gmail.com; gpascoal@fmh.utl.pt

N. Morais
Higher School of Health, University of Aveiro, Aveiro, Portugal
e-mail: nuno.morais@ua.pt

R.M.N. Jorge et al. (eds.), *Technologies for Medical Sciences*, Lecture Notes
in Computational Vision and Biomechanics 1, DOI 10.1007/978-94-007-4068-6_11,
© Springer Science+Business Media B.V. 2012

shoulder structures. Fortunately, musculoskeletal system has the ability to adapt to the high load activities in order to achieve the best performance and avoid injury. Not all the adaptations are considered beneficial and some of them have been involved in the pathomechanics of shoulder pain and disability.

The throwing shoulder poses major challenges to clinicians. It is a complex of great mobility in which static and dynamic stability depends on the synchronized position and motion between scapula and humerus. Understanding the role of the scapula in shoulder function and dysfunction is one of the recent directions in the scientific community. It is accepted that changes in scapular kinematics are related to shoulder pathology however clinical procedures to assess scapular contribution to total shoulder motion have been poorly developed. Here is presented the contribution of the scapula to one of the most acknowledged functional adaptations of the throwing shoulder – the external rotation gain.

1.1 Shoulder Structure and Function

1.1.1 Glenohumeral Joint Structure and Function

The glenohumeral joint is composed by static and dynamic stabilizers. The dynamic stabilizers of the glenohumeral joint include the rotator cuff, the scapulothoracic muscles, and the long head of the biceps tendon, while the static stabilizers include the osseous anatomy, the fibrocartilaginous labrum, and the glenohumeral joint capsule [1–4]. The stability demands on these structures are even higher during the practice of overhead sports such as tennis [5], volleyball [6], handball [7, 8], baseball [9–13], water polo [14] and swimming [5, 10].

The mobility of the shoulder joint is the result of motion in both the glenohumeral joint and scapulothoracic-gliding plane. Most of the thoracohumeral motion takes place in the glenohumeral joint, which itself allows for glenohumeral elevation up to 120° and in addition the humerus is able to axially rotate about 135° relative to the scapula [4, 15, 16].

Alterations in either the anatomy of the joint, e.g. glenoid version [17], or deficiencies in the intrinsic biomechanical properties of the ligamentous and/or capsular components can cause motion abnormalities and focal contact stresses or even develop instability [2, 18]. Depending on the injured structures involved, the direction of instability may be primarily anterior, inferior or posterior, or a combination of these. The degree of instability may range from mild subluxation to dislocation, with associated injuries to the bony (e.g. Hill Sachs lesion), capsulolabral structures (e.g. Bankart and SLAP lesions), or both, and surrounding musculature (e.g. rotator cuff tears and impingement). Isolated injuries are not very common and usually one problem may lead to other [19, 20].

1.1.2 The Shoulder Girdle Structure and Function

The shoulder girdle is a morphofunctional unit composed by the scapula and the clavicle bones, resting on the thorax. Scapula and clavicle are connected via acromioclavicular joint. Both bones are linked to the thorax via sternoclavicular joint and the functional scapulothoracic joint. In this context, the thorax acts as a stable base for the movements of the upper limb. Together the thorax and the shoulder girdle form a closed kinematic chain mechanism with some degree of interdependence. As consequence, the shoulder girdle moves with respect to the thorax at the same time that is used as a stable base for muscles acting on the humerus.

1.2 Overhead-Throwing Athletes

Thrower athletes also called overhead-throwing athletes include throwers (e.g. baseball pitchers), swimmers, water polo, handball, and volleyball players. From a functional standpoint, these sports require repetitive overhead motions, which are discontinuous and ballistic in nature, and where the throwing arm is forced forward from maximal external to near maximal internal rotation, while the arm is kept in an elevated position.

Kinematics of the throwing arm motion (with ball) is frequently described as a particular sequence of phases, the "*throwing cycle*" [1, 21], that includes the initial and late cocking phases, where the arm assumes an elevated-external rotated position, followed by an acceleration and a follow-through (deceleration) phases. At the end of the acceleration phase the object (ball) is released or stroked. On throwers, during the deceleration phase, the posterior rotator cuff musculature acts eccentrically in order to decelerate or "*brake*" the internal and horizontal adduction arm motion, generated during the acceleration phase. The act of throwing requires a coordinated motion that progresses from the toes to the fingertips. This sequence of events has been described conceptually as a kinetic chain. For the kinetic chain to work effectively, sequential muscle activity is required so that the energy that is generated in the lower body can be transmitted to the upper body through the arm, hand, and fingers, and finally to the ball. The speed of the ball is then determined by the efficiency of this process. Body rotation, timing and positioning of the scapula are key elements in the kinetic chain. Any physical condition that alters the components of the kinetic chain, especially one that affects the so called "*core*" (trunk, back and proximal parts of the lower limbs), will alter more distal segments and may result in the development of a dysfunctional shoulder [1].

The inherent contradiction for overhead athletes is the fact that the shoulder must be loose enough to perform overhead activity and yet stable enough to prevent the joint from "*giving way*" or sub-luxating [22]. In elite-level throwers, there is a delicate balance between shoulder mobility and stability. The shoulder needs to be mobile enough to reach extreme positions of rotation so that velocity can be imparted to the ball, but at the same time the shoulder needs to remain stable so that the humeral head remains within the glenoid socket, creating a stable fulcrum for rotation; this is known as the "*thrower's paradox*". With each pitch, the soft-tissue envelope that surrounds the shoulder is loaded at levels that approach the ultimate failure loads of the tissues, which are thus quite vulnerable to injury.

1.3 The "Throwing Shoulder"

Numerous studies have documented motion adaptations on the dominant shoulder of throwers either by comparing shoulders bilaterally or with the dominant shoulder of non-athletes [5, 6, 13, 23, 24]. One of the most visible and highlighted adaptations, imposed by the repetitive throwing cycle at high velocities over time, includes changes on shoulder rotational ROM pattern with increased external rotation (external rotation gain) and limited internal rotation (glenohumeral internal rotation deficit), while the range of the total arc of motion (external arc *plus* internal arc) is kept unchanged [22].

In general, the shoulder rotational adaptation on the asymptomatic dominant throwing shoulder of an elite-level athlete was described as an increased external rotation arc and a correspondent decrease in the internal rotation arc, while the amplitude of the total arc is kept unchanged, in a condition called the "*posterior shift*" [11, 25–27]. This adaptive pattern was mostly described through goniometric studies [28–30] where the athletes were assessed in a supine or a sitting position with the arm placed at 90° of abduction. The arm is then passively rotated from the extreme position (end-range) internal rotation until the end-range of external rotation, or vice-versa. Following this standard goniometry procedure, the shoulder rotation end-range is determined by the examiner according to the sensation of capsular end-feel, the scapular liftoff momentum or perceived pain. A few studies described the changes on the rotational pattern using an active end-range determination [31, 32] and no studies to date have specifically investigated how humeral rotational pattern is affected by active or passive end-range determination in overhead throwing athletes.

The posterior shift in the total arc of motion is considered to be a physiological adaptation of the shoulder joint to throwing. According to Wilk et al. [27] most throwers exhibit an obvious motion disparity, whereby shoulder external rotation (ER) is excessive and internal rotation (IR) is limited when measured at 90° of abduction. This loss of IR on the throwing shoulder, referred to as "*glenohumeral internal rotation deficit*" (GIRD) [8, 33, 34], is suggested to be caused by the retraction of the posterior capsule induced by the increased amplitude of external rotation in the late cocking phase. This allows hyper-external rotation as the posterior capsule reaches maximum length while the anterior capsule still allows for additional external rotation. Burkhart et al. [19] described the GIRD as an alternative mechanism for primary progression of "*internal impingement-like*" changes in the shoulder. The glenohumeral internal rotation deficit model is based on the high prevalence of posterior capsular contractures and contractures of the posterior band of the inferior glenohumeral ligament in thrower shoulders. When a posterior capsular contracture develops, the center of rotation of the humerus, or the contact point of the humerus on the glenoid, is shifted postero-superiorly. This shift functionally increases the length of the anterior aspect of the capsule, which provides more clearance for the greater tuberosity, diminishing the glenohumeral contact point of the anterior-inferior aspect of the capsule with proximal part of the humerus. As a result, the biceps anchor is peeled back under tension, causing injury to the postero-superior structures, especially the postero-superior aspect of the labrum (SLAP lesion). The so-called peel-back progression mechanism permits further laxity of the anterior aspect of the capsule [19, 35]. With the glenohumeral internal rotation deficit model, one attempts to identify throwers at risk for shoulder injury by quantifying the internal rotation deficit individuals are considered to have a clinically relevant glenohumeral internal rotation deficit when there is a loss of internal rotation of the throwing shoulder as compared with the non-throwing side. Such deficits are commonly found in overhead throwers, when compared with measurements on the contralateral side, as well as concomitant increases in external rotation.

Some studies suggested an osseous adaptation as a possible explanation for the increased external rotation observed on the throwing arm, namely an increase on the angle of the humeral head retroversion, or humeral torsion [33]. More external rotation range in the dominant arm could be seen as a strategy to improve performance, allowing increased cocking of the throwing arm which leads to higher ability to generate power and speed or release [36]. Other authors though do not look at these adaptations as single benefits but as abnormal stresses at the joints and the surrounding tissues which may cause shoulder pain, decreased performance or some unspecific shoulder disorders [37, 38]. Pieper [8] found an augmented angle of retroversion (up to 15°) in the dominant shoulder of 51 handball players, when compared with the non-dominant shoulder. This retroversion seems to increase the available external rotation range-of-motion (ROM) but at the same time reduced the ability of the rotator cuff to control high forces or velocities through the extremes to shoulder ROM which could lead to excessive humeral head translation and culminate in shoulder pain [31, 33]. Thus, it remains unclear whether there are benefits or disadvantages associated to changes in humeral torsion.

Humeral torsion may not be the only mechanism that explains the external rotation gain in throwers. It seems that the looseness of the connective that surrounds and stabilizes the glenohumeral joint may also play a role. The inferior glenohumeral ligament complex (IGHLC) is considered to be the most restraining structure at the late cocking position [39, 40] followed by the coracohumeral ligament [39]. It is likely that with the continuous excessive external rotation in throwing mechanics, the anterior capsule and the anterior band of the IGHLC may become looser than normal subjects [41, 42]. The link between looseness of the anterior band of the IGHLC, increased anterior and inferior humerus head translations and humeral external rotation was demonstrated in cadaveric models [42].

1.4   Problem

Despite advances in diagnostic and treatment interventions, shoulder injuries continue to plague throwing athletes [43]. These athletes are prone to shoulder injuries as a result of the high forces placed on the shoulder during the throwing motion. Overhead athletes require a delicate balance between shoulder mobility and stability in order to meet the functional demands of their respective sport. Altered mobility patterns, concerning rotational movement, as mentioned before, have been consistently reported in the dominant shoulder of throwers such as elite baseball pitchers [21], volleyball players [44] or handball players [45].

Commonly, clinical ROM testing includes the measurement of maximal external and internal rotation using a goniometric approach, i.e., placing patient in a supine or a sitting position, with the arm abducted to 90° and totally supported by the table. In this position, the examiner passively rotates the arm until the extreme position of internal or external rotation (end-range). In a sited position the examiner has to stabilize the inferior angle of the scapula, having the patient hold his/her elbow at a side while rotating the forearm around the long axis of the humerus [46, 47]. On both procedures the examiner passively sets the arm according to the capsular end-feel [28, 48, 49], or by scapular liftoff [47] or even by pain [46]. On the other hand, the goniometric protocol imposes that the scapular motion must be limited by a posterior force applied by the examiner on the coracoids process and clavicle, restricting arm motion to the glenohumeral joint.

From a biomechanical perspective the goniometric protocol has three key limitations: (1) the end-range is determined by clinical end-feel, as opposed to an objective assessment of torque; (2) goniometers were designed to assess glenohumeral motion, but they are really measuring both glenohumeral and scapulothoracic motion and scapula can have a significant effect on both goniometric and vertebral level measurements. Isolating glenohumeral motion typically requires a fixation technique to prevent unwanted scapular motion, but this approach is difficult to perform and may induce unwanted artifact into the measurement. Third, the effect of the plane of motion has not been well documented [26].

1.5   Purpose of the Study

The main purpose of the study was to clarify the scapular contribution to the amplitude of shoulder external rotation on thrower athletes. The assessment of internal and external rotation ROM is a standard part of a shoulder clinical examination. However, the contribution of shoulder girdle in the rotational motion pattern often is frequently not considered by clinicians. Additionally, the study looks to quantify the effects of the end-range determination and the speed of motion on the external rotation ROM. To date, no studies have specifically investigated how humeral rotational pattern is affected by active or passive end-range determination in overhead throwing athletes.

2 Methods

2.1 Sample

Twenty-four subjects ($n = 24$) divided in two groups were studied: the throwers group with three volleyball players (height $= 181 \pm 4{,}7$ cm; age $= 22 \pm 4{,}0$ years; body mass: $75 \pm 7{,}6$ kg) and six handball players (height $= 184 \pm 3{,}7$ cm; age $= 22 \pm 0{,}9$ years; body mass $= 81 \pm 5{,}6$ kg); and the non-thrower group with 12 non-thrower athletes (height $= 176 \pm 4{,}7$ cm; age $= 26 \pm 2{,}9$ years; body mass $= 73 \pm 7{,}5$ kg).

2.2 Kinematic Proceedings

Humeral and scapular 3D positions were recorded by means of a 6DOF electromagnetic tracking device (Hardware: "Flock of Birds system" Ascension Technology; Software: Motion Monitor v 7.0) which allowed simultaneous tracking of four sensors at a sampling rate of 100 Hz per sensor. This system allows the registration of the position and orientation of the sensors in space always when they are inserted in an extended electromagnetic field.

The static accuracy of these sensors with an Extended Range Transmitter is up to 0.76 cm RMS/0.5 degrees RMS at a 1.52 m distance from the transmitter. The static resolution is 0.08 cm/0.1 degrees RMS at 1.52 m from the transmitter. On data collection a four sensors setup was used. Thorax sensor was attached over T1 using double faced tape assuring its fixation. The arm sensor, placed just below the deltoid attachment, by mean of a cuff firmly adjusted to the arm. Finally the scapular sensor was attached to the superior flat surface of the acromion process, using the same kind of tape (Table 1).

Table 1 Bony landmarks used on the definition of the local coordinate system of the thorax, scapula and humerus, according with Wu et al. [50]

Segment	Bony landmark	Abbreviations
Thorax	T8 spinous process	T8
	Xiphoid process of the sternum	PX
	C7 Spinous process	C7
	Incisura Jugularis of the sternum	IJ
Scapula	Angulus acromialis	AA
	Trigonum Spinae Scapulae	TS
	Angulus Inferior Scapulae	AI
Humerus	Epicondylus medialis	EM
	Epicondylus lateralis	EL
	Glenohumeral rotation centre[a]	GH

[a]Estimated by motion recordings, calculating the pivot point of instantaneous helical axes of GH motion [51, 52]

Table 2 Bony landmarks used on the definition of the local coordinated system of the thorax, scapula and humerus, according with Wu et al. [50]

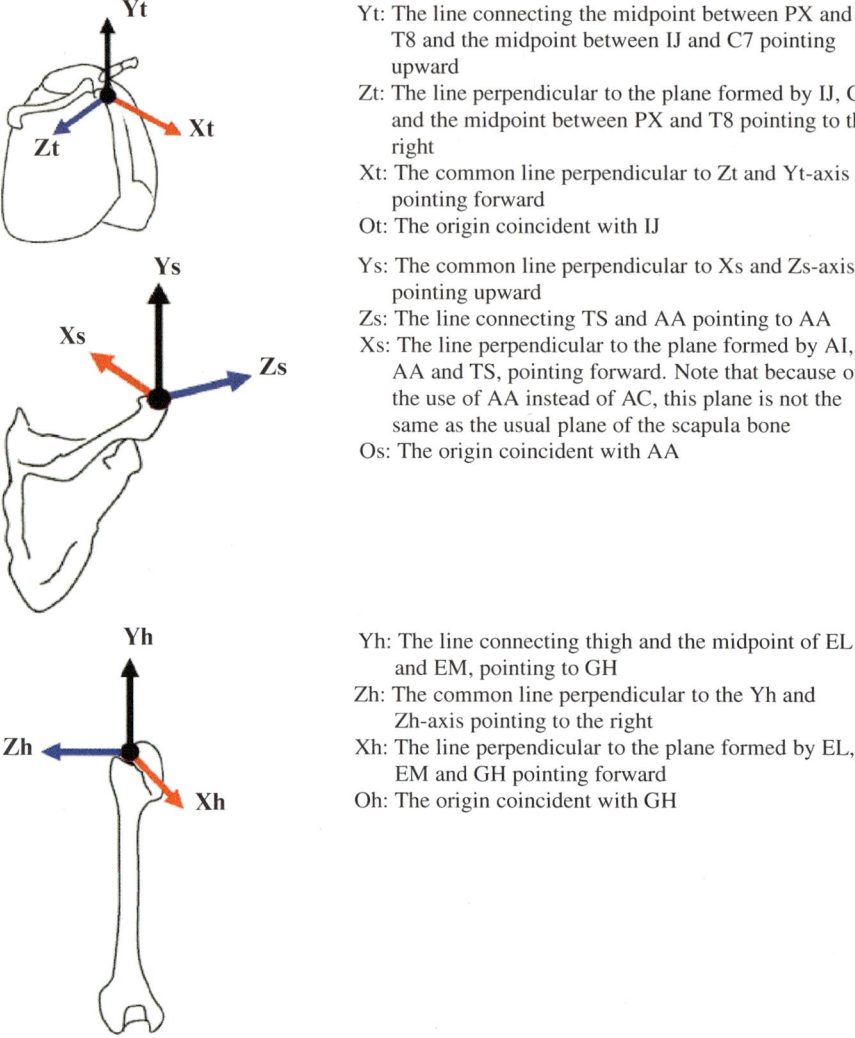

Yt: The line connecting the midpoint between PX and T8 and the midpoint between IJ and C7 pointing upward

Zt: The line perpendicular to the plane formed by IJ, C7 and the midpoint between PX and T8 pointing to the right

Xt: The common line perpendicular to Zt and Yt-axis pointing forward

Ot: The origin coincident with IJ

Ys: The common line perpendicular to Xs and Zs-axis pointing upward

Zs: The line connecting TS and AA pointing to AA

Xs: The line perpendicular to the plane formed by AI, AA and TS, pointing forward. Note that because of the use of AA instead of AC, this plane is not the same as the usual plane of the scapula bone

Os: The origin coincident with AA

Yh: The line connecting thigh and the midpoint of EL and EM, pointing to GH

Zh: The common line perpendicular to the Yh and Zh-axis pointing to the right

Xh: The line perpendicular to the plane formed by EL, EM and GH pointing forward

Oh: The origin coincident with GH

A fourth sensor mounted on a hand-held acrylic stylus (±6,5 cm) was used on bony landmarks digitalization in order to link sensors position to the local anatomical coordinate systems (LCS) (Table 2) and subsequently calculated segments and joint rotations by combining the LCSs with the sensor motions. Segments LCSs and joint rotations definition, expressed in Euler angles, were made according to the shoulder ISB standardization protocol [50].

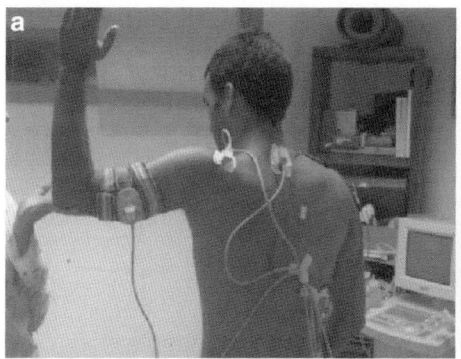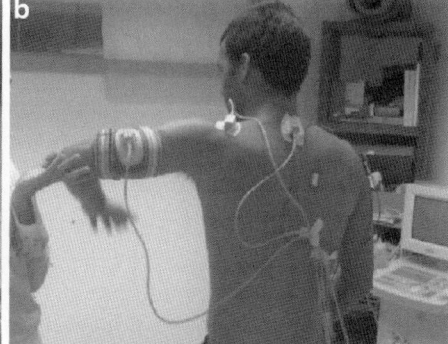

Fig. 1 (**a**) Subjects performing external and (**b**) internal rotation

2.3 Task

The subject was in a seated position, with supported feet, keeping the hips and knees at 90° flexion. The shoulder evaluated was at 90° of humeral elevation and in the scapular plane supported by the researcher. The subjects performed one task in two specific conditions concerning velocity: (1) slow axial rotation; (2) fast axial rotation (figure A). Subjects performed total axial rotation since maximal external (Fig. 1a) rotation until maximal internal rotation (Fig. 1b).

At the first condition, subjects were asked to perform slow motion, keeping the scapula stable. At the second condition, they performed the movement reproducing a ballistic one. Both conditions were repeated for three times each. Humeral axial rotation was described with respect to the scapula, the glenohumeral (HRs) angles, and with respect to thorax, the thoracohumeral (HRt). Scapular position was described with respect to the thorax as protraction (Syt), lateral rotation (Sxt) and spinal tilt (Szt). These angles were recorded at end-range of active fast and slow (subject self-selected end-of-range).

2.4 Statistics

A mixed-model two-way ANOVA was used to test the main effect of group (between-group factor) on the three scapular (Syt, Sxt and Szt) and the two humeral (HRt and HRs) dependent variables, as well as test for an interaction of group and speed motion (slow vs. fast; within-subjects factor). A bivariate correlation test was used to describe the relationships between HRt and scapular variables. Another bivariate correlation test was runned in order to describe the relationships between scapular spinal tilt (Szt) and shoulder external thoracohumeral and scapulohumeral rotation.

3 Results

No significant interaction was found between group and speed motion for any of the three scapular and the two humeral dependent variables.

On both groups, the increment of arm velocity imposed a decrease on the amplitude of the humeral external rotation. The throwers group showed at the end-range of the humeral external rotation, significantly less amplitude of HRs (23° difference; P = 0.04) and a scapula more in retraction (15° difference; P = 0.00). Considering the influence of the fast arm condition, amplitude of HRs was lower at the end-range of external rotation (13,6° difference; P = 0.04). Also on throwers, scapula was also kept more in retraction at the end-range of ER (Table 3).

Considering fast shoulder external rotation between spinal tilt (Szt) and thoracohumeral (TH) and glenohumeral (GH) arc a positive correlation was found on the control group.

Concerning volleyball players a negative correlation was found between Szt and TH and no correlation on handball players was realized. In the control group we found a linear relation, so, with higher external rotation, less scapular tilt is shown. At the non-throwers group movement occurs more in the GH while in volleyball we have movement in GH and scapula. At fast condition on volleyball players a negative correlation was shown (Fig. 2). On volleyball players, scapula assumes a position on posterior spinal tilt (acromion backwards) when humerus is positioned more in external rotation. No correlation was found between volleyball players and the slow arm condition.

Table 3 Humeral and scapular 3D position at the end-range of external rotation on both groups (throwers and non-throwers) during the fast condition. [Mean ± standard deviation (degrees)]

	Non-throwers	Throwers
Humeral external rotation w.r.t. Thorax	−96.3 ± 26.8	−77.5 ± 19.2
Humeral external rotation w.r.t. Scapula	−90.4 ± 29.2	−65.6 ± 19.5
Scapular protraction (*Syt*) (at end-range of humeral external rotation)	32.5 ± 14.0	17.4 ± 5.6
Scapular lateral rotation (*Sxt*) (at end-range of humeral external rotation)	42.1 ± 9.8	39.4 ± 12.1
Scapular spinal tilt (*Szt*) (at end-range of humeral external rotation)	8.3 ± 7.1	9.9 ± 6.5

w.r.t. with respect to

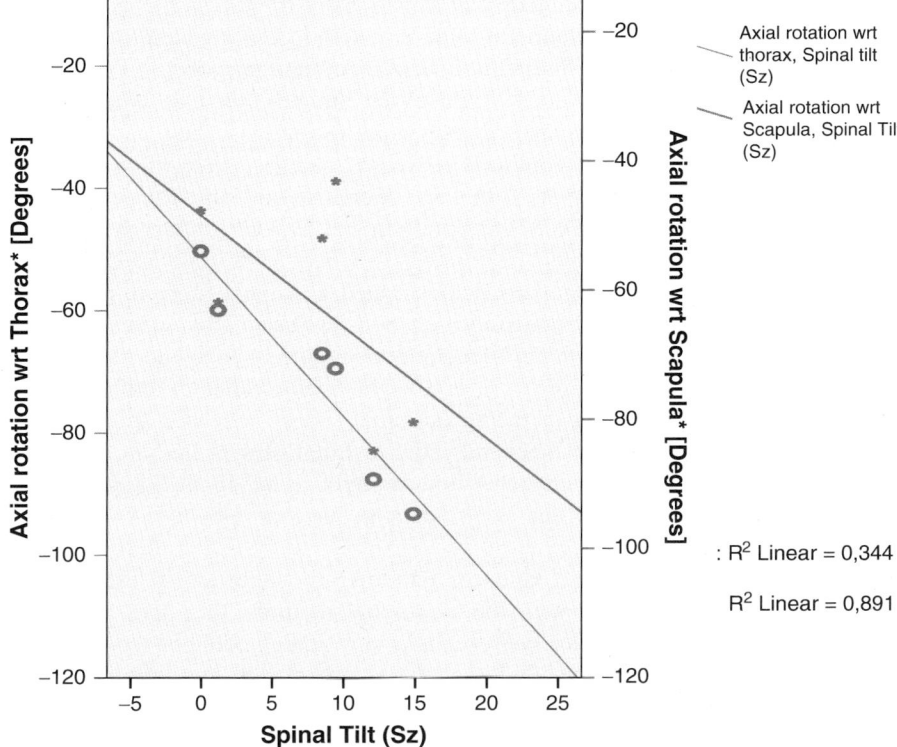

Fig. 2 Volleyball athletes: correlation between spinal tilt (degrees) (Szt) and shoulder axial rotation (degrees) **w.r.t.** thorax (TH) and **w.r.t.** scapula (degrees) (GH) in fast condition

4 Discussion

Several studies had identified several morphologic and functional adaptations on the dominant shoulder of overhead athletes, such as volleyball players [53], water polo players [54], baseball players [33, 45, 49, 55–57], swimmers [10] and body building [28].

In our study, throwers also showed a significant increase on glenohumeral external rotation and loss of internal rotation, while the rotational arch was maintained (External Rotation + Internal Rotation) as previously reported [28, 33, 49, 57–62].

In opposition to our study and considering glenohumeral rotational range of motion variation in overhead-athletes Dwelly et al. [23] demonstrated using a sample of 29 baseball male athletes and 19 softball female athletes, that there is a significant gain of shoulder external rotation amplitude at the dominant arm, and a significant raise of the total arch of motion. No changes were found at the amplitude of internal rotation during the season.

The analysis of the morphofunctional adaptations of the thrower athlete cannot be circumscribed to the glenohumeral joint, and should be extended to the other joints of the shoulder complex, particularly the scapulothoracic joint.

During the throwing cycle it is suppose that athletes, such as volleyball or handball players, keep their scapula stable while the arm is fastly moved from a full external position to a full internal position. Scapular stabilization could be challanged when the arm motion is to fast. Therefore, an innadequate scapular position at the end-range of glenohumeral motion will lead to shoulder dysfunction and pathology [21].

The results showed that throwers demonstrated a scapula more in retraction (acromion backwards) when compared with non-throwers. This seems to work as a protective mechanism for the glenohumeral joint. In fact, the inability to retract the scapula, appears to impart several negative biomechanical effects on the shoulder, including narrowing of the subacromial space, increased strain on the anterior-inferior glenohumeral ligament, reduced impingement-free arc of upper limb elevation, reduced isometric elevation strength tested in the sagital plane. Concerning this, throwers on our study seem to have developed an adaptation towards stability.

While in clinical trial these kinds of patterns are important to evaluate, to allow a better rehabilitation, with the traditional methods this does not seem possible. Using 3D kinematic analysis, scapular positioning could be recorded and morphofunctional adaptations could be identified, and also the specific movement of throwers. While using traditional goniometry this cannot be possible.

Concerning axial shoulder rotation, scapular contribution is crucial as it is well recognized that the external rotation needed to perform the throwing motion occurs not only at the glenohumeral joint but also with the participation of the scapula [21].

Excessive motion is required at the shoulder joint during throwing, yet the glenohumeral joint must remain stable to resist injury. We found that volleyball players show a more posterior tilted scapula when arm is positioned more in external rotation, while the control group showed less posterior scapula tilt. This seems to demonstrate that shoulder adaptation on volleyball players, while throwing, does not occur only at the glenohumeral joint, as it is commonly assumed in clinical practice, but instead it is supported by the trunk where the scapula in retraction and posterior tilt gives the necessary stability to achieve best performance. This seems the reason why proper 3D position of the scapula relative to the humerus and trunk is so relevant for muscle function. The scapula acts as the common point of attachment of the rotator cuff and primary humeral movers such as the biceps, deltoid and triceps, as well as several scapular stabilizers. Poor position of the scapula can lead to alterations to the relationship between length and tension of each muscle, thus adversely affecting muscle force generation [45]. An imbalance in external rotators will lead to alterations in scapular tilt. Concerning the movement, clinical trials use passive and active motion. But the active motion used is usually a slow motion [26], and not simulating the sports practice. In our study we looked for active motion. We have used an elevated arm position as the testing position, however the calibration one, was the same proposed in the ISB protocol [50] as mentioned in methods, with the arm at a side. While testing we hoped that when raising the arm to the elevated position (arm at 90° flexion and abduction) the zero stayed the same, we didn't expect to have any complementary rotation, and it happened that way. So the main reason to find more external rotation at non-throwers is possibly the fact that we were evaluating active motion and not passive one.

Knowledge of joint ROM and speeds of movement along with joint forces and moments will provide a scientific basis for improved and rehabilitative protocols for throwers.

5 Conclusions

Speed was not an interaction factor between groups. At the end-range of arm external rotation the volleyball players group showed a scapula more in retraction and in posterior tilt (acromion backwards). No such correlation was found in the control group or the handball players, possibly due to sports adaptation.

This group also showed less amplitude of external rotation in active motion.

As a limitation of this study we would include possible skin artifacts, especially at the arm sensor. To avoid this situation we used a sensor mounted on a cuff tiny adjusted to the arm just below the deltoid attachment, trying to ensure the position of the sensor towards the skin.

Acknowledgments The authors would like to thank to Vitoria Sport Club Guimarães, Portugal for allowing using their facilities and athletes and Pedro Miguel Ribeiro for all support on data collection.

References

1. Braun S, Kokmeyer D, Millett PJ (2009) Shoulder injuries in the throwing athlete. J Bone Joint Surg Am 91(4):966–978
2. Lee S-B, Kim K-J, O'Driscoll SW, MOrrey BF, An K-N (2000) Dynamic glenohumeral stability provided by the rotator cuff muscles in the mid-range and end-range of motion: a study in cadavera. J Bone Joint Surg Am 82
3. Matsen FA, Chebli C, Lippitt S (2006) Principles for the evaluation and management of shoulder instability. J Bone Joint Surg 88:647–659
4. Veeger HEJ, van der Helm FCT (2007) Shoulder function: the perfect compromise between mobility and stability. J Biomech 40(10):2119–2129
5. Gomes RRTaJLE (2009) Measurement of glenohumeral internal rotation in asymptomatic tennis players and swimmers. Am J Sports Med 37:1017–1023
6. Schwab LM, Blanch P (2009) Humeral torsion and passive shoulder range in elite volleyball players. Phys Ther Sport 10(2):51–56
7. Murachovsky J, Ikemoto RY, Nascimento L, Bueno R, Coelho J, Komeçu M, Wilson P (2007) Avaliação da retroversão da cabeça do úmero em jogadores de handebol. Acta Ortop Bras 15(5):258–261

8. Pieper HG (1998) Humeral torsion in the throwing arm of handball players. Am J Sports Med 26(2):247–253
9. Laudner KG, Stanek JM, Meister K (2007) Differences in scapular upward rotation between baseball pitchers and position players. Am J Sports Med 35(12):2091–2095. doi:10.1177/0363546507305098
10. Oyama S (2006) Profiling physical characteristics of the swimmer's shoulder: comparison to basebol pitchers and non-overhead atheletes. University of Pittsburg, Pittsburgh
11. Tokish JM, Curtin MS, Kim YK, Hawkins RJ, Torry MR (2008) Glenohumeral internal rotation deficit in the asymptomatic professional pitcher and its relationship to humeral retroversion. J Sport Sci Med 7(1):78–83
12. Tripp BL, Yochem EM, Uhl TL (2007) Functional fatigue and upper extremity sensorimotor system acuity in baseball athletes. J Athl Train 42(1):90–98
13. Warden SJ, Bogenschutz ED, Smith HD, Gutierrez AR (2009) Throwing induces substantial torsional adaptation within the midshaft humerus of male baseball players. Bone 45(5):931–941
14. Webster MJ, Morris ME, Galna B (2009) Shoulder pain in water polo: a systematic review of the literature. J Sci Med Sport 12(1):3–11
15. Magermans DJ, Chadwick EK, Veeger HE, van der Helm FC (2005) Requirements for upper extremity motions during activities of daily living. Clin Biomech (Bristol, Avon) 20(6):591–599
16. van der Helm FCT, Pronk GM (1995) Three dimensional recording and description of motions of the shoulder mechanism. J Biomech Eng 177:27–40
17. Nyffeler RW, Sheikh R, Atkinson TS, Jacob HAC, Favre P, Gerber C (2006) Effects of glenoid component version on humeral head displacement and joint reaction forces: an experimental study. J Shoulder Elbow Surg 15:625–629
18. Kelkar R, Wang VM, Flatow E, Newton PM, Ateshian GA, Bigliani L, Pawluk JR, Mow VC (2001) Glenohumeral mechanics: a study of articular geometry, contact and kinematics. J Shoulder Elbow Surg 10:73–84
19. Burkhart SS, Morgan CD, Kibler WB (2003) The disabled throwing shoulder: spectrum of pathology part I: pathoanatomy and biomechanics. Arthroscopy 19(4):404–420
20. Meister K (2000) Injuries to the shoulder in the throwing athlete. Part one: biomechanics/pathophysiology/classification of injury. Am J Sports Med 28(2):265–275
21. Werner SL, Guido JA, Jr., Stewart GW, McNeice RP, Vandyke T, Jones DG (2006) Relationships between throwing mechanics and shoulder distraction in collegiate baseball pitchers. J Shoulder Elbow Surg 29(3):354–358
22. Borsa PA, Laudner KG, Sauers EL (2008) Mobility and stability adaptations in the shoulder of the overhead athlete. Sports Med 38(1):17–36
23. Dwelly PM, Tripp BLP;, Tripp PAP, Eberman LEP, Gorin SD (2009) Glenohumeral rotational range of motion in collegiate overhead-throwing athletes during an athletic season. J Athl Train 44(6):611–616
24. Oyama S, Myers JB, Wassinger CA, Daniel Ricci R, Lephart SM (2008) Asymmetric resting scapular posture in healthy overhead athletes. J Athl Train 43(6):565–570
25. Borich MR, Bright JM, Lorello DJ, Cieminski CJ, Buisman T, Ludewig PM (2006) Scapular angular positioning at end range internal rotation in cases of glenohumeral internal rotation deficit. J Orthop Sports Phys Ther 36(12):926–934
26. McCully SP, Kumar N, Lazarus MD, Karduna AR (2005) Internal and external rotation of the shoulder: effects of plane, end-range determination, and scapular motion. J Shoulder Elbow Surg 14(6):602–610
27. Wilk KE, Obma P, Simpson CD, Cain EL, Dugas JR, Andrews JR (2009) Shoulder injuries in the overhead athlete. J Orthop Sports Phys Ther 39(2):38–54
28. Barlow JC, Benjamin BW, Birt PJ, Hughes CJ (2002) Shoulder strength and range-of-motion characteristics in bodybuilders. J Strength Cond Res 16:367–372
29. Downar JM, Sauers EL (2005) Clinical measures of shoulder mobility in the professional baseball player. J Athl Train 40(1):23–29

30. Ellenbecker TS, Roetert EP, Piorkowski PA, Schulz DA (1996) Glenohumeral joint internal and external rotation range of motion in elite junior tennis players. J Orthop Sports Phys Ther 24(6):336–341

31. Ellenbecker TS, Roetert EP (2002) Effects of a 4-month season on glenohumeral joint rotational strength and range of motion in female collegiate tennis players. J Strength Cond Res 16(1):92–96

32. Hayes K, Walton JR, Szomor ZR, Murrell GA (2001) Reliability of five methods for assessing shoulder range of motion. Aust J Physiother 47:289–294

33. Crockett HC, Gross LB, Wilk KE, Schwartz ML, Reed J, O'Mara J, Reilly MT, Dugas JR, Meister K, Lyman S, Andrews JR (2002) Osseous adaptation and range of motion at the glenohumeral joint in professional baseball pitchers. Am J Sports Med 30(1):20–26

34. Nakamizo H, Nakamura Y, Nobuhara K, Yamamoto T (2008) Loss of glenohumeral internal rotation in little league pitchers: a biomechanical study. J Shoulder Elbow Surg 17(5):795–801

35. Burkhart SS, Morgan CD, Kibler WB (2003) The disabled throwing shoulder: spectrum of pathology. Part II: evaluation and treatment of SLAP lesions in throwers. Arthroscopy 19(5):531–539

36. Wang HK, Cochrane T (2001) A descriptive epidemiological study of shoulder injury in top level english male volleyball players. Int J Sports Med 22:159–163

37. McClure P, Tate ARP, Kareha SD, Irwin DD, Zlupko ED (2009) A clinical method for identifying scapular dyskinesis, part 1: reliability. J Athl Train 44(2):160–164

38. Tsai NT, McClure PW, Karduna AR (2003) Effects of muscle fatigue on 3-dimensional scapular kinematics. Arch Phys Med Rehabil 84(7):1000–1005

39. Kuhn JE, Bey MJ, Huston LJ, Blasier RB, Soslowsky LJ (2000) Ligamentous restraints to external rotation of the humerus in the late-cocking phase of throwing: a cadaveric biomechanical investigation. Am J Sports Med 28(2):200–205

40. Turkel SJ, Panio MW, Marshall JL, Girgis FG (1981) Stabilizing mechanisms preventing anterior dislocation of the glenohumeral joint. J Bone Joint Surg Am 63(8):1208–1217

41. Herrington L (1998) Glenohumeral joint: internal and external rotation range of motion in javelin throwers. Br J Sports Med 32(3):226–228

42. Mihata T, Lee Y, McGarry MH, Abe M, Lee TQ (2004) Excessive humeral external rotation results in increased shoulder laxity. Am J Sports Med 32(5):1278–1285

43. Conte S, Requa RK, Garrick JG (2001) Disability days in major league baseball. Am J Sports Med 29(4):431–436

44. Forthomme B, Crielaard JM, Croisier JL (2008) Scapular positioning in athlete's shoulder - particularities, clinical measurements and implications. Sports Med 38(5):369–386

45. Myers JB, Laudner KG, Pasquale MR, Bradley JP, Lephart SM (2005) Scapular position and orientation in throwing athletes. Am J Sports Med 33(2):263–271

46. Boon AJ, Smith J (2000) Manual scapular stabilization: its effect on shoulder rotational range of motion. Arch Phys Med Rehabil 81(7):978–983

47. Ellenbecker TS, Bailie DS, Mattalino AJ, Carfagno DG, Wolff MW, Brown SW, Kulikowich JM (2002) Intrarater and interrater reliability of a manual technique to assess anterior humeral head translation of the glenohumeral joint. J Shoulder Elbow Surg 11(5):470–475

48. Awan R, Smith J, Boon AJ (2002) Measuring shoulder internal rotation range of motion: a comparison of 3 techniques. Arch Phys Med Rehabil 83(9):1229–1234

49. Reagan KM, Meister K, Horodyski MB, Werner DW, Carruthers C, Wilk K (2002) Humeral retroversion and its relationship to glenohumeral rotation in the shoulder of college baseball players. Am J Sports Med 30(3):354–360

50. Wu G, van der Helm FC, Veeger HE, Makhsous M, Van Roy P, Anglin C, Nagels J, Karduna AR, McQuade K, Wang X, Werner FW, Buchholz B (2005) ISB recommendation on definitions of joint coordinate systems of various joints for the reporting of human joint motion–Part II: shoulder, elbow, wrist and hand. J Biomech 38(5):981–992

51. Stokdijk M, Nagels J, Rozing PM (2000) The glenohumeral joint rotation centre in vivo. J Biomech 33(12):1629–1636

52. Veeger HE (2000) The position of the rotation center of the glenohumeral joint. J Biomech 33(12):1711–1715
53. Wang HK, Macfarlane A, Cochrane T (2000) Isokinetic performance and shoulder mobility in elite volleyball athletes from the United Kingdom. Br J Sports Med 34(1):39–43
54. Tainha C, Pascoal AG (2006) Alterações do padrão de rotação externa e abdução horizontal do braço em jogadoras de polo aquático. Revista Re(habilitar) - Revista da ESSA 2:3–21
55. Borstad JD (2006) Resting position variables at the shoulder: evidence to support a posture-impairment association. Phys Ther 86(4):549–557
56. Osbahr DC, Cannon DL, Speer KP (2002) Retroversion of the humerus in the throwing shoulder of college baseball pitchers. Am J Sports Med 30(3):347–353
57. Safran MR, Borsa PA, Lephart MS, Fu FH, Warner JJP (2001) Shoulder proprioception in baseball pitchers. J Shouder Elbow Surg 10:438–444
58. Benjamin M, Toumi H, Ralphs JR, Bydder G, Best TM, Milz S (2006) Where tendons and ligaments meet bone: attachment sites ('entheses') in relation to exercise and/or mechanical load. J Anat 208:471–490
59. Burkhart SS, Morgan CD, Kibler WB (2003) The disabled throwing shoulder: spectrum of pathology part III: The SICK scapula, scapular dyskinesis, the kinetic chain, and rehabilitation. Arthroscopy 19(6):641–661
60. Laudner KG, Myers JB, Pasquale MR, Bradley JP, Lephart SM (2006) Scapular dysfunction in throwers with pathologic internal impingement. J Orthop Sports Phys Ther 36(7):485–494
61. Myers JB, Laudner KG, Pasquale MR, Bradley JP, Lephart SM (2006) Glenohumeral range of motion deficits and posterior shoulder tightness in throwers with pathologic internal impingement. Am J Sports Med 34(3):385–391
62. Safran MR, Borsa PA, Lephart SM, Fu FH, Warner JJ (2001) Shoulder proprioception in baseball pitchers. J Shoulder Elbow Surg 10(5):438–444

Supercritical Solvent Impregnation of Natural Bioactive Compounds in *N*-Carboxybutylchitosan and Agarose Membranes for the Development of Topical Wound Healing Applications

A.M.A. Dias, M.E.M. Braga, I.J. Seabra, and H.C. de Sousa

Abstract Supercritical Solvent Impregnation (SSI) was used to load topical membrane-type wound dressing biomaterials with natural based bioactive compounds namelly quercetin as an antiinflammatory and thymol as anaesthetic and skin permeation enhancer. The biodegradable and biocompatible membranes where prepared as film- and foam-like structures of *N*-carboxybutylchitosan and agarose to study the influence of morphological structure on the fluid handling capacities of the materials. Results show that SSI is a feasible and advantageous process that permits to 'tune' the relative loaded amounts of the bioactive substances by changing the operational conditions. The process also promotes the size reduction of quercetin particles with a significant improvement in its solubility in aqueous solutions and consequently in its bioavailability. The prepared materials present a sustained delivery for quercetin and adequate fluid handling capacities that are in the typical and desired ranges for commercial wound dressings.

1 Wound Healing

A wound is defined as a break in the epithelial and/or sub-epithelial integrity of the tissues which can be caused accidentally, intentionally or be a part of a disease process [1]. Wounds can be classified as acute wounds (resulting from incision or trauma) or chronic wounds (venous leg ulcers, pressure and diabetic foot ulcers) being also usually distinguished as open wounds (incisions, lacerations,

A.M.A. Dias (✉) • M.E.M. Braga • I.J. Seabra • H.C. de Sousa
CIEPQPF, Chemical Engineering Department, FCTUC, University of Coimbra, Rua Sílvio Lima, Pólo II – Pinhal de Marrocos, 3030-790 Coimbra, Portugal
e-mail: adias@eq.uc,pt; marabraga@eq.uc.pt; hsousa@eq.uc.pt

I.J. Seabra
ESAC, Politechnic Institute of Coimbra, Bencanta, 3040-316 Coimbra, Portugal
e-mail: iseabra@esac.pt

R.M.N. Jorge et al. (eds.), *Technologies for Medical Sciences*, Lecture Notes in Computational Vision and Biomechanics 1, DOI 10.1007/978-94-007-4068-6_12, © Springer Science+Business Media B.V. 2012

abrasions, punctured and penetrating wounds) and closed wounds (contusions, hematoma and crush injuries) [2]. The healing of a wound requires a complex conjugation of biological and molecular actions of cell migration, cell proliferation and extracellular matrix deposition that result from the interaction of different cells, mediators and growth factors. This process usually involves four overlapping phases of coagulation, inflammation, migration–proliferation and remodeling [3]. Each one of these phases is normally characterized by several specific body response stimuli which are often identified by the generation of some characteristic tissues and/or secretions that may as well require specific treatment agents/conditions [4]. In most cases, wound healing is a natural process which leads to the restoration of tissue integrity but, in some cases, due to many local (infection, tissue ischemia, poor surgical technique, formation of hematomas, presence of foreign bodies and mechanical pressure) and systemic factors (ageing, nutritional status, underlying diseases, medication), wounds fail to heal and become a complex medical problem requiring specialized care and treatment [5]. In these cases, the use of wound dressings may help to promote healing by creating proper physiologic wound environment and acting as a barrier for microorganisms.

2 Wound Dressings

Wound healing is significantly affected by three main factors which include dehydration of exposed tissues, the status of the blood supply bringing oxygen and nutrients to the area, and sepsis [6]. The main function of wound dressings should be to help the body's own healing mechanism and to provide clean conditions in the wound. An *ideal* wound dressing prevents dehydration and scab formation, is permeable to oxygen, water vapor and CO_2, is sterilizable, absorbs excess blood and exudates, protects against secondary infections, supplies mechanical protection to the wound, is non-adherent, non-toxic, non-allergic and non-sensitizing, economic and present a long shelf-life [7]. The selection of the *best* wound dressing is not always a simple task as wound healing is a dynamic process in which wounds undergo different phases of healing. Instead, wounds require different dressings, depending on the type and dimension of the wound, its positioning on the body and, in particular, on the depth of tissue damage, stage of healing and level of exudate [8]. Careful monitoring of the exudate can provide information for the application of systemic and local therapies [9].

One of the most important requirements of any dressing system is the capacity to guarantee the optimal moisture content of a wound and the surrounding skin. The works published by Winter [10, 11] were the first showing that, under moist conditions, wounds healed 50% faster than those healed in open air (dry) conditions. In the case of medium or highly exuding wounds, the dressing should be able to remove the excess wound fluid but, in dry or lightly exuding wounds, the dressing should maintain the exposed tissue in the optimum state of hydration. This facilitates epithelialisation and promotes autolytic debridement also enhancing the viability of the epithelial cells by protecting them from dehydration and scab formation [12]. Commonly used wound dressings comprise cotton gauze, foams, sponges, wads or other fibrous materials. Gauze and other fibrous materials are efficient absorbing dressings but, when removed, they usually remove new tissue formed causing wound injury and disturbing new tissue growth, delaying the healing process and causing pain. Cotton gauze present good absorption properties and soft handle, but they do not maintain the moist environment that has proved to facilitate faster wound healing as it allows moisture to evaporate from the wound [12, 13]. Thus, there is a need for a dressing which is non-adherent while being absorbent and that can balance the moisture in the wound environment. This has been the driving force in the development of the large number of products that are currently available and that include [14]:

1. *Semipermeable film dressings* for low to medium exuding wounds: adhesive, elastic, thin transparent films (allow inspection of wound), permeable to gases but impermeable to liquid and bacteria. Film dressings are indicated as primary dressings in minor burns, simple abrasions and lacerations and as a post-operative layer over dry sutured wounds. Examples of these materials include Opsite, Flexiguard, Tegaderm, Melfilm and Bioclusive
2. *Foam dressings* for moderately exudating wounds: highly absorbent, cushioning and protective, and insulate and conform well to body surfaces. Foams facilitate a moist wound environment and absorb excess exudate to decrease the risk of maceration. Foams are generally nonadhesive and require a secondary dressing or tape/bandage to keep in place. Examples of these materials include Allevyn, Lyofoam, Tielle plus and Biatin Adhesive
3. *Alginate dressings* for medium to heavily exuding wounds and also good for bleeding wounds: highly absorbent, biodegradable dressings derived from seaweed. An active ion exchange of calcium ions for sodium ions at the wound surface forms soluble sodium alginate gel that provides a moist wound environment. Moreover, it was demonstrated that calcium ions released by this type of dressing are a natural co-factor in the coagulation therapy promoting haemostasis in bleeding wounds. Examples of these materials include Kaltostat, Sorbsan and Algisite
4. *Hydrocolloids* are moisture-retentive dressings, which contain gel-forming agents such as sodium carboxymethylcellulose, gelatin and pectin. Many products combine the gel-forming properties with elastomers and adhesives are applied to a carrier such as foam or film to form an absorbent, self adhesive, waterproof material. In the presence of wound exudates, hydrocolloids absorb liquid and form a gel. Examples of these materials include sheets such as Alione, Combiderm and Duoderm, paste such as GranuGel and hydrofibre such as Aquacel and Versiva
5. *Hydrogels* for wounds that range from dry to mildly exudating and that can be used to degrade slough on the wound surface: composed by complex hydrophyllic polymers have a high water content (90%) which creates a moist wound surface. Hydrogels are insoluble polymers that expand in water and

are available in sheet, amorphous gel or sheet hydrogel impregnated dressings. Hydrogels provide a moist environment for cell migration and absorb some exudate. As absorption of exudate is poor, they can cause maceration. Examples of these materials include Aquafoam, Intrasite, Nu-Gel, Purilon and Sterigel

Due to the complexity that characterizes the wound healing process, new materials, usually known as multi-layered wound dressings, are being developed. They are comprised by a combination of the different materials described above, where each layer has a distinct property to enhance the wound-healing process, maintains a proper moisture level, prevents adherence (consequently reducing the pain associated with wound treatment and dressing changes) and at a relatively reduced cost [15–17]. These multi-layer products are usually constituted by a physical bacterial barrier, an absorptive layer (alginate or other fiber-gelling dressing, foam, hydrocolloid or hydrogel) and a semi-adherent or non-adherent layer over the wound site. Examples of commercially available composite dressings include Stratasorb (Medline), 3M Tegaderm (3M), Alldress (Molnlycke health Care), Covaderm Plus (DeRoyal), Versiva (ConvaTech), Coversite plus (Smith & Nephew), Telfa Ventex (Kendall), MPM (MPM), Viasorb (Sherwood-davis & Geck), Silon Dual-Dress (Bio Med Sciences).

Recent research is centered on the use of biodegradable and biocompatible materials to be used in each of the above discriminated layers. Healing of dermal wounds with natural polymers is attractive mostly because these polymers (or their degradation products) are usually biocompatible and they present non-irritant and non-toxic properties, thus being their dermis application easy and safe [18]. Moreover, natural polymers are normally inexpensive, readily available from renewable sources, potentially biodegradable and capable of a multitude of possible chemical modifications [19]. These materials include alginates, collagens, chitosan, chitin, derivatives from chitosan or chitin and their blends as is the case of chitosan and alginate [20], alginate and water-soluble chitin [21] or collagen and chitosan blends [22]. So far, research has focused on studies with alginate based materials but the interest in chitin and its derivatives is growing due to the benefits that this biomaterial presents to the wound healing process.

Chitin, a naturally abundant polysaccharide obtained from crustaceans (shrimps, crabs and crawfish) and insects' shells is the second most abundant organic compound in nature, after cellulose. Studies demonstrated that chitin represents 14–27% and 13–15% of the dry weight of shrimp and crab processing wastes, respectively [23]. Chitin is highly hydrophobic and is insoluble in water and most organic solvents, while chitosan, obtained from chitin by removing sufficient acetyl groups ($-COCH_3$) from the molecule, is soluble in dilute acids such as acetic and formic acids. Several efforts have been reported in the literature to prepare functional derivatives of chitosan in order to make them soluble in aqueous systems [24]. The presence of the more or less bulky substituent weakens the hydrogen bonds of chitosan inducing changes in the swelling capacity of the matrix, depending on the hydrophobicity of the substituent, although retaining the film-forming property of chitosan [25].

Among others, the main benefits of using chitin based materials for wound healing are that they initiate fibroblast proliferation, help in ordered collagen deposition, and stimulate an increased level of natural hyaluronic acid synthesis at the wound site, leading to faster wound healing and scar prevention. Chitosan possesses ionic charges, which leads to the ability to chemically bind with negatively charged fats, lipids, cholesterol, metal ions, proteins and macromolecules. Chitosan based materials also proved to exhibit radical scavenging activity towards a number of radicals, being this activity directly related to the degree of deacetylation of the macromolecule [26]. This property is important to regulate the inflammatory process of the wound by reducing the reactive oxygen and reactive nitrogen species that are overproduced by inflammatory cells, especially in chronic wounds [27].

N-Carboxybutylchitosan, a modified and more water-soluble chitosan derivative, presents inhibitory and bactericidal/fungal activities and is able to prevent secondary infections leading to limited scar formation [28]. This biomaterial also presents relatively good mechanical properties for several biomedical applications and can be processed by different methods, originating materials in different forms and shapes such as particles, thin films and porous monolith structures [29]. This is an important issue when developing wound dressing materials as it will permit to control the membranes permeation to water vapor and oxygen, their swelling capacity, as well as the sustained rate-controlling release of drugs or bioactive species, by varying the thickness and the porosity of the processed layers. Besides its biocompatibility, it may also neutralize the wound alkalinity (pH ~ 8) and restore the natural pH of the wound or the skin. This happens due to its chemical inherent acidity (presence of an acidic carboxylic group in their chemical structure) or to the formation of acidic compounds during their hydrolysis by the action of skin enzymes [5]. Agarose is a non-charged neutral polysaccharide that is soluble in hot water and capable of forming thermoreversible physical or non-covalent hydrogels when cooled down below its gelation temperature [30]. Because of its non-toxicity, biocompatibility, favorable interactions with living cells and fast degradation into non-toxic metabolites, agarose-based physical hydrogels are widely implemented in many biological and medical fields [31–33] and, more recently, as natural polymer-based scaffolds [34, 35].

Based on intensive research, modern wound dressings are developed by taking into consideration two essential factors: that the dressing is able to provide a moist wound environment and able to stimulate the granulating process or protecting against the damage of a new formed tissue. This later can be enhanced by the impregnation of the dressing based materials with active substances like antibiotics and antimicrobial and antiseptic agents such as calcium, zinc or silver ions, framycetin, chlorhexidine acetate and povidone iodine. Zinc and copper ions in particular, besides being non-toxic, can be easily attached to wound dressings through chelation with fibres containing amine groups. In this respect, chitosan fibres treated with zinc and copper compounds have the combined antimicrobial properties of the chitosan as well as the metal ions. Commercially available examples of these impregnated materials include Acticoat, Aquacell Ag, Arglaes, Inadine, Iodoflex, Silverlon, Sofra-Tulle, Bactigras and Inadine [13, 36]. Recent studies have also focused on the impregnation of natural bioactive substances into wound dressings for wound infections as is the case of honey [37], tea tree oil (antimicrobial and antiinflammatory activities) being a promising adjunctive wound treatment [38], extract of cinnamon leaves [39], extract of grapefruit flesh or seeds (bactericidal, fungicidal, antiviral, antiparasitic and antiinflammatory agent) [40] and *Bletilla striata* herbal extract [41].

Studies of the topical application of compounds with free radical scavenging properties have shown to significantly improve healing and protect tissue from oxidative damage [42]. However, a too high concentrated application of antioxidants may result in toxic response in the wound. To obtain good results on wound healing, a slow release of the antioxidant is required. Moreover, and since wound dressings are directly in contact with damaged skin, there are strict toxicity/dose requirements for the type of applicable antioxidant/antimicrobial agents.

The incorporation of drugs or other bioactive species into polymeric matrices is usually done by physical mixing of these substances during polymeric synthesis, or by immersing and soaking the previously prepared polymeric materials into a solution which contains the bioactive substances to be impregnated. These methods are relatively simple to implement, but they also present some disadvantages like the use of organic solvents (which have to be removed to acceptable limits both for health/safety reasons and for product integrity maintenance), possible occurrence of undesired substances reactions and/or degradation, low incorporation yields and heterogeneous dispersion [43–45]. To overcome these issues, the use of supercritical fluid methodologies is being presented as a valuable alternative to prepare specialized materials for biomedical applications, for which restrictive toxicity/biocompatibility limits are imposed and need to be accomplished.

3   Supercritical Fluid Impregnation/Deposition

The use of supercritical fluids for chemical and physical polymer processing is an actual and growing research field supported by its broad range of possible applications which includes polymerization, fractionation, foaming, dyeing/impregnation, encapsulation and micronization (by different methods including supercritical antisolvent (SAS), rapid expansion of supercritical solutions (RESS), particles from gas saturated solution (PGSS), supercritical assisted atomization (SAA)), sterilization, crystal growth, and as mixing/blending aids for crystalline or viscous materials [46, 47].

A supercritical fluid or a dense gas is a substance that exists at or near its critical point, which is located at the end of the phase boundary between the gas and liquid phases of the substance (Fig. 1). When pressure and temperature increase beyond the critical point the phases become indistinguishable as either a gas or a liquid, and become a supercritical fluid (SCF) [48]. At this condition, the fluid can have density and solvent properties similar to those of the corresponding liquid but with lower viscosity and higher diffusion rate much closer to a gas, as listed in Table 1.

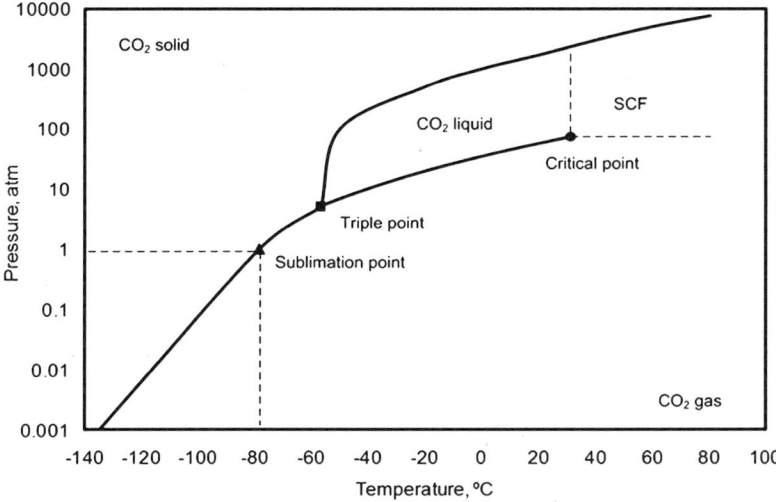

Fig. 1 Schematic phase diagram of CO_2 indicating the compound sublimation point (▲), triple point (■) and supercritical point (●), respectively, using experimental data from NIST Chemistry Webbook

Table 1 Typical ranges for some physical properties of gases, liquids and supercritical fluids [49]

Property	Gas	SCF	Liquid
Density (g cm^{-3})	6×10^{-4}–2×10^{-3}	0.2–0.9	0.6–1.6
Diffusion coefficient (cm^2/s)	0.1–0.4	2×10^{-4}–7×10^{-4}	2×10^{-6}–2×10^{-5}
Viscosity (cP)	0.01–0.03	0.01–0.09	0.2–3.0

Another important advantage of SCFs over conventional solvents includes their density-dependent solvent power which controls its ability to dissolve solutes [50]. Moreover, as the density is related to pressure and temperature and as a SCF is highly sensitive to changes in pressure, it is possible to control the solute-solvent interactions in SCFs by varying the process conditions. This high sensitivity induces an ability to tune the density and solvent strength of a SCF and consequently its selectivity to dissolve various compounds.

Any substance can be used as a supercritical fluid however, particular attention has been given to supercritical carbon dioxide (scCO$_2$) since it is an environmentally clean solvent with mild critical point value (Tc = 31.1°C and Pc = 73.8 bar) making its operation safe and cheap. Besides its intensive use as an alternative solvent in extraction of nutraceuticals from vegetal matrices [51], scCO$_2$ is being extensively used in the field of medical polymers and bioblends, which are very sensitive to residual solvents, benefiting from the use of a non-toxic, inert, and environmentally-friendly processing media [46]. The advantageous mass transfer properties of dense CO$_2$ allows it to impregnate amorphous polymers with various CO$_2$-soluble compounds, including monomers, catalysts, initiators, and various bio-actives that have affinity for CO_2. In pharmaceutical processing $scCO_2$ offers a particular advantage in that the polymer plasticization processing can be carried out at low temperatures [52] which is important for thermally sensitive drug or biomaterials (e.g. enzyme) formulations, where the incipient may degrade when exposed to high temperatures [53].

The development of sustained drug delivery based on the use of supercritical fluid assisted mixing of drug particles and biological materials in degradable/non-degradable polymers is an innovative application of the methodology and one of the main reasons for polymer processing in pharmaceutical field. This kind of pharmaceutical preparations permit to obtain fast release for drugs with low water solubilities, prolonged-delayed release for drugs with high water solubilities, protection of the active principle, minimization of haematic concentration peaks avoiding side effects and better patient compliance [54]. The resulting products can be used for tissue engineering applications such as scaffolds and controlled drug delivery devices using both biodegradable and non-biodegradable polymers. The above mentioned high diffusivity and low surface tension of dense CO_2 enables it to easily penetrate into the polymeric matrix, dispersing solutes throughout the polymer. Furthermore, this diffusion enhancement can be controlled ("tuned") just by changing the operational pressure and temperature. Upon depressurization the CO_2-soluble compounds become entrapped in the polymer substrate, and can also cause the polymer substrate to foam. When returning back to atmospheric temperature and pressure, dense CO_2 will return to its gaseous state without leaving any residual solvent, originating a highly pure final product [53, 55]. Therefore, impregnation using $scCO_2$ results from the equilibrium between CO_2 swelling and plasticizing capacity and CO_2 solubility for the additive(s) to be loaded, assuring the appropriate plasticization of the polymeric substrate as well as the appropriate solvent power for the additive(s). This will strongly favor the additive partition into the polymeric phase over the supercritical phase, yielding higher loadings and a more uniform distribution of the additives in the whole polymeric substrate [56–58].

Although CO_2 is the most frequently employed SCF, it also presents several limitations mainly due to its inability to dissolve high molecular weight compounds and to its non-polarity and lack of several specific solvent–solute and solvent–polymer interactions that would lead to high polymeric drug loading. A frequent strategy to increase drug solubility in $scCO_2$ is the addition of small amounts of specific co-solvents (like ethanol or water) which can change its solvent power, sometimes up to several hundred percent in terms of solubility enhancement [59, 60]. The efficacy of a dense CO_2 process to create a controlled drug delivery system is dependent on pressure, glass transition temperature (Tg) of the polymer and interactions between the polymer, bioactive substance and dense CO_2. The dispersion of the drug within the polymer matrix is dependent on the drug CO_2 solubility as well as on the drug affinity for the polymer. Two different impregnation mechanisms may occur. The first one is explained by the interaction of the drug molecules with the polymer active sites: the drug molecules leave the supercritical phase and reach the polymeric active sites, while the concentration of the drug in the fluid is kept constant by the progressive dissolution of other amounts of drug. The second mechanism is a simple physical entrapment of the drug molecules inside the polymeric matrix when the solvent is removed. The first mechanism, obviously, leads to higher impregnation amounts and usually prevents re-crystallization of the drug [61]. When polymer-SCF phase interactions are present and are favorable, high pressures usually facilitate the diffusion process mostly because they will allow more fluid absorption which will generate a higher swelling degree. This is the case when higher operational pressure determines higher drug loading in the polymeric matrix. On the other hand, when drug–SCF phase interactions are stronger than drug–polymer interactions, pressure usually will be an unfavorable factor because higher pressures will originate an increase in SCF phase density, thus leading to an increased solvating power of the mobile phase. At the same time, and if the polymer–SCF phase interactions are still appreciable, this increased density will also originate an increase in polymer swelling. As a result of these two combined factors, more drug will "choose" to diffuse out the polymeric matrix and stay in the mobile phase, originating a low polymeric loading [62–65].

A compilation of some of the works published over the last decade concerning the supercritical impregnation/loading of bioactive compounds into different polymeric matrices is resumed in Table 2. These works intended to develop optimized drug delivery systems (DDS) for different ophthalmic, topical, dental applications aiming to obtain sustained releases able to deliver the bioactive compound for longer periods of time at a constant rate, avoiding dose fluctuation, and excessive dosage. In some cases it was also attempted to reduce the cristallinity of the solute in order to improve its solubility in aqueous media and consequent bioavailability. The bioactive compounds impregnated include synthetic and natural based materials with different hydrophilicities. In the case of the more hydroplylic compounds, the effects of the use of safe co-solvents like water and ethanol was addressed proving to be an effective way to overcome the hydrophobic character of $scCO_2$.

4 Case Study

The incorporation of bioactive compounds like anti-inflammatories, anti-microbials and antiseptics into wound dressing materials can play an active role in the wound healing process to prevent inflammation and bacterial infection and to accelerate tissue regeneration, by stimulating body's healing responses with the minimum final scar formation [74, 75]. With this idea in mind, a recent work was carried out to study the possibility of developing potential hydrogel-type delivery systems based on natural-origin bioactive species envisaged for wound healing applications [45]. The impregnated wound dressing models were prepared using biodegradable and biocompatible natural-based polymeric matrices, namely N-carboxybutylchitosan (CBC) and agarose (AGA), that were impregnated/loaded with two natural-origin bioactive compounds, quercetin and thymol, separately or as mixture, by using a supercritical solvent impregnation (SSI) methodology.

Table 2 Examples of drug delivery systems prepared using supercritical fluid impregnation method

Impregnated polymer	Impregnated bioactive solute	Application	Reference
Poly(vinylpyrrolidone)	Ibuprofen	Antiinflammatory DDS	[61]
Poly(vinylpyrrolidone)	Indomethacin	Improve drug availability	[66]
Chitosan thermosets	Indomethacin	Improve drug availability	[67]
Poly(vinylpyrrolidone)	Ketoprofen	Improve oral availability	[68]
Poly(sebacic anhydride),	Indomethacin	Implant device	[69]
Porous methacrylate system	Chlorhexidine diacetate	Dental materials	[70]
Chitosan derivatives (N-carboxymethyl chitosan, N-carboxybutyl chitosan and N-succinyl chitosan)	Flurbiprofen and timolol maleate	Ophthalmic DDS	[44]
Hydroxypropylmethyl cellulose	Indomethacin	DDS using highly water swelled gel system	[71]
Poly(e-caprolactone) blends	Timolol maleate	Ophthalmic DDS	[63]
Poly(vinylpyrrolidone)	Piroxicam	Antiinflammatory DDS	[72]
Poly(methyl methacrylate)	Triflusal	Implant carrier as antiinflammatory DDS	[73]
Commercial silicone-based hydrogel contact lenses	Acetazolamide and timolol maleate	Ophthalmic DDS	[64]
Commercial contact lenses (nelfilcon A, omafilcon A, methafilcon A and hilafilcon B)	Flurbiprofen and timolol maleate	Ophthalmic DDS	[65]
N-carboxybutyl chitosan and agarose	Quercetin and thymol	Topical wound dressing	[45]

Biopolymer substrate materials were prepared in the shape of films and as foams in order to understand how their different physical-chemical characteristics may influence their final loading, release and barrier properties. The advantages of using chitosan and agarose based biomaterials as support for the wound dressing materials were previously mentioned and justified. Quercetin and thymol were chosen mainly due to their important biological activities that can contribute to enhance the wound healing process as will be described in what follows.

The potential of polyphenols or flavonoids as antioxidant natural based compounds is well studied and demonstrated [76–78]. All flavonoids have the same basic chemical structure – a three-ringed molecule with hydroxyl (OH) groups attached but depending on the type and number of other substitutions more than 4,000 flavonoids, with different activities can be obtained. Quercetin, one of the most abundant of the flavonoid molecules, is widely distributed in the plant kingdom being found in many usually consumed foods, including apple, onion, tea, berries, and brassica vegetables, as well as many seeds, nuts, flowers, barks, and leaves. It is also found in medicinal botanicals, including *Ginkgo biloba*, *Hypericum perforatum* (St. John's Wort), *Sambucus canadensis* (elder), and many others, and is often a component of the medicinal activity of the plant [79]. Among other properties, quercetin is recognized as an intra-arterial pressure reducer preventing cardiovascular disease [80] also presenting strong antioxidant [81–84], antiinflammatory [85] and antiviral activities [86]. Despite its wide spectrum of potential pharmacological properties, the use of quercetin in the pharmaceutical field is quite limited and few human quercetin absorption studies exist due to its low aqueous solubility and to its easy degradation in aqueous intestinal fluids [87]. It appears that only a small percentage of about 2% of quercetin is absorbed after an oral dose [88]. In order to make the administration effective, high oral doses of about 400–500 mg three times per day is typically used in clinical practice. In order to overcome this issue, quercetin chalcone, a water soluble derivative, is usually administrated and it might be used in smaller doses; typically 250 mg three times per day [89]. Topical and transdermal administration may provide an efficient alternative for quercetin delivery in order to enrich the endogeneous cutaneous protection system, which would represent a successful strategy for diminishing ultraviolet radiation oxidative damages as well as any involved inflammation processes of the skin [90].

The transdermal delivery of relatively high molecular weight compounds is usually enhanced by the simultaneous administration of skin permeation enhancers like terpenes of which L-menthol is a successful reported example [91]. These compounds reduce the diffusional penetration barrier by inducing a temporary and reversible increase on its permeability by disrupting the hydrogen-bonding network and increasing the hydration levels of the lipid system, probably by forming new aqueous channels [91–93]. Thymol is a monoterpenic phenol usually found in thyme oil with chemical structure similar to L-menthol that can in principle be used as permeation enhancer. Besides, it presents strong antioxidant, anaesthetic, antiseptic and antiinflammatory activities [94, 95] being also an anti-bacterial and/or anti-microbial agent showing a broad-spectrum of biological activities against bacteria, yeasts and fungi [96, 97]. These properties strengthen the potential applicability of this substance as an active compound for impregnated wound dressing materials.

5　Materials and Processes

The molecular structures of employed bioactive substances and polymeric biomaterials are represented in Fig. 2. N-carboxybutylchitosan (CBC) and agarose (AGA) solutions were prepared according to the procedure already described in the literature and references therein [45]. Films of CBC and foams of CBC and AGA were prepared by the solvent casting method and by freeze-drying, respectively. The average thickness of all obtained sample materials was 95 ± 5 μm

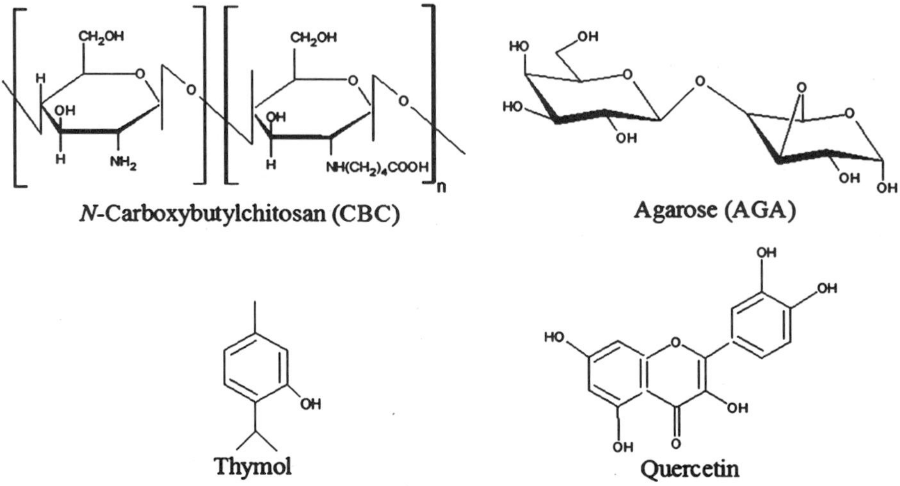

Fig. 2 Structural formula of employed bioactive substances and polymeric biomaterials

(for films) and 250 ± 15 μm (for foams). After drying, polymeric samples were cut in rectangular pieces of approximately 10×5 mm and weighing approximately 3 ± 0.5 mg and 5 ± 1 mg, for foams and films, respectively.

The supercritical impregnation apparatus used in this work was already described in the literature [44, 63–65]. A schematic representation of its main components is given in Fig. 3. In general terms, it is comprised of a compressed air-operated CO_2 liquid pump, a visual high-pressure stainless steel impregnation cell, a thermostatic controlled water bath and a magnetic stirring plate as an auxiliary tool to dissolve and to homogenize the high pressure mixture (bioactive compounds plus $scCO_2$/co-solvent).The procedure consists in placing weighed samples of CBC (or AGA) foams or films into the high-pressure cell that already contained known amounts of quercetin and/or thymol. The amounts of employed bioactive compounds were established by taking into account the available cell volume and the compounds solubility in $scCO_2$ (at the tested experimental conditions) and by using amounts that corresponded to 10% of the saturation solubility limit. Ethanol (EtOH), 10% v/v, was used as the co-solvent for the quercetin system and in order to increase its solubility in $scCO_2$. The system is then closed and pressurized up to the pre-established operational pressure and after bath temperature stabilization. Two different operational conditions (10 MPa/303 K and 20 MPa/323 K) were tested in order to study their influence on the amounts of loaded bioactive compounds. The system is then maintained in static conditions for 3 h allowing the diffusion of the solvent (pressurized CO_2 or CO_2/co-solvent mixture), saturated with quercetin and/or thymol, through the polymeric matrix. After this period, the solvent is removed by slow depressurization (1 $MPa.min^{-1}$) in order to not alter or damage the processed polymeric samples.

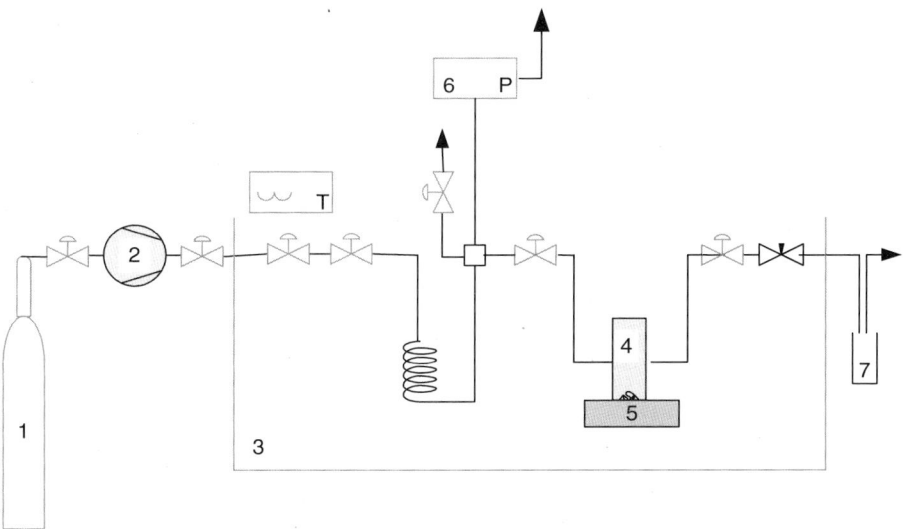

Fig. 3 Schematic diagram of the experimental supercritical impregnation apparatus: (*1*) CO$_2$ reservoir; (*2*) high pressure CO$_2$ pump; (*3*) water bath; (*4*) high pressure stainless steel impregnation cell; (*5*) magnetic stirrer; (*6*) pressure transducer and (*7*) glass trap

6 Effect of the Process Conditions on the Polymeric Matrices

As previously mentioned, one of the advantages of using SCF technology is the possibility to change the matrix porosity by changing process conditions like pressure, residence time and depressurization rate. This is an important factor when developing wound dressing materials as it can influence the permeability of the dressing to gases and moisture and also the kinetic release of a bioactive compound to the wound in the case of impregnated materials. The porosity of the CBC films and foams and AGA foams was measured by mercury porosimetry (Micromeritics, Pore Sizer 9320). Table 3 presents the relative variation induced by the process on the porosity, pore size and apparent density of the three samples studied. As expected the pore diameter of the foam like structure is higher (10–500 μm) than that of the film (0–10 μm). This difference is illustrated in Fig. 4 which compares the pore size distribution of the samples before and after processing at 323 K and 20 MPa for 3 h. The processing of the materials followed an experimental procedure similar to the one previously described except that in this case any bioactive compound was included in the high pressure cell. The vertical axis in Fig. 4, (−dV/dlogD) is a differential of the volume of mercury intruded at each pore diameter (D) and is therefore related to the volume of macropores of each diameter. As can be seen, scCO$_2$ processing increased sample porosity, acting as a morphological and porogenic agent for all the samples being this effect most pronounced for CBC films with a porosity increase of over 40% and only slightly for CBC foam. When comparing CBC and AGA foams it can be seen that processing has a higher effect on the number and size of the pores of AGA foams.

Table 3 Effect of supercritical CO_2 processing (323 K and 20 MPa) on the morphology of the samples

	Relative variation (%)[a]		
	CBC film	CBC foam	AGA foam
Total intrusion volume (mL/g)	+169.9	+4.1	+23.6
Total pore area (m²/g)	+266.3	+33.5	+102.4
Average pore diameter (μm)	−26.3	−22.0	−38.9
Apparent (skeletal) density (g/mL)	−10.6	+19.3	+0.6
Porosity (%)	+39.6	+1.6	+1.5

[a]Relative variation (%) = (after processing-before processing)/before processing × 100

7 Fluid Handling Properties of Prepared Polymeric Samples

The ability to control the loss of moisture from a wound is commonly determined by the moisture vapor permeability of the dressing or dressing system. As already mentioned, excessive exudate can cause maceration of the periwound skin, which in turn can lead to infection, and therefore the wound dressing material should be highly absorbent to prevent fluid from spreading over the surrounding healthy tissue and simultaneously permeable to water vapor and thus permitting the passage of a significant quantity of the aqueous component of exudate from the wound to the environment by evaporation. The fluid handling capacity (FHC) of a material is given by the following equation:

$$FHC = Absorbency + Moisture\ Vapor\ Loss \tag{1}$$

where the absorbency and the moisture vapor loss represent the mass of water vapor absorbed and permeated by the dressing material. These parameters were measured for the CBC and AGA membranes following standard procedures and as described in the literature [45]. The absorbency of the membranes was measured at 305 K with the membranes exposed to a 95% relative humidity (RH) atmosphere. The moisture vapor loss was determined according to a modified ASTM standard (inverted-cup, E96-90, Procedure D) by monitoring the amount/mass of evaporated water through the test-sample membrane and by measuring the weight loss from a water-filled homemade modified Payne Cup at 305 K filled with 5 g of de-ionized and distilled water and the test-sample membrane was fixed onto its opening, with an exposed central circular aperture of 3.14×10^{-4} m² exposed to a relative humidity (RH) of approximately 20% at 305 K. By way of illustration, Fig. 5 compares the fluid handling capacity of CBC and AGA membranes with some commercial materials over 24, 48 and 96 h. The results show that different materials present different rates of hydration with time. Some products reach full absorbency after 24 h, others are still absorbing after 96 h. These differences clearly have potentially important clinical implications for the use of the products concerned. The studied materials reach equilibrium absorbency after 12 h with values equal to 50%, 45% and 30% for CBC film, CBC foam and AGA foam, respectively. The values obtained for the

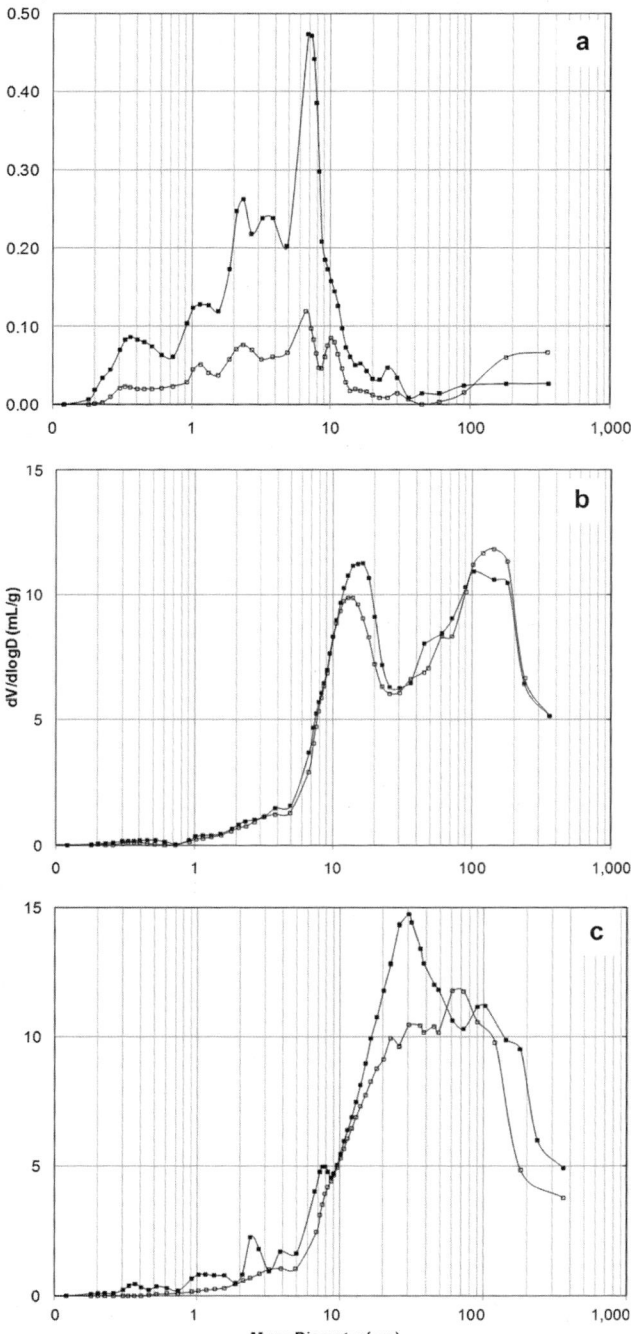

Fig. 4 Interconnected macropore size distribution for CBC films (**a**), CBC foams (**b**) and AGA foams (**c**) before (open symbols) and after processing at 323 K and 20 MPa (full symbols), obtained from mercury porosimetry

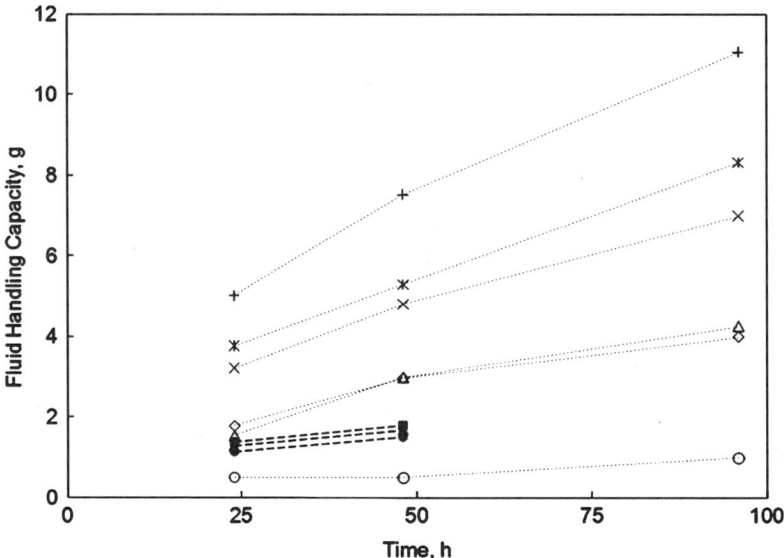

Fig. 5 Comparison of the fluid-handling capacities of CBC film (■), CBC foam (▲), AGA foam (●) with commercially available hydrocolloid dressings after 24, 48 and 96 h: Tegasorb (+), Comfeel Plus (*), Cutinova Hydro (×), Algoplaque (△), Granuflex (◇) and Askina Biofilm Transparent (○)

FHC of these materials are between the ones observed for Algoplaque, Granuflex and Askina Biofilm Transparent. These membranes consist in sterile and transparent semi-permeable hydrocolloid dressing composed by an inner layer containing a dispersion of gelatin, pectin and/or carboxy-methylcellulose incorporated in an elastomeric mesh and an outer layer of polyurethane which is impermeable to exudate and micro-organisms. In contact with the wound, it absorbs progressively the exudates, forms a moist gel and creates the condition that favors the healing process regarding moisture, temperature and pH (according to manufacturer indications). They are indicated in the treatment of chronic exuding wounds such as leg ulcers, pressure sores, minor burns, donor sites, (after haemostasis has been achieved), and other types of granulating wounds. If applied to wounds containing dry slough or necrosis, the dressing prevents the loss of water vapor from the surface of the skin, and this effectively rehydrates the dead tissue, which is then removed by autolysis.

8 Influence of Process Parameters on the Amount of Quercetin and Thymol Loaded

The effect of process conditions on the total amount of quercetin and thymol loaded into the different polymeric matrices is shown in Fig. 6. The results permit to conclude that:

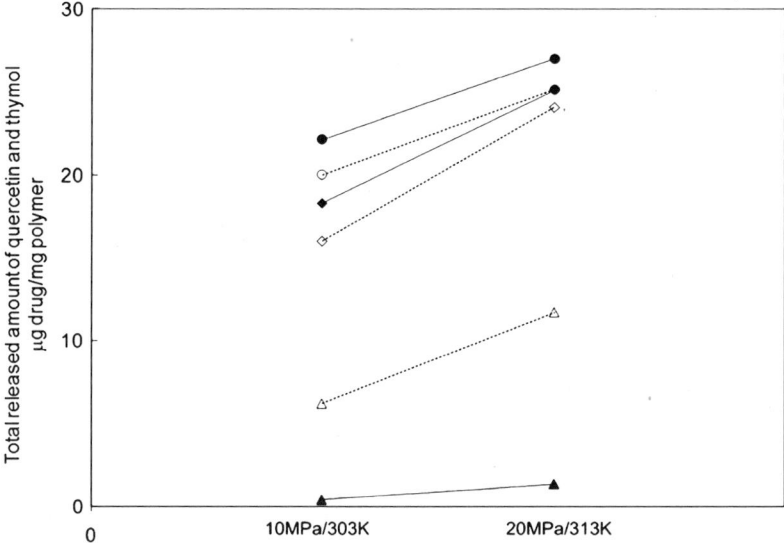

Fig. 6 Quercetin (full symbols) and thymol (open symbols) total loaded amounts into CBC foams (●), AGA foams (♦) and CBC films (▲) at 10 MPa and 303 K and 20 MPa and 323 K. Lines serve only as guides for the eye

1. Higher pressure and higher temperature led to higher quercetin and thymol loaded amounts for all the employed polymeric samples. Despite both working conditions (10 MPa/303 K and 20 MPa/323 K) correspond to similar solvent densities (17.5 mol/L), in this case, the different transport properties (viscosity and diffusivity) characterizing each condition, as well as the higher scCO$_2$ swelling and plasticization of most polymers that is usually favored at this conditions led to an improve in the impregnation/loading efficiency [45, 48, 98];

2. Foam like structures permit to load higher amounts of quercetin and thymol (15–30 μg/mg polymer) when compared to CBC films (<12 μg/mg polymer) due to their higher porosities, in the range from 10 to 500 μm as confirmed by mercury porosimetry, which has as main consequence the significant increase in diffusivity and in the available surface area of this porous structures;

3. Contrary to foams, CBC film structures permit to load higher amounts of thymol when compared to quercetin due to shape/molecular volume factors that limit the amount of loaded quercetin;

4. Specific and favorable interactions between quercetin and CBC (enhancing quercetin polymer/mobile phase partition coefficient) and the higher solubility of thymol in scCO$_2$ justifies the similar amounts loaded for each compound in CBC foams [45]. In fact, the higher affinity of thymol for the solvent phase also promotes its removal during the depressurization step, being this effect more pronounced in foam-like structures.

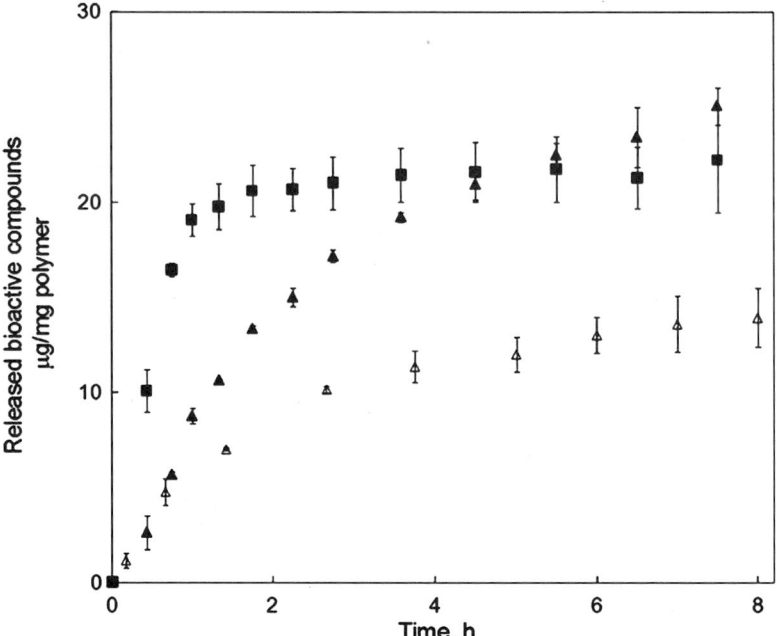

Fig. 7 Release profiles for CBC samples loaded with quercetin (▲) and thymol (■) at 20 MPa and 323 K for 3 h and soaked into an ethanolic solution at 2 mg/mL for 3 h (△)

The release profiles of CBC membranes, simultaneously impregnated with quercetin and thymol, at 20 MPa/313 K is shown in Fig. 7. The results show a more sustained release profile for quercetin that the authors justified due to its higher molecular volume, lower solubility in water and also, and most important, due to specific interactions between the –OH groups of the molecule with –NH$(CH_2)_4$COOH groups from CBC and still some unmodified -NH$_2$ groups (from chitosan) and –NHCOCH$_3$ groups (from chitin) [45, 87, 99, 100]. The lower molecular volume of thymol together with its higher aqueous solubility justifies its faster release. Fig. 7 also presents the release profile for a CBC sample soaked into an ethanolic solution of quercetin at 2 mg/mL (maximum solubility at room temperature) for 3 h. It is clear that the SSI process significantly enhances the amount of quercetin that can be loaded into the polymeric matrix (almost duplicates its value) also avoiding the ethanol evaporation step. This improvement in quercetin loading, releasing and consequently on its bioavailability is most probably due to quercetin particle sizes reduction during SSI processing what was confirmed by SEM analysis [45].

Finally, the antioxidant capacity of the CBC membrane loaded with quercetin and thymol at 20 MPa/323 K was tested using a method based on the coupled oxidation of β-carotene/linolenic acid system [101] optimized by Braga et al. [102]. This colorimetric based method consists in evaluating the capacity of a potential

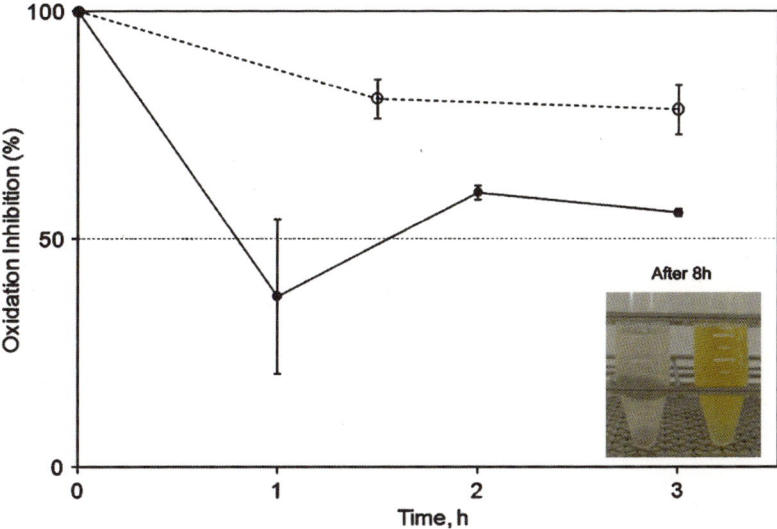

Fig. 8 Antioxidant activities of quercetin (○) and CBC membrane loaded with quercetin and thymol by SSI at 20 MPa and 323 K (●). Enclosed picture represents the control and the membrane system after 8 h of oxidative reaction

antioxidant system by measuring its capacity to be oxidized preferentially avoiding the oxidation of β-carotene. After starting the oxidative reaction, the oxidation of β-carotene is followed by measuring the color of the solution at specific time intervals at 470 nm. The samples presenting higher color intensity correspond to the ones that have higher antioxidant capacity. The method was applied in this work to investigate the antioxidant activity of the CBC membranes impregnated at 20 MPa and 313 K. The procedure was similar to the one reported in the literature, where the extract was substituted by a sample of impregnated membrane. Figure 8 compares de results obtained for an ethanolic mixture of quercetin and thymol with the ones obtained for the CBC loaded membranes. Results show that for the monitored period, the impregnated membrane is able to inhibit the oxidation of β-carotene by almost 50%. The trend is dependent on the release of quercetin from the membrane what justifies the lower value observed at the first hour where only 40% of the total loaded amount was delivered to the reaction medium. Unfortunately, the method did not permit to follow the reaction for longer periods as the slow dissolution of the polymeric matrix causes dispersion that interferes with the colorimetric method. However, visual observation after 8 h (photo attached to Fig. 8) permits to conclude that the membrane presents a prolonged antioxidant activity what can be advantageous for long term wound healing processes.

References

1. Robson MC (1997) Wound infection: a failure of wound healing caused by an imbalance of bacteria. Surg Clin North Am 77:637–650
2. Attinger CE, Janis JE, Steinberg J, Schwartz J, Al-Attar A, Couch K (2006) Clinical approach to wounds: Débridement and wound bed preparation including the use of dressings and wound-healing adjuvants. Plast Reconstr Surg 117(7S):72S–109S
3. Falanga V (2005) Wound healing and its impairment in the diabetic foot. Lancet 366: 1736–1743
4. Wiseman DM, Rovee DT, Alvarez OM (1992) Wound dressings: design and use. In: Cohen IK, Diegelmann RF, Lindblad WJ (eds) Wound healing: biochemical and clinical aspects. Saunders, Philadelphia, pp 562–580
5. Rajendran S (2009) Advanced textiles for wound care. Woodhead Publishing Limited/CRC Press LLC, Oxford/Boca Raton
6. Winter GD (2006) Some factors affecting skin and wound healing. J Tissue Viability 16:20–23
7. Ovington LG, Peirce B (2001) Wound dressings: form, function, feasibility, and facts. In: Krasner DL, Rodeheaver GT, Sibbald RG (eds) Chronic wound care: a clinical source book for healthcare professionals, 3rd edn. HMP Communications, Wayne, pp 311–319
8. Cutting KF, White RJ (2002) Maceration of the skin: 1: the nature and causes of skin maceration. J Wound Care 11:275–278
9. White RJ, Cutting KF (2004) Maceration of the skin and wound bed by indication. In: White RJ (ed) Trends in wound care III. Quay, Dinton
10. Winter GD (1962) Formation of the scab and the rate of epithelialisation of superficial wounds in the skin of the young domestic pig. Nature 193:293–294
11. Winter GD (1963) Effect of air exposure and occlusion on experimental human skin wounds. Nature 200:378–379
12. Weller C, Sussman G (2006) Wound dressings update. J Pharm Pract Res Geriatr Ther 36:318–324
13. Aramwit P, Muangman P, Namviriyachote N, Srichana T (2010) In vitro evaluation of the antimicrobial effectiveness and moisture binding properties of wound dressings. Int J Mol Sci 11:2864–2874
14. Jones V, Grey JE, Harding KG (2006) Wound dressings. BMJ 332:777–780
15. Mi FL, Wu Y, Shyu SS, Schoung JY, Huang YB, Tsai YH, Hao JY (2002) Control of wound infections using a bilayer chitosan wound dressing with sustainable antibiotic delivery. J Biomed Mater Res 59:438–449
16. Mi FL, Wu YB, Shyu SS, Chao AC, Lai JY, Su CC (2003) Asymmetric chitosan membranes prepared by dry/wet phase separation: a new type of wound dressing for controlled antibacterial release. J Membr Sci 212:237–254
17. Sripriya R, Kumar MS, Sehgal PK (2004) Improved collagen bilayer for the controlled release of drugs. J Biomed Mater Res B Appl Biomater 70B:389–396
18. Sezer AD, Hatipoglu F, Cevher E, Ogurtan Z, Bas AL, Akbuga J (2007) Chitosan film containing fucoidan as a wound dressing for dermal burn healing: preparation and in vitro/in vivo evaluation. AAPS Pharm Sci Tech 8:E1–E8
19. Prabu SL, Shirwaikar AA, Shirwaikar A, Kumar A, Jacob A (2008) Design and evaluation of matrix diffusion controlled transdermal patches of diltiazem hydrochloride. Ars Pharm 49:211–227
20. Knill CJ, Kennedy JF, Mistry J, Miraftab M, Smart G, Groocock MR, Williams HJ (2004) Alginate fi bres modifi ed with unhydrolyzed and hydrolyzed chitosans for wound dressings. Carbohydr Polym 55:65–76
21. Fan L, Du Y, Zhang B, Yang J, Cai J, Zhang L, Zhou J (2005) Preparation and properties of alginate/water-soluble chitin blend fibres. J Macromol Sci, A 42:723–732
22. Chen JP, Chang GY, Chen JK (2008) Electrospun collagen/chitosan nanofibrous membrane as wound dressing. Colloids Surf A: Physicochem Eng Aspects 313–314:183–188

23. D'Ayala GG, Malinconico M, Laurienzo P (2008) Marine derived polysaccharides for biomedical applications: chemical modification approaches. Molecules 13:2069–2106
24. Skjak-Braek G, Anthonsen T, Sandford PA (1989) Chitin and chitosan: sources, chemistry, biochemistry, physical properties, and applications. Elsevier, New York
25. Yang H, Zhou S, Deng X (2003) Preparation and properties of hydrophilic–hydrophobic chitosan derivatives. J Appl Polym Sci 92:1625–1632
26. Moseley R, Stewart JE, Stephens P, Waddington RJ, Thomas DW (2004) Extracellular matrix metabolites as potential biomarkers of disease activity in wound fluid: lessons learned from other inflammatory diseases? Br J Dermatol 150:401–413
27. James TJ, Hughes MA, Cherry GW, Taylor PT (2003) Evidence of oxidative stress in chronic venous ulcers. Wound Repair Regen 11:172–176
28. Muzzarelli RR, Tarsi O, Filippini E, Giovanetti G, Biagini PE (1990) Antimicrobial properties of N-carboxybutyl chitosan. Antimicrob Agents Chemother 34:2019–2023
29. Öztürk E, Agalar C, Keçeci K, Denkbas EB (2006) Preparation and characterization of ciprofloxacin-loaded alginate/chitosan sponge as a wound dressing material. J Appl Polym Sci 101:1602–1609
30. Wang N, Wu XS (1997) Preparation and characterization of agarose hydrogel nanoparticles for protein and peptide drug delivery. Pharm Develop Techn 2:135–142
31. Cascone MG, Barbani N, Cristallini C, Giusti P, Ciardelli G, Lazzeri L (2001) Bioartificial polymeric materials based on polysaccharides. J Biomat Sci Polym 12:267–281
32. Hoffman AS (2002) Hydrogels for biomedical applications. Adv Drug Deliv Rev 54:3–12
33. Drury JL, Mooney DJ (2003) Hydrogels for tissue engineering: scaffold design variables and applications. Biomaterials 24:4337–4351
34. Lozinsky VI, Damshkaln LG, Bloch KO, Vardi P, Grinberg NV, Burova TV, Grinberg VY (2008) Cryostructuring of polymer systems. XXIX. Preparation and characterization of supermacroporous (spongy) agarose-based cryogels used as three-dimensional scaffolds for culturing insulin-producing cell aggregates. J App Polym Sci 108:3046–3062
35. Roman JMV, Cabanas JP, Doadrio JC, Vallet-Regi M (2008) An optimized b-tricalcium phosphate and agarose scaffold fabrication technique. J Biomed Mater Res 84A:99–107
36. Borkow G, Okon-Levy N, Gabbay J (2010) Copper oxide impregnated wound dressing: biocidal and safety studies. Wounds Compend Clin Res Pract 22:301–310
37. Moore OA, Smith LA, Campbell F, Seers K, McQuay HJ, Moore RA (2001) Systematic review of the use of honey as a wound dressing. BMC Complement Altern Med 1:2
38. Halcón L, Milkus K (2004) Staphylococcus aureus and wounds: a review of tea tree oil as a promising antimicrobial. Am J Infect Control 32:402–408
39. Ebert D (1998) Dressing for promoting wound healing contains a viscous oily extract of cinnamon leaves. Patent DE19849017-C1
40. Steinhauser T, Haering L (1999) Wound dressing containing dilute solution of grapefruit flesh or seed extract, as active agent having e.g. bactericidal, antiinflammatory and healing promoting action. Patent DE19929298-A1
41. Liu BS, Huang TB (2010) A novel wound dressing composed of nonwoven fabric coated with chitosan and herbal extract membrane for wound healing. Polym Compos 31:1037–1046
42. Sen CK, Khanna S, Gordillo G, Bagchi D, Bagchi M, Roy S (2002) Oxygen, oxidants, and antioxidants in wound healing: an emerging paradigm. Ann N Y Acad Sci 957:239–249
43. Li X, Jasti BR (2006) Design of controlled release drug delivery systems. McGraw-Hill, New York
44. Braga MEM, Pato MTV, Silva HSRC, Ferreira EI, Gil MH, Duarte CMM, de Sousa HC (2008) Supercritical solvent impregnation of ophthalmic drugs on chitosan derivatives. J Supercrit Fluids 44:245–257
45. Dias AMA, Braga MEM, Seabra IJ, Ferreira P, Gil MH, de Sousa HC (2011) Development of natural-based wound dressings impregnated with bioactive compounds and using supercritical carbon dioxide. Int J Pharm 408:9–19
46. Quirk RA, France RM, Shakesheff KM, Howdle SM (2004) Supercritical fluid technologies and tissue engineering scaffolds. Curr Opin Solid State Mater Sci 8:313–321

47. Kikic I (2009) Polymer–supercritical fluid interactions. J Supercritical Fluids 47:458–465
48. Kikic F, Vecchione F (2003) Supercritical impregnation of polymers. Curr Opin Solid St Mat Sci 7:399–405
49. Yoganathan RB, Mammucari R, Foster R (2010) Dense gas processing of polymers. Polymer Reviews 50:144–177
50. Pereda S, Bottini SB, Brignole EA (2008) Supercritical fluid extraction of nutraceuticals and bioactive compounds: fundamentals of supercritical fluid technology. CRC Press, Boca Raton
51. Mukhopadhyay M (2000) Natural extracts using supercritical carbon dioxide. CRC Press, Boca Raton
52. Darr JA, Poliakoff M (1999) New directions in inorganic and metal-organic coordination chemistry in supercritical fluids. Chem Rev 99:495–541
53. Howdle SM, Watson MS, Whitaker MJ, Popv VK, Davies MC, Mandel FS, Wang JD, Shakesheff KM (2001) Supercritical fluid mixing: preparation of thermally sensitive polymer composites containing bioactive materials. J Chem Soc Chem Commun 1:109–110
54. Reverchon E, Adami R, Cardea S, Della Porta G (2009) Supercritical fluids processing of polymers for pharmaceutical and medical applications. J Supercritical Fluids 47:484–492
55. Ginty PJ, Whitaker MJ, Shakesheff KM, Howdle SM (2005) Drug delivery goes supercritical. Mater Today 8:42–48
56. Shieh Y, Su J, Manivannan G, Lee PH, Sawan SP, Dale Spall W (1996) Interaction of supercritical carbon dioxide with polymers II. Amorphous polymers. J Appl Polym Sci 59:707–714
57. West BL, Kazarian SG, Vincent MF, Brantley NH, Eckert CA (1998) Supercritical fluid dyeing of PMMA films with azo-dyes. J Appl Polym Sci 69:911–919
58. Wang Y, Yang C, Tomasko D (2002) Confocal microscopy analysis of supercritical fluid impregnation of polypropylene. Ind Eng Chem Res 41:1780–1786
59. Knox DE (2005) Solubilities in supercritical fluids. Pure Appl Chem 77:513–530
60. Duarte ARC, Santiago S, de Sousa HC, Duarte CMM (2005) Solubility of acetazolamide in supercritical carbon dioxide in the presence of ethanol as a cosolvent. J Chem Eng Data 50:216–220
61. Kazarian SG, Martirosyan GG (2002) Spectroscopy of polymer/drug formulations processed with supercritical fluids: in situ ATR-IR and Raman study of impregnation of ibuprofen into PVP. Int J Pharm 232:81–90
62. Kazarian SG, Vincent MF, West BL, Eckert CA (1998) Partitioning of solutes and cosolvents between supercritical and polymer phases. J Supercrit Fluids 13:107–112
63. Natu MV, Gil MH, de Sousa HC (2008) Supercritical solvent impregnation of poly(ε-caprolactone)/poly(oxyethylene-b-oxypropylene-b-oxyethylene) and poly(ε-caprolactone)/poly(ethylene-vinyl acetate) blends for controlled release applications. J Supercrit Fluids 47:93–102
64. Costa VP, Braga MEM, Guerra JP, Duarte ARC, Duarte CMM, Leite EOB, Gil MH, de Sousa HC (2010) Development of therapeutic contact lenses using a supercritical solvent impregnation method. J Supercrit Fluids 52:306–316
65. Costa VP, Braga MEM, Duarte CMM, Alvarez-Lorenzo C, Concheiro A, Gil MH, de Sousa HC (2010) Anti-glaucoma drug-loaded contact lenses prepared using supercritical solvent impregnation. J Supercrit Fluids 53:165–173
66. Gong K, Viboonkiat R, Rehman IU, Buckton G, Darr JA (2005) Formation and characterization of porous indomethacin-PVP coprecipitates prepared using solvent-free supercritical fluid processing. J Pharm Sci 94:2583–2590
67. Gong K, Darr JA, Rehman IU (2006) Supercritical fluid assisted impregnation of indomethacin into chitosan thermosets for controlled release applications. Int J Pharm 315:93–98
68. Manna L, Banchero M, Sola D, Ferri A, Ronchetti S, Sicardi S (2007) Impregnation of PVP microparticles with ketoprofen in the presence of supercritical CO_2. J Supercrit Fluids 42:378–384

69. Gong K, Rehman IU, Darr JA (2007) Synthesis of poly(sebacic anhydride)-indomethacin controlled release composites via supercritical carbon dioxide assisted impregnation. Int J Pharm 338:191–197

70. Gong K, Braden M, Patel MP, Rehman IU, Zhang Z, Darr JA (2007) Controlled release of chlorhexidine diacetate from a porous methacrylate system: supercritical fluid assisted foaming and impregnation. J Pharm Sci 96:2048–2056

71. Gong K, Rehman IU, Darr JA (2008) Characterization and drug release investigation of amorphous drug–hydroxypropyl methylcellulose composites made via supercritical carbon dioxide assisted impregnation. J Pharmaceut Biomed Anal 48:1112–1119

72. Banchero M, Manna L, Ronchetti S, Campanelli P, Ferri A (2009) Supercritical solvent impregnation of piroxicam on PVP at various polymer molecular weights. J Supercrit Fluids 49:271–278

73. Lopez-Periago A, Argemi A, Andanson JM, Fernandez V, Garcia-Gonzalez CA, Kazarian SG, Saurina J, Domingo C (2009) Impregnation of a biocompatible polymer aided by supercritical CO_2: evaluation of drug stability and drug–matrix interactions. J Supercrit Fluids 48:56–63

74. Cabodi M, Cross V, Qu Z, Havenstrite KL, Schwartz S, Stroock AD (2006) An active wound dressing for controlled convective mass transfer with the wound bed. J Biom Mat Res Part B 13:210–220

75. Seydim AC, Sarikus G (2006) Antimicrobial activity of whey protein based edible films incorporated with oregano, rosemary and garlic essential oils. Food Res Int 39:639–644

76. Alvarez M, Zarelli VEP, Pappano NB, Debattista NB (2004) Bacteriostatic action on synthetic polyhydroxylates chalcones against escherichia coli. Biocell 28:31–34

77. Manach C, Williamson G, Morand C, Scalbert A, Rémésy C (2005) Bioavailability and bioefficacy of polyphenols in humans. I. Review of 97 bioavailability studies. Am J Clin Nutr 81:230S–242S

78. Perron NR, Brumaghim JL (2009) A review of the antioxidant mechanisms of polyphenol compounds related to iron binding. Cell Biochem Biophys 53:75–10

79. Boots AW, Haenen GR, Bast A (2008) Health effects of quercetin: from antioxidant to nutraceutical. Eur J Pharmacol 582:325–337

80. Pace-Asciak CR, Hahn S, Diamandis EP (1995) The red wine phenolics trans-resveratrol and quercetin block human platelet aggregation and eicosanoid synthesis: implications for protection against coronary heart disease. Clin Chim Acta 235:207–219

81. Saija A, Scalese M, Lanza M (1995) Flavonoids as antioxidant agents: importance of their interaction with biomembranes. Free Radic Biol Med 19:481–486

82. Miller AL (1996) Antioxidant flavonoids: structure, function and clinical usage. Altern Med Rev 1:103–111

83. Kuhlmann MK, Burkhardt G, Horsch E (1998) Inhibition of oxidant-induced lipid peroxidation in cultured renal tubular epithelial cells (LLC-PK1) by quercetin. Free Radic Res 29:451–460

84. O'Reilly JD, Sanders TA, Wiseman H (2000) Flavonoids protect against oxidative damage to LDL in vitro: use in selection of a flavonoid rich diet and relevance to LDL oxidation resistance *ex vivo*? Free Radic Res 33:419–426

85. Raso GM, Meli R, Di Carlo G (2001) Inhibition of inducible nitric oxide synthase and cyclooxygenase 2 expression by flavonoids in macrophage J774A.1. Life Sci 68:921–931

86. Kaul TN, Middleton E Jr, Ogra PL (1985) Antiviral effect of flavonoids on human viruses. J Med Virol 15:71–79

87. Zhang Y, Yang Y, Tang K, Hu X, Zou G (2008) Physicochemical characterization and antioxidant activity of quercetin-loaded chitosan nanoparticles. J Appl Polym Sci 107:891–897

88. Gugler R, Leschik M, Dengler HJ (1975) Disposition of quercetin in man after single oral and intravenous doses. Eur J Clin Pharmacol 9:229–234

89. Manach C, Regerat F, Texier O (1996) Bioavailability, metabolism and physiological impact of 4-oxoflavonoids. Nutr Res 16:517–534

90. Casagrande R, Georetti SR, Verri WA Jr, Borin MF, Lopez RFV, Fonseca MJV (2007) In vitro evaluation of quercetin cutaneous absorption from topical formulations and its functional stability by antioxidant activity. Int J Pharm 328:183–190

91. Olivella MS, Lhez L, Pappano NB, Debattista NB (2007) Effects of dimethylformamide and L-menthol permeation enhancers on transdermal delivery of quercetin. Pharm Dev Tech 12:481–484

92. Sunil TK, Narishetty RP (2005) Effect of l-menthol and 1,8-cineole on phase behavior and molecular organization of SC lipids and skin permeation of zidovudine. J Control Release 102:59–70

93. Chantasart D, Kevin LS (2010) Relationship between the enhancement effects of chemical permeation enhancers on the lipoidal transport pathway across human skin under the symmetric and asymmetric conditions in vitro. Pharm Res 27:1825–1836

94. Priestley CM, Williamson EM, Wafford KA, Sattelle DB (2003) Thymol, a constituent of thyme essential oil, is a positive allosteric modulator of human GABAA receptors and a homo-oligomeric GABA receptor from *Drosophila melanogaster*. British J Pharmacol 140:1363–1372

95. Braga PC, Sasso MD, Culici M, Bianchi T, Bordoni L, Marabini L (2006) Anti-inflammatory activity of thymol: inhibitory effect on the release of human neutrophil elastase. Pharmacol 77:130–136

96. Nobile MA, Di Benedetto N, Suriano N, Conte A, Lamacchia C, Corbo MR, Sinigaglia M (2009) Use of natural compounds to improve the microbial stability of Amaranth-based homemade fresh pasta. Food Microbiol 26:151–156

97. Hu Y, Du Y, Wang X, Feng T (2009) Self-aggregation of water-soluble chitosan and solubilization of thymol as an antimicrobial agent. J Biomed Mater Res 90A:874–881

98. Fleming OS, Kazarian SC (2005) Polymer processing with supercritical fluids. In: Kemmere MF, Meyer T (eds) Supercritical carbon dioxide: in polymer reaction engineering. Wiley, Weinheim, pp 205–234

99. Xia Y, Guo T, Zhao H, Song H, Song M, Zhang B, Zhang B (2007) A novel solid phase for selective separation of flavonoid compounds. J Sep Sci 30:1300–1306

100. Pasanphan W, Chirachanchai S (2008) Conjugation of gallic acid onto chitosan: an approach for green and water-based antioxidant. Carbohydr Polym 72:169–177

101. Hammerschmidt PA, Pratt DE (1978) Phenolic antioxidants of dried soybeans. J Food Sci 43:556–559

102. Braga MEM, Leal PF, Carvalho JE, Meireles MAA (2003) Comparison of yield, composition, and antioxidant activity of turmeric (Curcuma longa L.) extracts obtained using various techniques. J Agric Food Chem 51:6604–6611

Improving Post-EVAR Surveillance
with a Smart Stent-Graft

Isa C.T. Santos, Alexandra T. Sepulveda, Júlio C. Viana, António J. Pontes,
Brian L. Wardle, S.M. Sampaio, R. Roncon-Albuquerque,
João Manuel R.S. Tavares, and L.A. Rocha

Abstract Abdominal aortic aneurysms (AAA or triple A's) are indolent and
deadly diseases. Their treatment options involve either an invasive procedure or
a minimally invasive one. When the minimally invasive procedure, endovascular
aneurysm repair (EVAR), was introduced, it revolutionized the treatment of AAA's
due to advantages such as shortened hospital stays and reduced costs. As EVAR
requires periodic imaging exams, questions are nowadays being raised regarding the
procedure's long-term cost-benefit relation. In order to reduce follow-up costs, new
technological solutions are being pursued, namely EVAR stent-grafts with sensing
capabilities. In this chapter, the suitability of aneurysm sac pressure measurement
for EVAR surveillance is evaluated using an AAA computer model. In addition the
design drivers underlying EVAR stent-grafts are reviewed and the development of a
new flexible pressure sensor integrated into a stent-graft is described.

I.C.T. Santos (✉) • J.M.R.S. Tavares
Faculdade de Engenharia da Universidade do Porto/Instituto de Engenharia Mecânica e Gestão
Industrial, Porto, Portugal
e-mail: isa.santos@fe.up.pt; tavares@fe.up.pt

A.T. Sepulveda • J.C. Viana • A.J. Pontes • L.A. Rocha
Institute for Polymers and Composites/I3N, University of Minho, Guimarães, Portugal
e-mail: xanasepulveda@dep.uminho.pt; jcv@dep.uminho.pt; pontes@dep.uminho.pt;
lrocha@dei.uminho.pt

B.L. Wardle
Technology Laboratory for Advanced Materials and Structures, Department of Aeronautics
and Astronautics, Massachusetts Institute of Technology, Cambridge, MA 02139, USA
e-mail: wardle@mit.edu

S.M. Sampaio • R. Roncon-Albuquerque
Vascular Surgery Hospital S. João, Faculdade de Medicina, Universidade do Porto,
Porto, Portugal
e-mail: sampaio@med.up.pt; roncon@med.up.pt

R.M.N. Jorge et al. (eds.), *Technologies for Medical Sciences*, Lecture Notes
in Computational Vision and Biomechanics 1, DOI 10.1007/978-94-007-4068-6_13,
© Springer Science+Business Media B.V. 2012

1   Introduction

In 1948, Albert Einstein was diagnosed with an abdominal aortic aneurysm (AAA), i.e., his aorta had a permanent and irreversible localized dilatation having at least a 50% increase in diameter compared with the normal one [1], Fig. 1. Like him, currently, it is estimated that more than 12 per 100,000 persons-year [2] are affected by this relatively indolent but serious condition.

In an attempt to reinforce the aortic wall and delay the inevitable rupture that took Einstein's life in 1955, Dr. Rudolph Nissen wrapped the visible anterior portion of the aneurysm with polyethene cellophane. Nowadays, two more effective treatments are available: open surgery and endovascular aneurysm repair (EVAR). While the first is an invasive procedure, the second is a minimally invasive one whose main advantages are decreased blood loss, less early morbidity and mortality, and shorter hospitalization [2].

When EVAR was introduced, it revolutionized the treatment of aortic aneurysms. However, and in spite of major advances in EVAR techniques, adverse reactions still occur [3] and lifelong surveillance is recommended [4]. Due to these complications, currently, questions are being raised regarding the follow-up costs [5] and alternative approaches, such as a smart stent-graft, are being pursued.

A stent-graft is an endoprosthesis composed of a metallic scaffold and a polymeric covering membrane. Its use and the technological background for the development of a new device with sensing capabilities are described in this chapter.

After describing the current treatment options for aortic aneurysms, stent-graft complications are presented as well as their surveillance techniques. Following, the

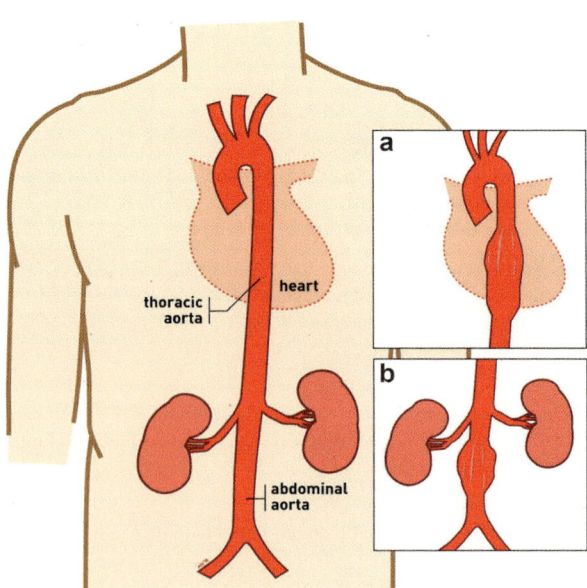

Fig. 1 Representation of a normal aorta, (**a**) a thoracic aortic aneurysm (TAA), and (**b**) an abdominal aortic aneurysm (AAA)

devices to measure pressure inside the aneurysm sac are described. The future trends for stent-graft's are also addressed highlighting the features of a smart stent-graft. A model of an AAA is presented along with a description of the development of a flexible pressure sensor.

2 Endovascular Aneurism Repair

Since the early 1950s, aneurysms' standard treatment has consisted of an open surgery (done under general anesthesia) and the replacement of the diseased segment of the aorta by a synthetic prosthetic graft [6], Fig. 2. In spite of its invasiveness and the fact of being limited to fit patients, this treatment is still a current practice and less invasive techniques, namely total laparoscopy and assisted laparoscopy, are being studied to minimize its disadvantages [7].

In the beginning of the 1990s, Volodos (in Ukraine) and Parodi (in Argentina) demonstrated that endovascular aneurysm repair (EVAR) was a safe and feasible practice [8]. This surgical procedure is done percutaneously and it is minimally invasive, Fig. 3. Typically, a small incision is made in each groin to expose the femoral arteries. Then, with the aid of catheters and guidewires, a stent-graft is guided to the affected artery segment allowing blood to pass without exerting pressure in the aneurysm sac and, thus, preventing wall rupture.

The first procedures resulted in several complications, some due to the inherent learning process, while others were due to the devices' inefficiency. With time, many of the problems have been solved due to the accumulation of experience and the introduction of better devices but, nevertheless, some problems still occur. These

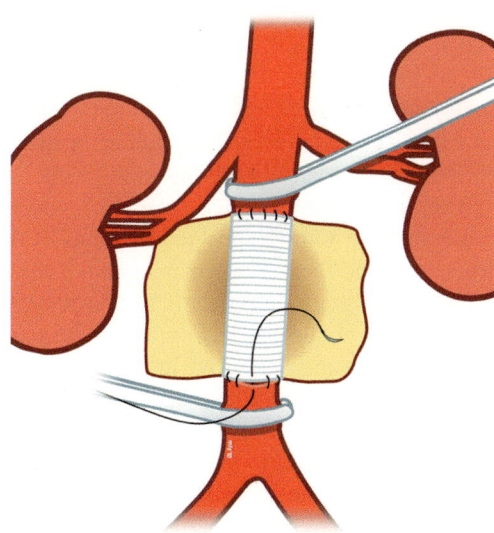

Fig. 2 Conventional treatment of AAA's, open surgery to insert a synthetic graft

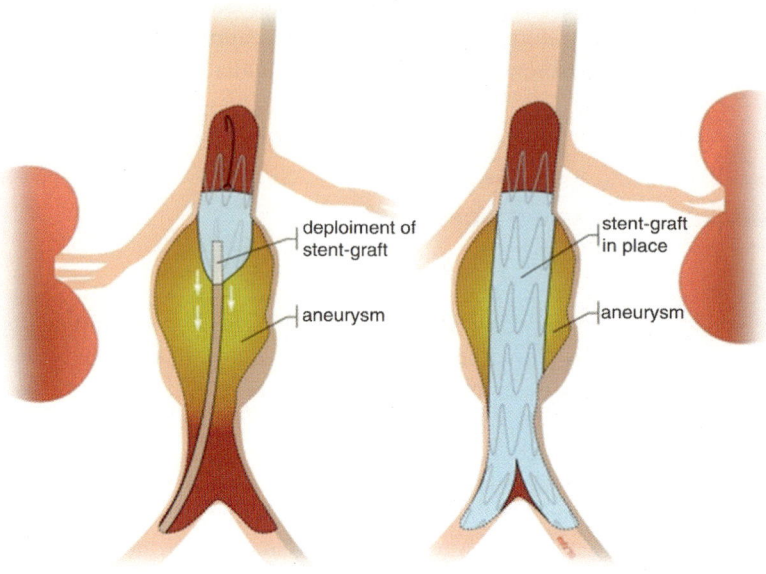

Fig. 3 Endovascular aneurysm repair (EVAR), stent-graft deployment sequence

Table 1 Complications involving stent-grafts (Adapted from [3])

Early complications	Late complications
Graft kink	Graft migration
Endoleaks	Neck dilatation
Graft explantation	Endoleaks
Structural failure	Structural failure: component separation, fabric tears, hook fractures
Graft infection	

complications can be classified as early or late and further detailed as systemic or related with the delivery, deployment, or the device itself [3]. Table 1 presents some of EVAR's problems involving stent-grafts.

The current surveillance protocol involves imaging exams, namely ultrasound and computed tomography angiography (CTA), at 1, 6, and 12 months after the procedure, and thereafter, on an annual basis [9].

Device migration and stent fractures or other indication of device fatigue are clear in plain abdominal radiography. Ultrasonography, besides allowing measuring the aneurysm sac, is effective in the detection of endoleaks but, even with enhanced sensitivity obtained with the use of contrast agents, requires a skilled technician to interpret the exams. CTA, MRI (magnetic resonance imaging) and MRA (magnetic resonance angiography) are sensitive tools to detect endoleaks but cannot be repeated often due to radiation and/or the use of nephrotoxic contrast agents. Furthermore, these exams are considered time consuming and expensive.

2.1 Measurement of Aneurism Sac Pressure

None of the medical imaging exams presently used provides measures of the pressure inside the aneurysm sac. This information is important because can be evidence of low-flow endoleaks or endotension [10].

Published data describe the use of catheters to measure pressure in the residual aneurysm sac [11]. However, although these methods provide precise measurements [4], they are invasive and bear multiple risks.

An alternative method for the measurement of the aneurysm sac's pressure is the implant of remote pressure transducers during EVAR. This solution is advantageous since measurements can be done when needed (hourly, weekly, etc.) in the patient's home or office instead of a hospital once or twice a year. Another important feature is the possibility to measure both the mean pressure and the pulsatile pressure without increasing risks for the patients. Following, the three telemetric pressure sensors currently available will be addressed.

3 Impressure AAA Sac Pressure Transducer

In 2003, the Impressure AAA Sac Pressure Transducer or RemonAAA from Israeli Remon Medical Technologies was the first permanently implantable, ultrasound-activated remote pressure transducer to measure intrasac pressure after EVAR [12].

The transducer, hand sewn to the outside of a stent-graft, contains a piezoelectric membrane that energizes a capacitor when actuated by ultrasound waves from a hand-held probe. Once charged, the aneurysm sac pressure is measured followed by the generation of an acoustic signal that is relayed to the hand-held probe. The probe then converts the acoustic signal to a pressure waveform that is presented on a computer screen.

In spite of ultrasound being safe and widely used for medical imaging, the measurement requires the use of an ultrasonic gel and direct contact between the skin and the transducer. Another drawback of this sensor is the impossibility of ultrasound to travel through air or bone, which may lead to difficulties communicating with the aneurysm sac.

The ImPressure sensor is the smallest (3 mm × 9 mm × 1.5 mm) of the three sensors described here, is the least radiopaque but still visible. As the sensor is sewn to the stent-graft, the fixation location must be carefully chosen in such a way that the sensor will measure the pressure inside the excluded aneurysm sac without being pushed against the aneurysm wall.

In October 2006, Remon Medical Technologies announced the first European implant of the sensor.

4   EndoSure Wireless Pressure Sensor

The EndoSure Wireless Pressure Sensor (CardioMems, Inc., USA) is made of two coils of copper wire within a fused silica matrix with a pressure sensitive surface. Passive telemetry is used for the signal transfer between the external device and the implant. Through inductive coupling, changes on the internal LC network (capacitor plus inductor) resonance frequency are detected on the external coil. The resonance frequency is related to the ambient pressure in which the sensor is located, and specially-designed software transforms the frequency shift between systolic and diastolic pressures into a wave form and pressure reading [13].

As the measurements are acquired via RF, there is no need for contact with the patient's skin or even the removal of the clothes, potentially allowing daily/weekly sampling at home.

The EndoSure sensor is deployed through its own delivery catheter (diameter 14 Fr/4.7 mm) during the EVAR procedure and has radiopaque markers to clearly define its location within the aneurysm sac.

The EndoSure sensor is cleared by the FDA for the measuring of intrasac pressure during endovascular abdominal aortic aneurysm repair and during endovascular thoracic aneurysm repair but is not yet approved for use in chronic surveillance.

5   TPS Telemetric Pressure Sensor

The TPS Telemetric Pressure Sensor was developed by the Helmholtz-Institute for Biomedical Engineering, RWTH Aachen in cooperation with the Institute of Materials in Electrical Engineering, RWTH Aachen [13, 14].

The TPS sensor consists of an implantable sensor capsule and an external readout station. The capsule comprises a capacitive absolute pressure sensor and an in-capsule signal-processing microchip including an inductive telemetry unit. The measured data is fully preprocessed to a digital data stream in the implant, so that errors during the transmission or from interferences between the sensor and the external readout station can be minimized. Moreover, the additional integrated temperature sensor allows errors caused by temperature variations to be noted and numerically corrected. In keeping with the requirements of medical implants, the pressure capsule has a two-layer encapsulation: a biocompatible, capsule-shaped silicone form and a Parylene-C layer creating an enclosed covering and ensuring the required stiffness.

The TPS sensor has fixation holes in both ends allowing to be sutured to the outer wall of stent-graft or be introduced separately.

This device has only been tested in an *in vitro* model but the results demonstrate that this is a promising technology [15]. Nonetheless, further clinical studies are required to evaluate the TPS Telemetric Pressure Sensor's durability and accuracy.

6   EVAR Cost Benefit

Comparing EVAR with conventional surgery, the first is preferable due to the fact of being less stressful and reducing significantly systemic complications [16], as well as having lower costs of inpatient stay and less or no need for intensive care facilities during recovery [6, 17]. While a number of early studies appeared to support this claim, nowadays, data shows otherwise [16]. Shorter stays at intensive care units and the hospital, reduced use of blood, fewer laboratory studies and fewer resources lead to cost savings, but later, additional costs exist for EVAR due to surveillance procedures.

The durability of open surgery, established with long-term follow-up studies, is excellent [16], so good that there is little or no requirement for long-term surveillance. Hayter [17] compared both hospital and follow-up costs of patients who had undergone EVAR or open surgery and concluded that EVAR costs were higher. One of the justifications presented was the endograft's high price.

When EVAR was introduced, it was thought to be more economical than open surgery because the price of the first stent-grafts was lower and the surveillance costs were not included in the analysis. Nowadays, EVAR can be considered cost-effective only for very elderly patients or those with a reduced life expectancy and doubtful for young patients, those who would benefit more from the short hospital stay and early return to full activity offered by open surgery.

Considering the longer life expectancies and the rising public expectations for quality of life, EVAR is an attractive treatment. However, its cost-benefit relation can be jeopardized by the requirement of long-term surveillance. In order to reduce and even eliminate these exams, new surveillance technologies are being investigated and the most promising technique identified thus far is remote pressure sensing [9].

The authors believe that including sensing capabilities in a stent-graft will benefit EVAR's future. Yet, that may not be enough. Preliminary results of a recent survey regarding the ideal features of a stent-graft show that attention should be given to the devices adaptability and delivery profile.

7   Future Trends for Stent-Grafts

Innovations on mechanisms for pressure detection within the aneurysm sac are being developed concurrent with novel architectures and materials for the construction of stent-grafts. Two original proposals that indicate future alternatives for stent-graft design are presented next.

7.1   Origami Stent-Graft

In 2006, Kuribayashi [18] described the design, the manufacture and the properties of an origami stent-graft. The new device received this designation because the paper folding patterns used in the Japanese art of origami was employed to fold it.

This prosthesis is made from a sheet that is folded dividing a cylindrical tube into a series of identical elements with hill and valley folds. The folding pattern used is responsible for the decrease and increase of both the diameter and the length when the device is folded and deployed, respectively. In addition, the folded configuration of each element makes the stent-graft flexible.

Unlike other devices, the origami stent-graft is made of a single component. A nickel titanium alloy is used that not only is biocompatible, but also has a shape memory effect that is used for the deployment of the device. Its main disadvantage is the price; the origami stent-graft is made using a foil that requires complex rolling and annealing methods to be produced.

7.2   Rigberg's Stent-Graft

The major determinant of the stent-graft's diameter when folded is the graft, not the stent itself. Thus, in order to reduce the pre-deployment diameter and the size of the delivery components, Rigberg presented in 2009 a feasibility study for a novel aortic stent-graft material [19]. In his work, the author proposes the replacement of currently used graft materials by a nickel titanium alloy (NiTi) thin-film. This material presents several advantages, such as biocompatibility, superelastic qualities, shape memory properties, and a tensile strength greater than 500 MPa. This last feature is of major importance since it enables the development of thinner devices with the same, or even higher, mechanical resistance. Moreover, the cost of thin-film NiTi is expected to be similar to the cost of ePTFE. Nonetheless, further studies regarding thrombogenicity, resistance to infection, and permeability are still required. Some design issues, such as the attachment of the stent to the graft or complex shapes, also need to be more deeply studied.

7.3   Smart Stent-Graft

A smart stent-graft can be defined as a stent-graft with some in-device mechanism to perform a given function with communication capabilities to an external element.

Although there is still no commercial device available, a smart stent-graft could be decomposed in three elements: a stent-graft, a sensing element and a display. The stent-graft, besides shielding the aneurysm from the blood pressure, has built-in sensing elements that are able to gather information concerning the patient's health and/or the prosthesis performance. The information gathered is then sent to an external element – a display – and can be used to diagnose the patient's or in the comprehension of the aneurysm's sac behavior after the implementation of the stent-graft.

Like a conventional stent-graft, such a device will be classified as a class III medical device and, as such, will have to be biocompatible, biostable, non-toxic, non-allergic and non-carcinogenic. Furthermore, it will have to be tolerated by the human body without causing a foreign body reaction or an inflammatory reaction.

Regarding the mechanical requisites, the device should be flexible and tough. Its components should also be mechanically durable, as well as excellent corrosion resistance. For a successful protection of the blood vessel, the device should have a design as less invasive as possible in order to minimize flow resistance and pressure drops. Radial force is another relevant feature, not only for stent-grafts to stay open without being crushed with muscular activity, but also to provide a good seal and to ensure fixation.

The deployment of the device is a critical step for the procedure's success, thus, the stent-graft should have a low profile to facilitate the deployment and minimize lesions in the access arteries. At this stage, radiopacity is also crucial to ensure the correct positioning of the prosthesis.

From the commercial point of view, the device must be capable of being adequately sterilized and stored as an "off-the-shelf" product. A broad range of sizes is desirable since it allows the treatment of a wider array of aneurysm anatomies.

One of the key questions in the design of a smart stent-graft regards the instrumentation capabilities required. Ideally, the device should be able to detect migration and leakages and possibly also monitor any of the device's material or structural degradation. Regarding the transmission of the measured data, the device must be able to transmit the data without any internal power. Moreover, the data cannot interfere with other implants nor be influenced by other electronic signals.

To assure patient's comfort and even reduce costs, the measurement protocol should be done during the doctor's appointment or at home and the results transmitted to the doctor's office. Regardless of where measurements are taken, the procedure should be quick, the least invasive as possible and avoid any kind of pain or even discomfort.

For a correct interpretation of the information measured, it is crucial to know the location where the data is being gathered.

8 Abdominal Aortic Aneurysm Model

Thus far, to measure the aneurysm sac's pressure, sensors are placed randomly and provide information regarding a single point. This data is insufficient to characterize the pressure distribution inside the aneurysm sac. Therefore, AAA models using finite elements can become a means to understand the medical condition and predict the optimal location to place the sensors.

Several studies using AAA models composed of a stent-graft, the aorta and the aneurysm sac have been presented in the literature [20–22], but they mainly studied the drag forces on the stent-graft, or the stresses on the vessel that can lead to rupture. Even though this information is important to improve existing knowledge about aneurysms, it conveys no detail about the pressure distribution, or the influence of AAA geometry on the aneurysm sac pressure.

Using computer-aided design (CAD) software, it is possible to implement parametric models to construct tridimensional (3D) models of the desired AAA in a

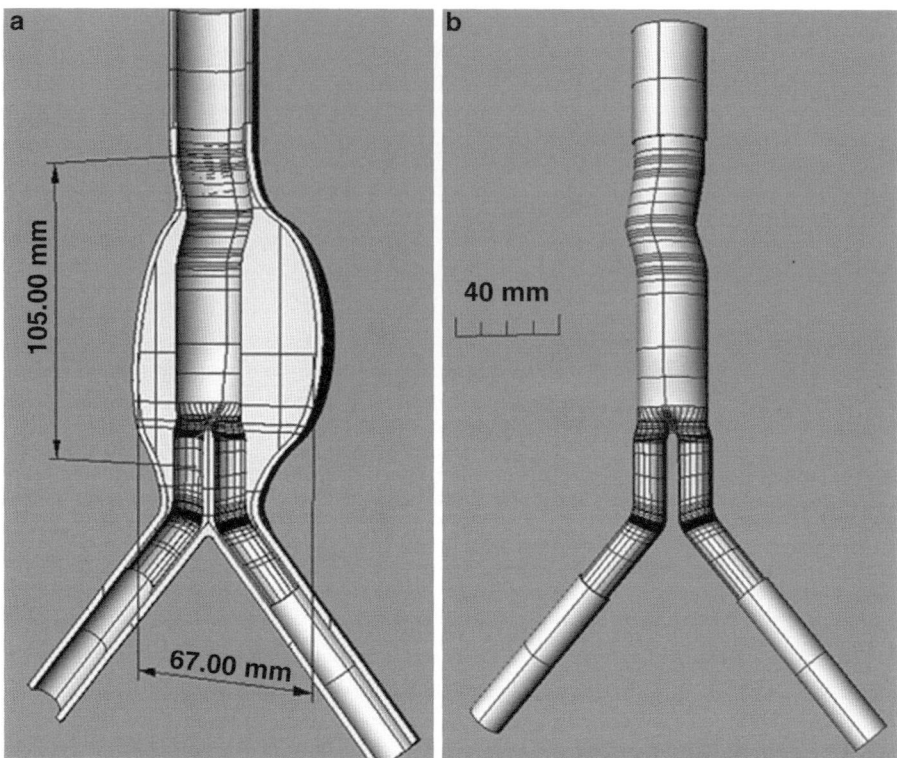

Fig. 4 3D models of an AAA. (**a**) Mechanical model and (**b**) fluidic model

fast and efficient manner, as in Fig. 4. For an accurate representation, the model must include the blood flow, the bifurcated stent-graft, the aorta wall motion (including the aneurysm wall) and the stagnant blood inside the aneurysm sac (essential for the pressure simulation inside the sac).

Due to the pulsatile nature of blood flow, transient simulations are often used to model the blood flow. Aneurysms can have several geometries and sizes [20, 23], but AAAs present most commonly a fusiform geometry. The aorta radius ranges from 2 to 2,5 cm and the wall thickness presents typical values around 2–2,5 mm [20, 23].

Figure 5 presents the main parameters of the 3D model implemented by the authors to assess the pressure distribution inside the aneurysm sac. The ANSYS multiple code coupling (MFX) with Fluid Solid Interface (FSI) coupling between ANSYS and CFX was used to solve the model.

The blood flow is considered newtonian, laminar and incompressible; the density is equal to 1.05 g/cm^3 and the viscosity is 0.0035 Pa.s.

The model uses an aorta radius and aorta wall thicknesses of 2.5 cm and 2.5 mm respectively, and an aneurysm length of 10.5 cm and main radius of 6.7 cm.

Fig. 5 Main modeling
parameters of an AAA

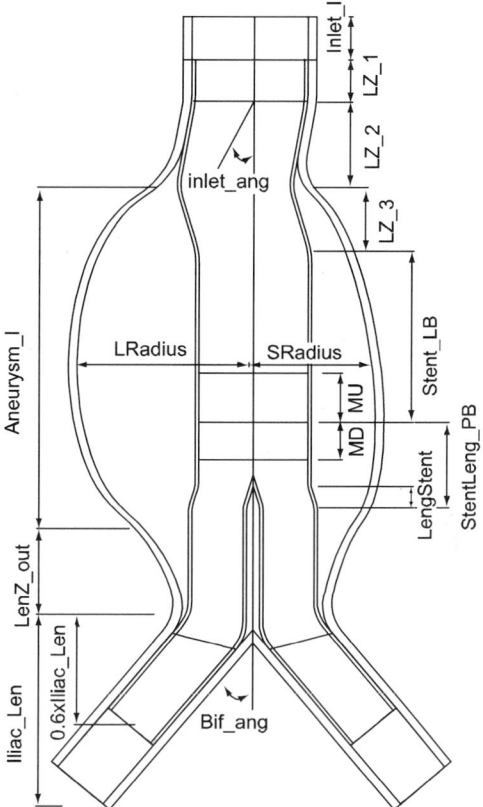

The diseased AAA wall is modeled as a linear, isotropic, elastic material with a density $\rho = 1.2$ g/cm^3, a Young's Modulus E $= 4.6$ MPa and a Poisson's ratio of 0.49 [20].

The healthy part of the aorta (AAA neck) and iliacs are also modeled as a linear, isotropic, elastic material with a density $\rho = 1.2$ g/cm^3, a Young's Modulus E $= 2$ MPa and a Poisson's ratio of 0.45.

The stent-graft model presented uses SHELL elements, and is modeled as a linear, isotropic material with a Young's Modulus E $= 10$ MPa and a Poisson's ratio of 0.3.

The aneurysm sac, an important part of the model for the pressure analysis, is modeled as a stagnant liquid by using FLUID80 element from the ANSYS element library. This element allows the simulation of stagnant fluids in containers with no flow. Figure 6 gives an overview of the meshed mechanical model.

The mechanical domain of the simulation assumes zero displacement at the top of the AAA neck and at the bottom of the iliacs, while a time dependent uniform velocity is applied at the inlet of the fluidic domain (Fig. 7a) and a time dependent normal traction (due to luminal pressure) on the outlet (Fig. 7b). The transient analysis is performed during a full cardiac cycle (1.1 s).

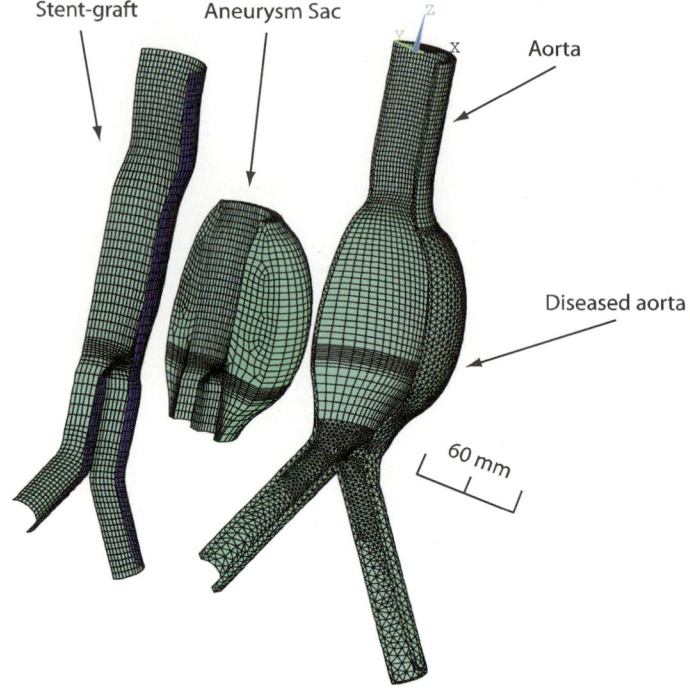

Fig. 6 Mechanical model mesh

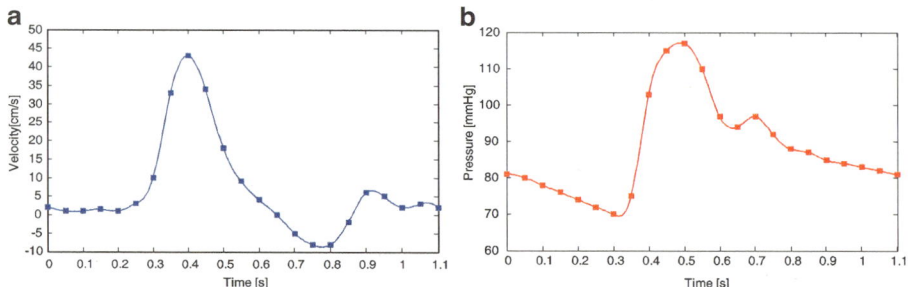

Fig. 7 Fluidic boundary conditions: (**a**) inlet velocity and (**b**) outlet pressure

To validate the FSI solver, simulations using a simpler AAA model without stent-graft were performed. The results showed a maximum aorta displacement of 1.9 mm and a maximum stress (von Mises) around 0.4 MPa, which were in good agreement with the data from [20] (using a similar geometry size).

Simulation results of the pressure distribution within the aneurysm sac at systolic pressure (t = 0.5 s) using the full AAA model with stent-graft are shown in Fig. 8a. The simulation results show some small pressure variations along the aneurysm sac,

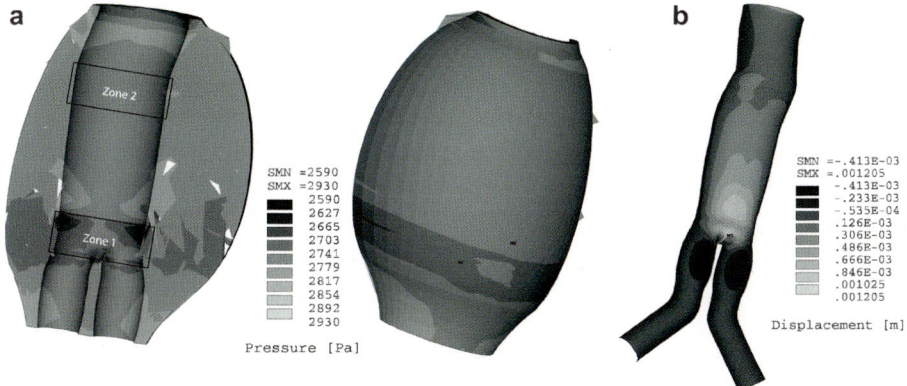

Fig. 8 Simulation results at systolic pressure (t = 0.5 s). (**a**) Aneurysm sac pressure and (**b**) stent-graft displacement

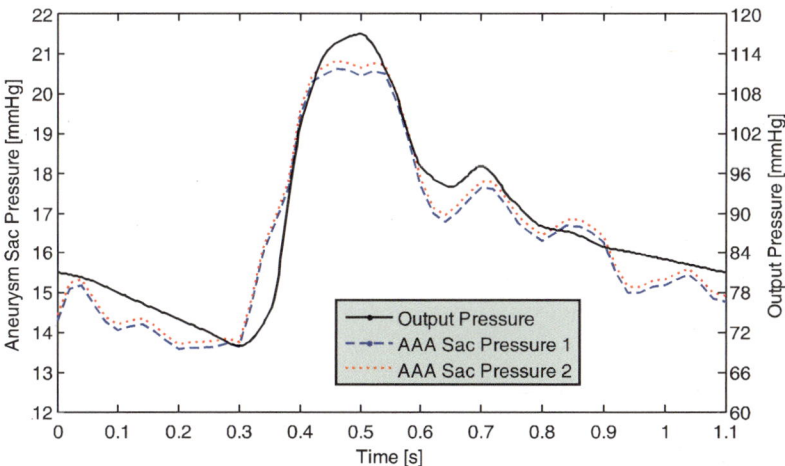

Fig. 9 Pressures inside aneurysm sac (zone 1 and 2 in Fig. 8a) and pressure boundary condition at the outlet

with the minimum pressure occurring close to the stent-graft bifurcation. A closer look to the stent-graft displacement at the same simulation time (Fig. 8b) suggests that the minimum pressures are related to the maximum stent-graft displacements.

The results from Fig. 8a show that the pressure within the aneurysm sac is almost uniform but do not give any information about the aneurysm sac pressure variation during a full cardiac cycle. Therefore, if two zones are defined (zone 1 and 2 in Fig. 8a) the mean pressures within those regions can be computed. The mean pressures in the two zones along with the pressure boundary condition at the outlet are depicted in Fig. 9.

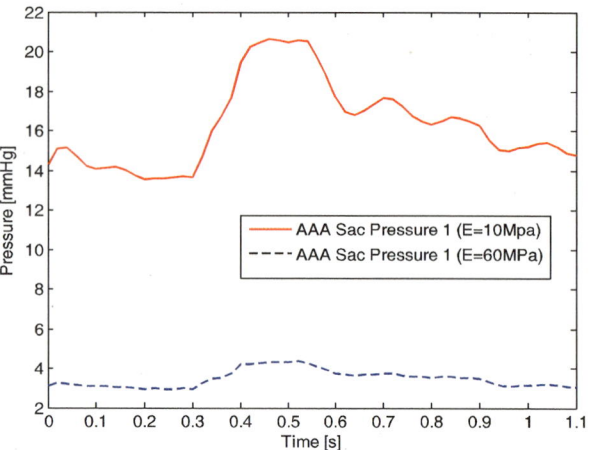

Fig. 10 Pressures inside aneurysm sac on zone 1 (see Fig. 8a) for different stent-graft material properties

These simulation results imply that the pressure variations within the aneurysm sac are related to the displacement of the stent-graft caused by the luminal pressure. If this is the case, the placement of one sensor on the region with less structural stability (higher displacement) might be a good indicator, when compared to another sensor placed elsewhere within the aneurysm sac, of the structural integrity of the stent-graft. These results also suggest that the pressure variations inside the aneurysm sac are related to the stent-graft material (structural behavior). Results for the same simulation boundary conditions but using a higher Young's Modulus for the stent-graft material, $E = 60$ MPa, Fig. 10, confirm the assumption that the pressure within the aneurysm sac depends on the structural behavior of the stent-graft material. In fact, simulations reveal that a large drop on the pressure within the aneurysm (>10 mmHg) sac occurs when the Young's Modulus is increased from 10 MPa to 60 MPa.

The abdominal aortic aneurysm CFD (Compute Fluid Dynamics) model with FSI is a suitable tool to study pressure changes within the aneurysm and indicates that pressure sensors can be used to detect post-EVAR complications. Pressure sensing in the aneurysm sac can be used both for leakage detection and to measure systolic and diastole blood pressures. If more than one sensor is used, model results suggest that the differences in pressure within the aneurysm sac can be an indicator of the stent-graft material integrity.

9   Development of a Flexible Pressure Sensor

A key component for the smart stent-graft is the pressure sensor. The sensing element must be flexible to enable its conformability to the stent-graft and thus the aorta. Such features allow the attachment of the sensor to the stent-graft and their deployment in a single step (as opposed to the requirement of two catheters as in the EndoSure device). Furthermore, it enables the placement of more than one sensor (a sensor cluster) contributing to a more comprehensive study of post-EVAR aneurysm evolution that, currently, is not possible.

9.1 Capacitive Sensor Design

Research on implantable pressure sensors is very active and has been supported and justified by the need of continuous pressure monitoring for patients with congestive heart failure, as an early diagnostic mechanism for some risk patients and for post-EVAR surveillance [24, 25].

Implantable pressure sensors are typically categorized into extra-arterial blood pressure devices and intra-arterial blood pressure devices [25]. The firsts are placed around the blood vessel and perform an indirect pressure measurement through the wall or through the expansion and contraction of the artery. They require an invasive surgical procedure for their implant while, on the other hand, the intra-arterial devices are in contact with the blood stream inside of the blood vessels.

After stent-graft placement, the aneurysm sac gets depressurized and the pressure drops down to a few mmHg as indicated by the simulations (12–22 mmHg according to Fig. 9). Therefore, if one wants to sense the luminal pressure value (ranges typically between 50 and 160 mmHg) through the aneurysm sac pressure, the sensor must be able to measure pressures between 6 and 26 mmHg. In addition, it needs a high dynamic range in order to detect stent-graft complications (in this case the sac gets pressurized and pressure increases to the luminal pressure values).

Typical configurations of capacitive pressure sensors use square-plate (diaphragm) electrodes separated by a dielectric (oftentimes of air) at a pressure P_0. Changes on the outside pressure (P_{out}) deform the square plate and consequently generate a capacitive change. A schematic of a square-plate (side length of 2a) pressure sensor is shown in Fig. 11. The sensor involves two coupled domains, mechanical and electrical, that define the sensor behavior.

A cross section of the square plate sensor is shown in Fig. 12 (section cut B-B) where only the mechanical domain is considered. The side length is 2a, t is the thickness and w_0 the deflection. The diaphragm is clamped at the edges. For a clamped diaphragm under a uniform load (like pressure), the angle of deflection, φ, is equal to zero at the center (r = 0) and at the edge (r = a) of the diaphragm. For these boundary conditions, the deflection of an isotropic square diaphragm under a pressure load can be modeled as [26]:

$$P_0 - P_{out} = \frac{Et^4}{(1-v^2)a^4}\left[4.20\frac{w_0}{t} + 1.58\frac{w_0^3}{t^3}\right] \tag{1}$$

where v is the Poisson's ratio, E is the Young's modulus, and $\Delta P = P_0 \text{-} P_{out}$ is the pressure load.

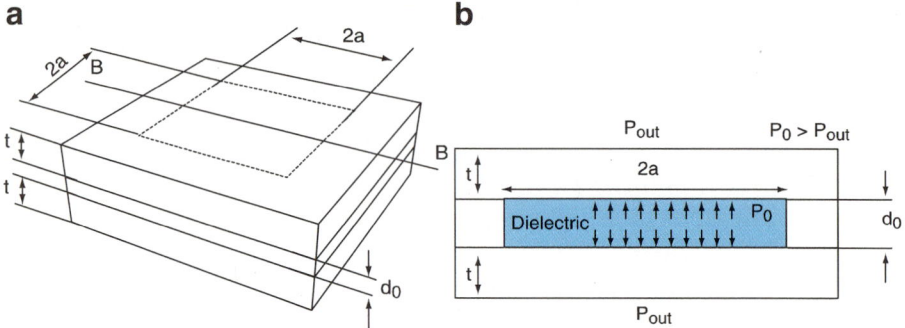

Fig. 11 Schematic of the pressure square (side length = 2a) sensor (**a**) 3D view and (**b**) section cut B-B

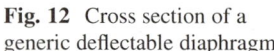

Fig. 12 Cross section of a generic deflectable diaphragm

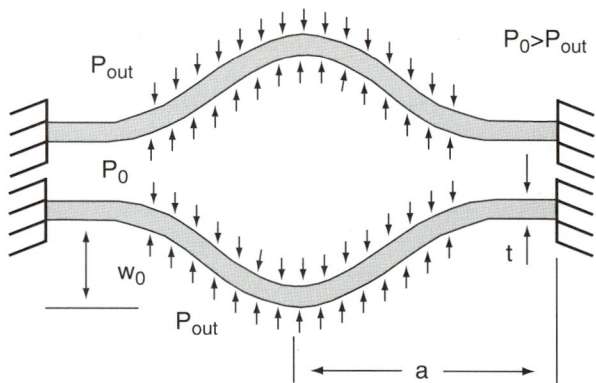

Equation 1 allows the calculation of the deflection at the center of the diaphragm for a given pressure load but the deflection along the diaphragm is still required to model the capacitive changes due to gap variation. Due to the complexity of the mechanical deflection calculation, trial functions that describe the deflection of the entire diaphragm are usually used [27]. Figure 13 shows the normalized deflection for a square diaphragm of side-length 2a when the following trial function for large deflection is used [27]:

$$w(x, y) = w_0 \left[\left(\cos \left(\frac{\pi x}{2a} \right) \right) \left(\cos \left(\frac{\pi y}{2a} \right) \right) \right] \tag{2}$$

Mechanical deflections caused by pressure changes will originate changes at the capacitor (electrostatic domain). A capacitor is an electronic component with two electrodes that are separated by a dielectric. For the simple case of a parallel plate capacitor, and in the absence of displacements, the model for the capacitor is (neglecting fringe fields):

$$C = \varepsilon_0 \varepsilon_r \frac{wl}{d_0} \tag{3}$$

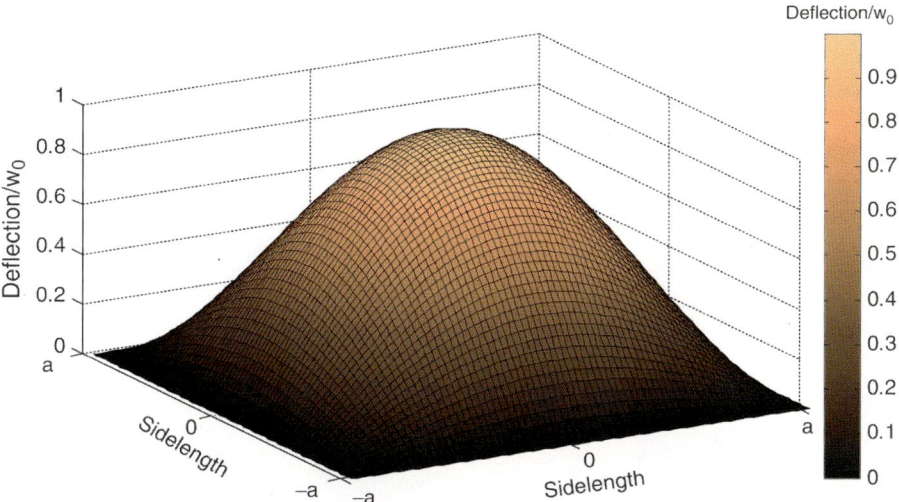

Fig. 13 Displacement profile along the square diaphragm using the trial function of (2)

where ε_0 is the permittivity of free space ($8.8546 \times 10{-}12$ F/m), ε_r is the relative permittivity, w and l are the width and length of the capacitor electrodes, and d_0 is the gap between the electrodes.

Since the capacitive sensor uses diaphragm electrodes with a complex bending profile, integration over the effective area of the electrodes is required to compute the total capacitance:

$$C = \int \int \frac{\varepsilon_0 \varepsilon_r}{d_0 + 2w(x,y)} dx dy \qquad (4)$$

where $w(x,y)$ is the distance between electrodes due to the diaphragm bending at position x, y. The integration in (4) can easily be solved numerically, enabling the computation of the capacitance for a given pressure change.

9.2 Fabrication Process

Given the characteristics of the application (the sensor will be attached to the stent-graft) the capacitive sensor must be foldable, extremely flexible and characterized by a very small profile. In addition, the technology should be simple and biocompatible. Silicon based micro technologies are widely used in implantable medical devices [24], but due to the application specifications, there are other technologies that can deliver better design approaches and results.

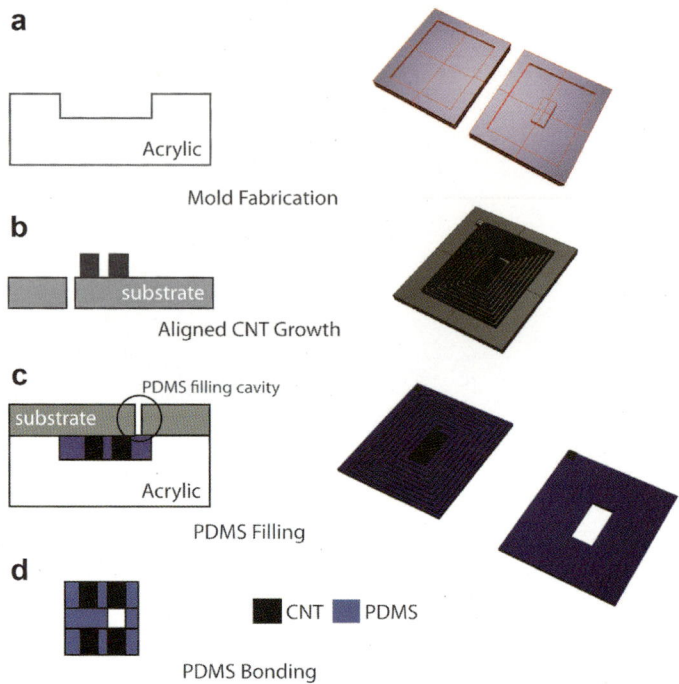

Fig. 14 Fabrication process flow for the development of a flexible pressure sensor with aligned-CNT/PDMS nanocomposites

A suitable candidate is the technology proposed by Sepúlveda [28], in which aligned carbon nanotubes (CNTs) are used to implement the conductive elements in a flexible substrate of polydimethylsiloxane (PDMS), a transparent, nontoxic and biocompatible silicone elastomer.

The technology process flow enabling the fabrication of a flexible pressure sensor is schematically presented in Fig. 14. Acrylic moulds are produced by CNC milling (Fig. 14a) for posterior fabrication of the PDMS membranes. This technique has low costs and fast production times, but it is associated with poor dimensional control (dimensions less than 50 μm are difficult to achieve) and more traditional micromachining may achieve the required tolerances.

The electrical components are based on aligned CNTs, as shown in Fig. 14b. Chemical vapor deposition (CVD) is used to grow forests or "carpets" of vertically-aligned CNTs [29]. A silicon substrate with patterned Fe/Al_2O_3 catalyst is placed on a horizontal quartz tube furnace at atmospheric pressure at 750°C [29] for the CNT growth. This method has the advantage of allowing the growth of high purity, high yield and vertically aligned CNTs. Next, the CNTs are embedded into the polymer matrix (PDMS). This step is schematically represented in Fig. 14c. The substrate is

Fig. 15 Cross section of a CNT/PDMS flexible pressure sensor

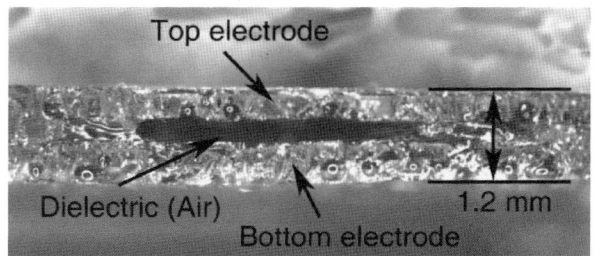

placed against the moulds, and the PDMS is introduced in the cavities through a hole to create an aligned-CNT/PDMS nanocomposite as described previously for epoxies using capillarity-assisted wetting [30], followed by the curing of the elastomer.

Three flexible membrane layers are required to fabricate the sensor, with the top and bottom layers defining the inductor and the electrodes, and the middle one defining the dielectric (air). This configuration requires bonding of PDMS membranes. Eddings [31] tested five different bonding techniques and the highest reported bond strength was obtained for both partial curing and uncured PDMS adhesive techniques. The latter approach is used to build the sensors, Fig. 15.

9.3 Material Properties and Results

The key step of the fabrication process is the CNT-PDMS impregnation and respective mechanical and electrical properties (that will govern the sensor response). Aligned CNTs are oriented in the out-of-plane (or normal to the wafer plane) direction such that the polymer nanocomposite can be presumed transversly isotropic, i.e., isotropic in the plane of the sensor. Furthermore, the modulus enhancement due to CNTs is likely minimal as the long axis of the CNTs are oriented perpendicular to the loading direction, such that the PDMS polymer dominates the response. Work on nanocomposites has shown significant increase in modulus due to aligned CNTs in polymer (PDMS) [32] and epoxy [33] in the CNT axis direction, but little reinforcement effect in the transverse direction as used here. This result is expected from composite micromechanics analyses and experimental results.

Experimental results using a prototype PDMS/CNT flexible pressure sensor are presented in Fig. 16. The tested sensors have a mechanical layer thickness of 670 μm and a dielectric thickness of 260 μm resulting in a total sensor thickness of 1.6 mm (670 μm + 260 μm + 670 μm). The area of the electrodes is 3.4 x 9 mm^2 (W x L). Despite the coarse sensor resolution (the geometry was not optimized since the devices are at a proof-of-concept stage), capacitive changes were measured when the sensor was placed inside a controlled pressure chamber (the dielectric is hermetically sealed at ambient pressure).

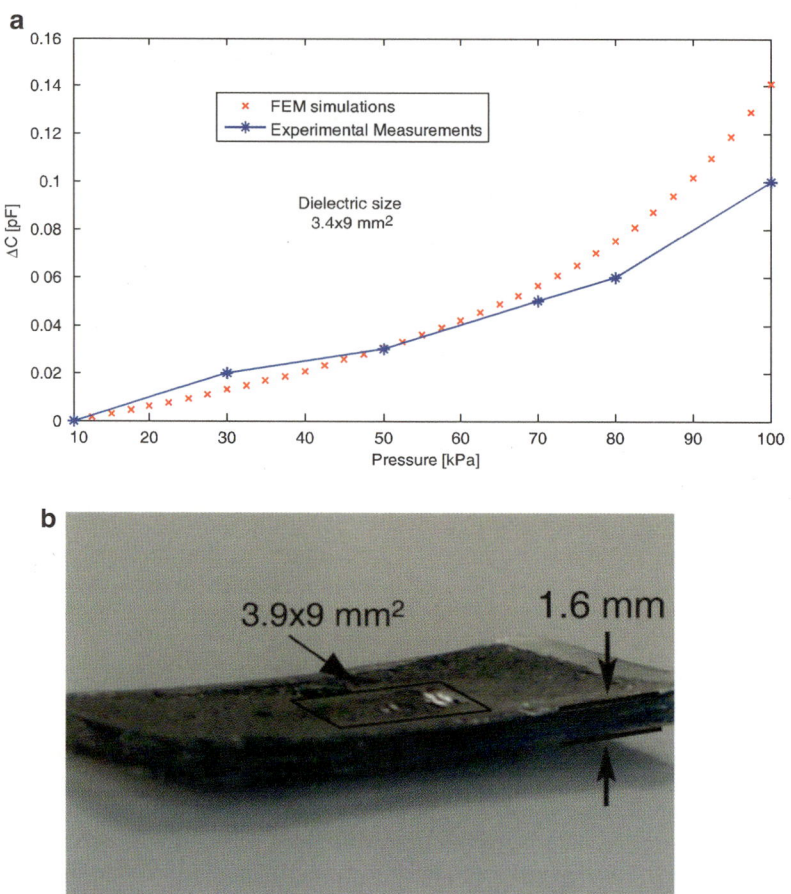

Fig. 16 Experimental results of a prototype CNT/PDMS flexible pressure sensor for a smart stent-graft. (**a**) Capacitive changes versus pressure and (**b**) image of the sensor with 10 kPa external pressure

10   Conclusions

Since its introduction, in the beginning of the 90s, EVAR became a viable alternative for the treatment of aneurysms. Despite the benefits of being a minimally invasive technique, recent cost-benefit analyses indicate that EVAR becomes more expensive on the long-term since it requires surveillance mechanisms to detect eventual post-EVAR problems, such as endoleaks and stent-graft migration.

Alternatives are currently being pursued to minimize the surveillance costs, and pressure measurements in the aneurysm sac are an attractive solution. Some stand alone pressure sensors are already available but the future will evolve to smart stent-grafts, i.e., stent-grafts with embedded pressure sensors for post-EVAR surveillance.

The use of pressure changes as a surveillance mechanism still requires a better understanding from the medical community. Nevertheless, AAA model simulation results validate the use of pressure sensors to detect post-EVAR complications. Although more data is required, multiple pressure measurements within the aneurysm sac can also enable the detection of stent-graft structural failure.

In order to place the sensors in the stent-graft, they must be thin and highly flexible. A newly developed technology based on CNTs has proven successful in the development of flexible pressure sensors and might enable the next generation of smart stent-grafts.

Acknowledgments The first and second authors wishes to thank FCT – Fundação para a Ciência e Tecnologia in Portugal, for the financial support provided by the PhD grants with reference SFRH/BD/42967/2008 and SFRH/BD/42922/2008 respectively.

This work is supported by FEDER through COMPETE and national funds through FCT – Foundation for Science and Technology in the framework of the project MIT-Pt/EDAM-EMD/0007/2008 (http://sensecardiohealth.wordpress.com).

The authors wish to thank Miguel Marafuz for the illustrations, Fabio Fachin for helpful discussions in the CNT-based MEMS device designs, and Dr. Roberto Guzman de Villoria for fabrication and testing assistance of the CNT-reinforced PDMS materials.

CNT-based polymer composite materials were developed with funding from Airbus S. A. S., Boeing, Embraer, Lockheed Martin, Saab AB, Spirit AeroSystems, Textron Inc., Composite Systems Technology, and TohoTenax Inc. through MIT's Nano-Engineered Composite aerospace STructures (NECST) Consortium.

References

1. Johnston KW, Robert BR, Tilson MD, Dhiraj MS, Larry H, James CS (1991) Suggested standards for reporting on arterial aneurysms. J Vasc Surg 13(3):452–458
2. Ricotta JJ II, Malgor RD, Oderich GS (2009) Endovascular abdominal aortic aneurysm repair: part I. Ann Vasc Surg 23(6):799–812. doi:10.1016/j.avsg.2009.03.003
3. Katzen BT, MacLean AA (2006) Complications of endovascular repair of abdominal aortic aneurysms: a review. Cardiovasc Intervent Radiol 29(6):935–946. doi:10.1007/s00270-005-0191-0
4. Baril DT, Kahn RA, Ellozy SH, Carroccio A, Marin ML (2007) Endovascular abdominal aortic aneurysm repair: emerging developments and anesthetic considerations. J Cardiothorac Vasc Anesth 21(5):730–742. doi:10.1053/j.jvca.2007.03.001
5. Young KC, Awad NA, Johansson M, Gillespie D, Singh MJ, Illig KA (2010) Cost-effectiveness of abdominal aortic aneurysm repair based on aneurysm size. J Vasc Surg 51(1):27–32. doi:10.1016/j.jvs.2009.08.004
6. Myers K, Devine T, Barras C, Self G (2001) Endoluminal versus open repair for abdominal aortic aneurysms. Paper presented at the 2do. Congreso Virtual de Cardiología - Congreso Internacional de Cardiología por Internet, Argentina, Set 1 - 30 Nov 2001
7. Dion Y-M, Joseph T (2010) Laparoscopic aortic surgery. In: Fogarty TJ, White RA (eds) Peripheral endovascular interventions. Springer, New York, pp 397–409, doi:10.1007/978-1-4419-1387-6_27
8. Greenhalgh RM (2004) Comparison of endovascular aneurysm repair with open repair in patients with abdominal aortic aneurysm (EVAR trial 1), 30-day operative mortality results: randomised controlled trial. Lancet 364(9437):843–848. doi:10.1016/S0140-6736(04)16979-1

9. Milner R, Kasirajan K, Chaikof EL (2006) Future of endograft surveillance. Semin Vasc Surg 19(2):75–82. doi:10.1053/j.semvascsurg.2006.03.002

10. Gilling-Smith G, Brennan J, Harris P, Bakran A, Gould D, McWilliams R (1999) Endotension after endovascular aneurysm repair: definition, classification, and strategies for surveillance and intervention. J Endovasc Surg 6:305–307

11. Carnero L, Milner R (2007) Aneurysm sac pressure measurement with a pressure sensor in endovascular aortic aneurysm repair. In: Lumsden AB, Lin PH, Chen C, Parodi JC (eds) Advanced endovascular therapy of aortic disease., pp 209–215, doi:10.1002/9780470988930.ch27

12. Ellozy SH, Carroccio A, Lookstein RA, Minor ME, Sheahan CM, Juta J, Cha A, Valenzuela R, Addis MD, Jacobs TS, Teodorescu VJ, Marin ML (2004) First experience in human beings with a permanently implantable intrasac pressure transducer for monitoring endovascular repair of abdominal aortic aneurysms. J Vasc Surg 40(3):405–412. doi:10.1016/j.jvs.2004.06.027

13. Schlierf R, Gortz M, Rode TS, Mokwa W, Schnakenberg U, Trieu K (2005) Pressure sensor capsule to control the treatment of abdominal aorta aneurisms. In: The 13th international conference on solid-state sensors, actuators and microsystems. Digest of technical papers. TRANSDUCERS '05. vol 1652, pp 1656–1659, doi:10.1109/SENSOR.2005.1497407

14. Springer F, Schlierf R, Pfeffer J-G, Mahnken A, Schnakenberg U, Schmitz-Rode T (2007) Detecting endoleaks after endovascular AAA repair with a minimally invasive, implantable, telemetric pressure sensor: an *in vitro* study. Eur Radiol 17(10):2589–2597. doi:10.1007/s00330-007-0583-4

15. Springer F, Günther R, Schmitz-Rode T (2008) Aneurysm sac pressure measurement with minimally invasive implantable pressure sensors: an alternative to current surveillance regimes after EVAR? Cardiovasc Intervent Radiol 31(3):460–467. doi:10.1007/s00270-007-9245-9

16. Rutherford RB, Krupski WC (2004) Current status of open versus endovascular stent-graft repair of abdominal aortic aneurysm. J Vasc Surg 39(5):1129–1139. doi:10.1016/j.jvs.2004.02.027

17. Hayter CL, Bradshaw SR, Allen RJ, Guduguntla M, Hardman DTA (2005) Follow-up costs increase the cost disparity between endovascular and open abdominal aortic aneurysm repair. J Vasc Surg 42(5):912–918. doi:10.1016/j.jvs.2005.07.039

18. Kuribayashi K, Tsuchiya K, You Z, Tomus D, Umemoto M, Ito T, Sasaki M (2006) Self-deployable origami stent grafts as a biomedical application of Ni-rich TiNi shape memory alloy foil. Mater Sci Eng A 419(1–2):131–137. doi:10.1016/j.msea.2005.12.016

19. Rigberg D, Tulloch A, Chun Y, Mohanchandra KP, Carman G, Lawrence P (2009) Thin-film nitinol (NiTi): a feasibility study for a novel aortic stent graft material. J vasc surg: official publication, the Society for Vascular Surgery [and] International Society for Cardiovascular Surgery, North American Chapter 50(2):375–380. doi:10.1016/j.jvs.2009.03.028

20. Li Z, Kleinstreuer C (2006) Analysis of biomechanical factors affecting stent-graft migration in an abdominal aortic aneurysm model. J Biomech 39(12):2264–2273. doi:10.1016/j.jbiomech.2005.07.010

21. Frauenfelder T, Lotfey M, Boehm T, Wildermuth S (2006) Computational fluid dynamics: hemodynamic changes in abdominal aortic aneurysm after stent-graft implantation. Cardiovasc Intervent Radiol 29(4):724–724. doi:10.1007/s00270-005-8227-z

22. Scotti CM, Finol EA (2007) Compliant biomechanics of abdominal aortic aneurysms: a fluid–structure interaction study. Comput Struct 85(11–14):1097–1113, doi:10.1016/j.compstruc.2006.08.041

23. Vorp DA (2007) Biomechanics of abdominal aortic aneurysm. J Biomech 40(9):1887–1902. doi:DOI: 10.1016/j.jbiomech.2006.09.003

24. Rogier AMR et al (2007) Microsystem technologies for implantable applications. J Micromech Microeng 17(5):R50. doi:10.1088/0960-1317/17/5/R02

25. Potkay J (2008) Long term, implantable blood pressure monitoring systems. Biomed Microdevices 10(3):379–392. doi:10.1007/s10544-007-9146-3

26. Chau H, Wise K (2005) Scaling limits in batch-fabricated silicon pressure sensors. IEEE Trans Electron Devices 34(4):850–858. doi:10.1109/T-ED.1987.23006

27. Senturia SD (2000) Microsystem design. Springer, New York

28. Sepúlveda AT, Moreira A, Fachin F, Wardle BL, Silva JM, Pontes AJ, Viana JC, Rocha LA (2010) Inductive-coupling system for abdominal aortic aneurysms monitoring based on pressure sensing. In: MME'2010 (21th MicroMechanics Europe), Enschede, 26–29 Sept 2010
29. Hart AJ, Slocum AH (2006) Rapid growth and flow-mediated nucleation of millimeter-scale aligned carbon nanotube structures from a thin-film catalyst. J Phys Chem B 110(16):8250–8257. doi:10.1021/jp055498b
30. Wardle BL, Saito DS, García EJ, Hart AJ, de Villoria RG, Verploegen EA (2008) Fabrication and characterization of ultrahigh-volume-fraction aligned carbon nanotube–polymer composites. Adv Mater 20(14):2707–2714. doi:10.1002/adma.200800295
31. Eddings MA, Johnson MA, Gale BK (2008) Determining the optimal PDMS–PDMS bonding technique for microfluidic devices. J Micromech Microeng 18(6):067001. doi:10.1088/0960-1317/18/6/067001
32. Ajayan PM, Schadler LS, Giannaris C, Rubio A (2000) Single-walled carbon nanotube–polymer composites: strength and weakness. Adv Mater 12(10):750–753. doi:10.1002/(sici)1521-4095(200005)12:10<750::aid-adma750>3.0.co;2-6
33. Cebeci H, Villoria RGd, Hart AJ, Wardle BL (2009) Multifunctional properties of high volume fraction aligned carbon nanotube polymer composites with controlled morphology. Compos Sci Technol 69(15–16):2649–2656. doi:10.1016/j.compscitech.2009.08.006

Synergic Multidisciplinary Interactions for Design and Development of Medical Devices

Ricardo Simoes

Abstract The development of medical devices is becoming increasingly complex, with the advent of information technologies and continuous advances in micro and nanotechnologies. Moreover, the demands in terms of performance, costs and other requisites of these devices have also become stricter. If, on the one hand, the results are clearly positive for society in terms of better health services (and the arguable improvement of the quality of life), on the other hand, there is the need to involve people from a variety of fields in the development process, and the tasks of planning and coordinating the implementation of a development strategy are ever more paramount.

This chapter presents some considerations about the product development cycle and the need for multidisciplinary teams in the product design and development processes of medical devices. The work methods and communication channels within the team, and the organization and coordination of that team are discussed. Opinions regarding different aspects of the development process, collected from individuals involved in medical devices development projects, are described and analyzed. Finally, a case-study is presented of a university-industry project, involving healthcare providers, for the development of a new health support system comprised of different types of medical devices. This project encompassed all the stages of PDD up to the laboratory-stage and establishing the main requisites for industrial productification. The developed system was implemented and field-tested (some of the individuals involved in the field test have answered the previously mentioned questionnaire).

R. Simoes (✉)
School of Technology, Polytechnic Institute of Cávado and Ave,
Campus do IPCA, 4750-810 Barcelos, Portugal

Institute for Polymers and Composites - IPC/I3N, University of Minho,
4800-058 Guimarães, Portugal
e-mail: rsimoes@ipca.pt; rsimoes@dep.uminho.pt

R.M.N. Jorge et al. (eds.), *Technologies for Medical Sciences*, Lecture Notes
in Computational Vision and Biomechanics 1, DOI 10.1007/978-94-007-4068-6_14,
© Springer Science+Business Media B.V. 2012

1 Introduction

As products are becoming increasingly complex, the product design and development (PDD) processes are also evolving into collaborative multidisciplinary team processes. This creates new challenges, both for product development, but also in project management. In the case of medical devices, this is further complicated by rigorous specifications and regulatory requirements [1], as well as the fact that the development process requires strong interaction with multiple individuals, with the concept of end-user depending on the specific device. It is this important to understand how the PDD process can be planned for and managed in the case of medical devices, whether they are a single biometric device or a complex information coordination system [2]. This chapter follows previous studies on product design specifications [3], wireless networks for health monitoring [4], evaluation of vital signs monitoring systems [5], communication platforms for medical data [6], embedded microelectronics [7], and performance evaluation of ZigBee networks [8].

The first section describes the life cycle of novel medical devices in the current context of increased complexity and performance demands.

The second section focuses on the laboratory development stage, with the goal of obtaining a fully functional product, although typically not optimized for production and not sufficiently competitive for the market. The actors and their respective roles are described, namely in the framework of user-centered design, with emphasis on the development team. In fact, for a successful outcome, a plethora of different people have to become involved in the project.

It is also important to establish how to get from user wants and needs to partial product design specifications (PDS). These need to be understood by people from different areas, requiring agile and effective communication among team members. The PDS are partial due to the fact that many specifications only need to be defined (and in fact, can only be defined due to insufficient knowledge) at the industrial productification stage.

Some specifications must even be jointly specified by team members of different expertise. Thus, an analysis is provided in the third section on the multidisciplinary integration within the development team and communication between this team and the different other actors that are essential for a successful product development process.

In large projects, and particularly when multidisciplinary teams are involved, the role of coordination becomes pivotal, and it is very important to understand some of the characteristics of how that can be effectively achieved. This is the goal of Sect. 14.4.

Section 14.5 describes a survey conducted with several people involved in medical devices development projects. These individuals were selected in order to cover the different profiles that are established in Sect. 14.3 (researchers, practitioners, managers). Although the number of surveyed professionals is small, the survey provides some interesting information on their different perspectives.

Finally, in Sect. 14.6, a case-study is succinctly described, where several different areas of expertise were brought together in a multidisciplinary team, working close together with different healthcare professionals, resulting in a health support system that includes biometric devices, communication networks, and information systems technology.

2 Life Cycle of Novel Products

Developing new products is a complex process, and multiple methodologies have been proposed over the years by different authors on how to approach this systematically. However, a major obstacle is the highly variable nature of the process. In the specific case of medical devices, new products usually take considerable time before reaching the market, not only due to the development stage, but also certification, setting up distribution channels, and many other necessary steps. Despite the wide range of possibilities, in most cases there are two main phases within the development process.

2.1 Main Phases

Medical devices are typically developed either by:

- Companies within the scope of their business plan;
- Research teams at Universities or R&D Centers within the scope of their ongoing research activities on healthcare or a specific research project.

These two cases may appear very different at first sight. However, in both cases there are, almost inevitably, two different development stages; see Fig. 1. The first stage results in a fully functional device but not optimized to be market competitive. A second stage is required, where many specifications and product features are revised, and several aspects which could (or had to) be left open are defined.

The difference between these two stages being conducted wholly within a single company or the first stage in a research unit and the second in a company (either through patenting or through a spin-off or a start-up) pertains essentially to:

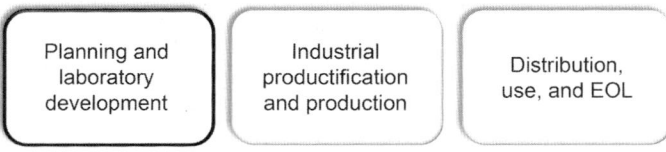

Fig. 1 Stages in the life cycle of novel medical devices

The extent of communication between the teams intervening in those two stages;

- Agility of the transfer process;
- Ability to retain members of the first stage team in the second stage team.
- After the industrial productification stage, come all other stages of a product life cycle, such as distribution, end-of-life handling, etc., undoubtedly important, but outside the scope of this chapter. Obviously, these later stages may have a large impact into decisions made for the development of subsequent versions of the product or future related products.

2.2 Focus of This Study

This work focuses on the first development stage, conducted by a research team, in cooperation with different clinical professionals, pursuing a fully functional, albeit laboratory-state, prototype.

3 The Laboratory Development Process

Only within the scope of laboratory development, there is much to understand regarding the different actors involved and what their role is in the process of going from the market needs to product concepts and subsequently product specifications.

3.1 Actors and Roles

One of the key features of current development practices in the field of medical devices is the involvement of health professionals from the start. This type of collaborative development, following widespread approaches such as living labs, translational research, or the most traditional sub-contracting the advice of expert healthcare professionals, is currently regarded as most effective and followed by the major companies in the field.

Independently of the degree of interaction between the development team and the end-users, these two main groups are vital elements of the process, as shown in Fig. 2.

Thus, on one side, we have the development team, responsible for the scientific development and technical implementation of the prototype solution.

For most medical devices, development teams have to incorporate researchers from a variety of fields, such as electronic engineering, computer science, biomedical engineering, materials engineering, design, and social sciences. The formation and inner working of these teams is further explored in §3.2.

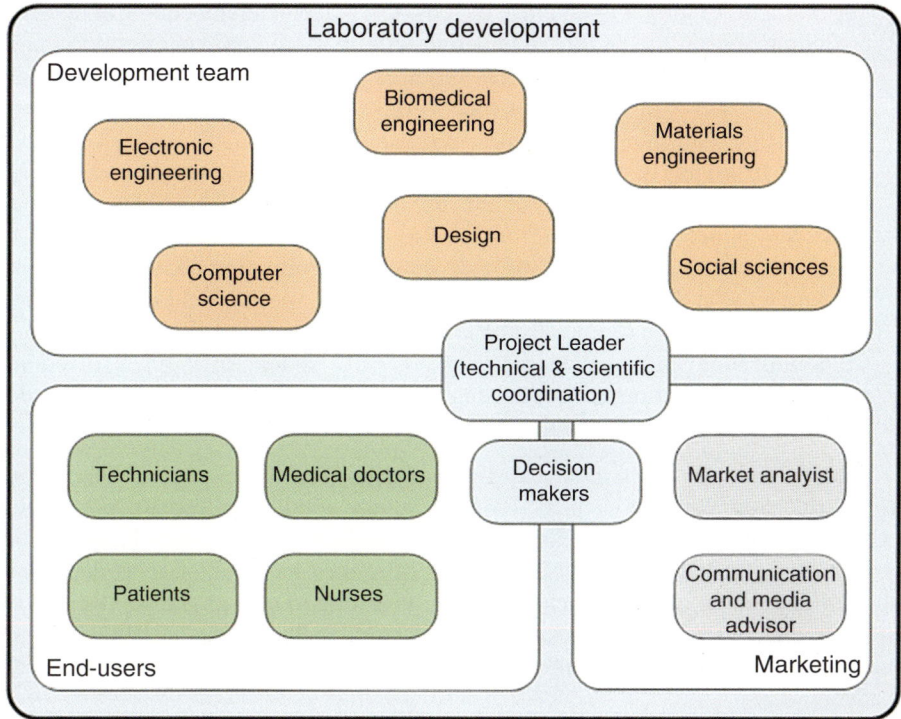

Fig. 2 Typical actors involved in the laboratory-stage product development cycle of novel medical devices

On the other side, we have end-users (various healthcare professionals and patients), marketing professionals, and decision makers (e.g. health provider facilities administrators):

- Medical doctors. They are the key interface between scientific research and field practice. Thus, they must be an integral part of the development, from concept development and selection, setting PDS (including technical and non-technical requirements), and product validation (including field trials). Their opinions will be collected by decision makers and thus they must find added value in the new products compared to previous solutions (if they exist). Their level of involvement and contribution to the project will naturally affect their opinion of the product.
- Nurses. Very often they will be the ones using the device. Even if not, they will be responsible for one of the following: setting it up, making it available to doctors, or giving it to patients. Their role is pivotal and their opinions should be collected from early development stages. It is important for them to validate the device.

- Technicians. Important to establish the physical placement/embedding of devices and equipment in the facility, interacting with existing computer networks and communication grids. Any changes required on the existing infrastructure or service practices will be difficult (due to the strict requisites and certifications in healthcare) and should be planned well in advance.
- Patients. It is vital to develop medical devices in a user-centered approach. In many cases, users are doctors or nurses, but often they are patients. In these cases, they should be involved from the earliest development stages.
- Market analysts. They should provide detailed information about current and upcoming technologies and solutions, trends in the specific field of the product being developed, and should also be involved in setting some PDS (e.g. cost).
- Communication and media advisors. Not only should they be involved in planning dissemination and advertising of the developed product, but they should create a plan for enticing the media, particularly for highly innovative devices.

On the end-user side, all these professionals are coordinated essentially by a few decision makers, such as hospital administrators (or board), or private healthcare facilities owners. These decision makers often have a technical or medical background, but will collect advice from their key staff on most decisions about the selection of health technologies or investing in new products. The bridge between the development team and all other actors, including the decision makers, marketing, and healthcare professionals, has to be coordinated by the project leader.

3.2   The Development Team

As previously stated, development teams have to incorporate researchers from a variety of fields:

- Electronic engineering: sensors, actuators, communication hardware/protocols, data processing.
- Computer science/Information Systems: data communication, data storage, data mining, security protocols, user interfaces.
- Biomedical engineering: usability, hardware, medical data acquisition and interpretation.
- Materials engineering: materials selection, device housing/casing, user interfaces.
- Design: user profiles, concept development, ergonomics, aesthetics, interfaces, device housing.
- Social sciences; user-perception of devices, user needs, questionnaires and interpretation, epidemiological aspects.

Obviously, the composition of the team is highly dependent on the specific device, but currently most devices will require tackling at least some of the competences listed for each of the fields of expertise above. It is thus not surprising to find teams will be based on the above listed competences, in some cases complemented by others with specific expertise.

One should notice that the only reason the development team roster above does not include clinical staff and medical doctors is because this discussion assumes the team is working cooperatively in close collaboration with those professionals, following the development approaches listed in §3.1.

3.3 Understanding Wants and Needs

On the earlier stages of the development process, methods such as Ethnographic Research and Voice of the Costumer can be employed to assess and understand user wants and user needs. These methods can help translating the 'needs and wants' of the user into product requirements and features. If the project is planned and implemented following a user-centered approach, identifying the best methods to be used for this purpose should not be a problem.

3.4 Product Design Specifications (PDS)

Pugh is one of the key authors dealing with this issue in depth [9]. He compiled a comprehensive list of types of specifications, in a wide range of aspects of the product development process. In this work, namely in §4, we analyze and classify the PDS, based on Pugh's list, which we believe helps in selecting specifications for a particular project. A better understanding of specifications and their role on the product development process is required, particularly in the current trend of faster obsolescence and increasing complexity of products [10].

The team will have to define a set of PDS at the early laboratory development stage. However, this will only be a partial PDS, since: (a) the team does not have sufficient understanding of the problem and sufficient definition of the solution to set some of the specifications at this stage, and (b) there is no need to establish specifications that will not affect the final output of the laboratory development process.

During the laboratory development stage, the key PDS to set are those that have a direct impact on the selection of concepts and solutions, selection of technologies (such as a communication standard), or usability. This is shown schematically in Fig. 3.

In Fig. 3, PDS are represented with respect to when they are set along the development process, considering two large stages: laboratory development and industrial productification. A bold PDS border implies a primary PDS, whereas dashed lines imply secondary PDS. Also, some PDS are shown stretching between

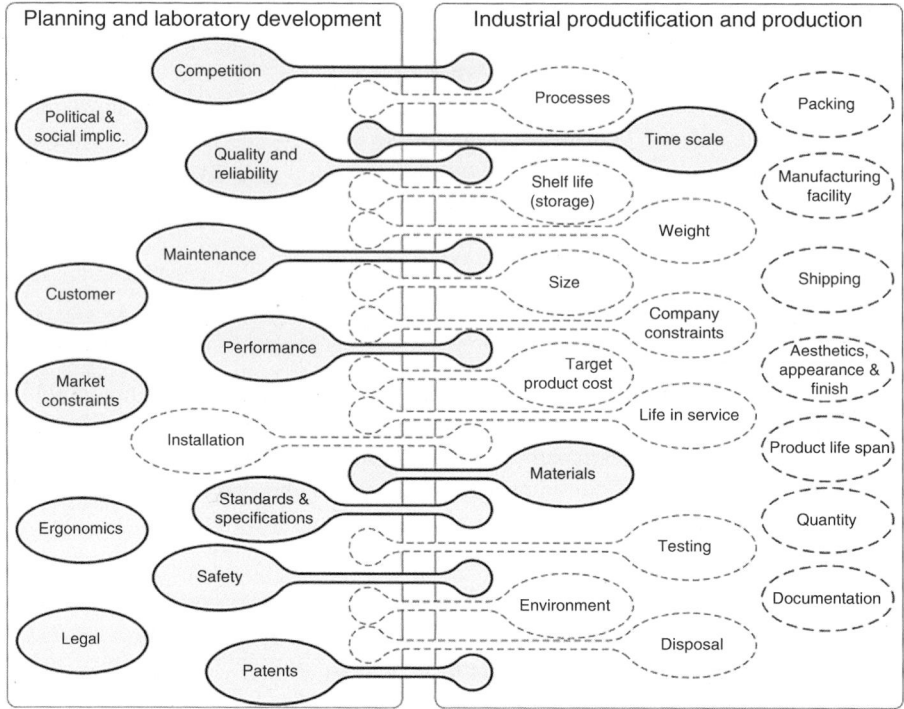

Fig. 3 Setting product design specifications at different development process stages. See text for interpretation and discussion

phases, which implies they are either: (1) set in the first stage and revised in the second, or (2) preliminarily considered in the first stage, but only fully defined in the second stage.

As an example, while ergonomics is important at an early stage, since it will come into play in concept selection and in the validation of the conceptual solution with end-users, aesthetics and finish can only be specified when materials, manufacturing processes, and cost are being defined.

Note that although the assessment in Fig. 3 categorizes PDS as being of primary or secondary importance in the specific framework of medical devices, this is quite subjective and dependent on the specific product. It also does not mean the secondary PDS do not require considerable attention. The assessment was essentially based on personal interpretation of current trends in development of medical devices from the analysis of multiple recent and ongoing projects in the area [11].

From the analysis of Fig. 3, one can state that the majority of what were labeled the most important PDS are set during the first stage of development, even though a little over half of them have to be revised in the second stage. Conversely, only a couple of the most important PDS are set in the second stage. It is also

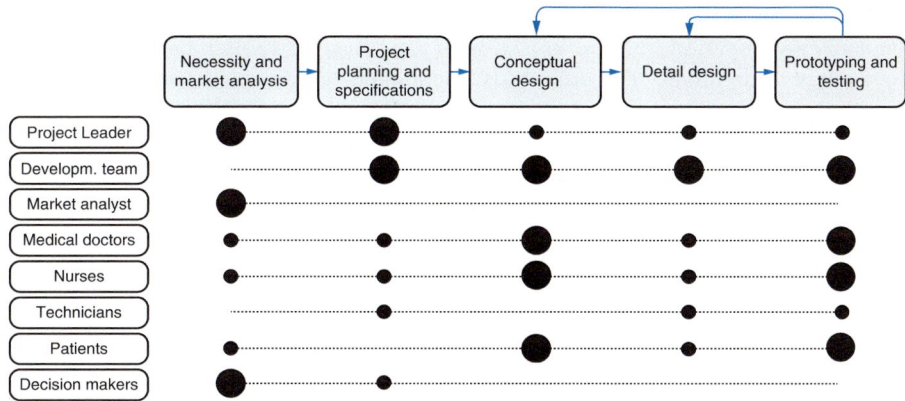

Fig. 4 Simplified product development cycle for the laboratory-stage development of medical devices and involvement of different actors along the development cycle. Circle size represents the level of involvement in each stage

interesting that only about one third of second phase PDS can be left open during the first stage, while the others must be at least preliminarily considered in the first stage. Finally, about three fifths (circa 60%) of the PDS fall in the second phase, which means they can only be fully set during that stage of the development process.

3.5 The Product Development Cycle

Within the laboratory development stage, a full product development cycle will take place. In the framework of this chapter, the important aspects to consider are the involvement of end-users early and throughout the process, as represented in Fig. 4.

4 Multidisciplinarity

4.1 Multidisciplinary Integration Within the Development Team

Working in multidisciplinary teams offers several advantages to the researcher. One of these is the quick access to expertise in complementary areas of knowledge. Another is the possibility to debate decisions with colleagues that have different perspectives (and possibly, conflicting opinions). Equally important is the ability to tackle much more complex challenges than those which could be handled by a single individual, even if highly gifted.

However, such teams do not always work well, and it is frequent to observe personal incompatibilities develop between team members, often creating the need to replace individuals. As previously mentioned, communication among team members is a key factor. Aside from personality traits which can inexorably lead to conflicts, the main pitfalls have to do with team coordination, namely the need to:

- Clearly establish roles/responsibilities in the team;
- State the expertise each member adds to the team;
- Have team members frequently describe their individual work in (also frequent) team meetings.

One of the important aspects of multidisciplinary team interaction is language. Here we consider essentially technical terminology. It is vital to ensure that all team members are aware of specific technical terminology used by others. Also, some consensus must be reached regarding adoption of technical terms which might vary among scientific areas. It can be mitigated by frequent meetings and formally setting the terminology to be used by the team.

4.2 Tasking and Scheduling

Stating that tasking and scheduling is important in this type of development projects is redundant. However, having multidisciplinary teams increases the complexity of the planning effort. First, as previously described, tasks must be very well defined and the role of each individual explicitly set for each task. Second, responsibilities must be assigned for every task, and it falls on the project leader to monitor task progress and intervene when necessary. Team members should not have to police each other. Last, while some tasks can be developed simultaneously, many will require input from other tasks. Almost any delay may cause other tasks to be put on-hold, possibly affecting the overall project schedule, and consequently, the predicted time to market.

Thus, compared to traditional project tasking and scheduling efforts, multidisciplinary teams for development of medical devices require additional care both in initial planning and in workflow monitoring.

4.3 Communication with Actors Outside the Development Team

There are clearly two different levels of communication here. On the one hand, multiple channels of communication are beneficial for the development process, namely between researchers and end-users. Examples are frequent meetings between the people responsible for collecting medical data (electronics or biomedical engineers) and doctors. Similarly, researchers working on devices with which healthcare professionals have to physically interact, need to meet with nurses, conduct brainstorming sessions, and perform preliminary tests with nurses, doctors, and possibly patients. These communication channels must work very effectively, and thus should be formally established jointly by the project leader and decision makers (e.g. hospital administrators).

On the other hand, the project leader is also responsible for communicating with the decision makers, market analysts, and media advisors. By having an overall view of the development project and being able to decide which information to release at each moment, the project leader has a pivotal role in lubricating the flow of information, simultaneously ensuring that confidential or sensitive information is not released untimely or unintentionally. There should be no direct independent communication between researchers and the decision makers and media advisors. Otherwise, their incomplete knowledge of the overall project, coupled with the fact that they are usually not aware of the long-term plans and strategy behind the development process, can lead to complicated communication mishaps.

4.4 Coordinating the Development Team

Following the discussion in §4.1 through §4.3, it becomes obvious that coordination of the development team requires a particular profile. The project leader has to supervise the development work, which makes a technical background highly desirable so he can articulate with the researchers and make decisions when necessary. He should be actively engaged in the development, but not supervise any of the tasks himself (e.g. brainstorming, field tests).

One of his main activities is coordination of the development team. This implies monitoring progress, but more importantly establishing boundaries, rules, roles, and responsibilities. He should assume a little more than his share of the blame for delays or the inability to fully reach intended development goals, and accept a little less than his share of the credits, recognizing the researchers' effort and congratulating individual achievements.

He must ensure team members learn to value the input of others, that they work cooperatively rather than competitively, and to be humble in their work. He should ensure no team member leaves questions unasked simply for fear of appearing ignorant.

Finally, it is often possible to delegate coordination of specific aspects of the development to the second most senior researcher (with extreme care to ensure that roles and responsibilities are understood by all), freeing the project leader for other tasks.

4.5   Coordinating the Overall Project

The role of coordinating the overall project is not trivial. This essentially includes:

- Monitor individual task progress, making swift changes to the workplan or redefining goals;
- Coordinate the research team, ensuring effective and efficient cooperation and communication channels (within the team and also external);
- Balance laboratory-stage development with the need to move on to productification to achieve a useful product time-to-market;
- Maintain frequent contact with decision makers and, when appropriate, with media advisors;
- Solve the plethora of problems that unexpectedly appear during development of medical devices (many common to any engineering project).

In the case of medical devices, the two main challenges relate to obtaining results within useful timeframes and usability issues (whether the device is employed by medical doctors, nurses, or patients).

5   Survey

The discussion so far in this chapter follows from the individual experience of the author in a series of research & development projects in this field. Despite the fact that this discussion has attempted to be unbiased and provide a bird's eye view of the entire process, it inexorably conveys a personal perspective. In order to provide a wider and even more unbiased outlook, a survey was conducted based on a questionnaire answered by people involved in different medical devices development projects. These individuals were selected in order to cover the different profiles previously described in Sect. 14.3 (researchers, practitioners, managers).

5.1   Survey Model

The questionnaire was purposefully made very simple. It contained only 4 questions. It is important to note that no statistical significance will be derived from this preliminary study; the number of people who answered the survey was small, since its main purpose was to validate if there are significant asymmetries in the perspective of the different people involved in the process.

The survey was conducted face-to-face with each of the individuals listed; names were omitted and only profiles are listed for each person inquired. First, the Fig. 2 diagram was shown, with indication to identify if any relevant profiles were missing. All those inquired have indicated no additional profiles, with the single exception of

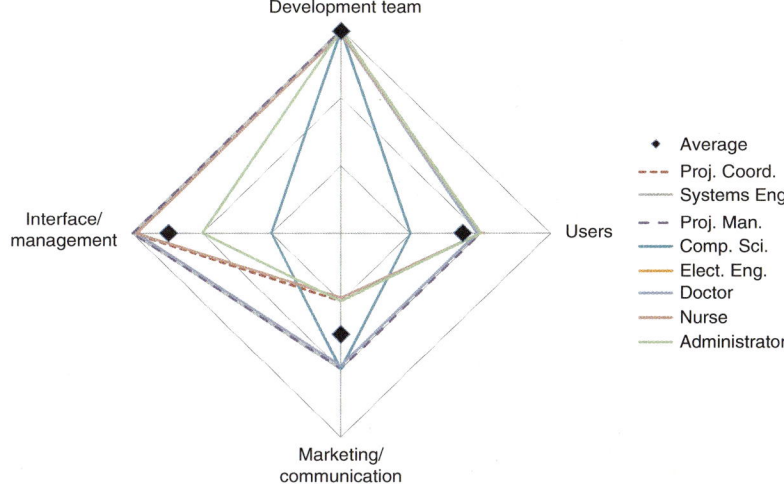

Fig. 5 Assessment of the degree of challenges, in a 1 to 4 scale, facing each of the 4 key groups typically involved in the development of medical devices. Each line corresponds to one inquired individual. The diamond symbols represent the average value for each group

a healthcare provider, who pointed out that investors and insurance companies are vital parts of the creation of new medical devices, although the latter only become key actors at the productification stage.

Subsequently, the questionnaire included three questions, each to be answered in a matrix with multiple options. These questions pertained to:

- Which of the groups (development team, medical staff, marketing, and coordinators/managers) have to deal with the most critical challenges in the process?
- Who has to become convinced by the developed solution?
- At which point of the development process (early or late stage) should each actor become involved?

The answers to each of these three questions were analyzed and the respective results are shown in the following section.

5.2 Survey Results

The first question aimed at identifying the level of challenges that each of the the four identified groups (development team, medical staff, marketing, and coordinators/managers) have to deal with the most critical challenges in the process. In the survey, a rating between 1 and 4 had to be assigned to each of these groups. The results of the survey for different individuals, covering a range of professional profiles, are shown in Fig. 5. These profiles were, respectively, the global project coordinator, a systems engineer, a project scientific manager,

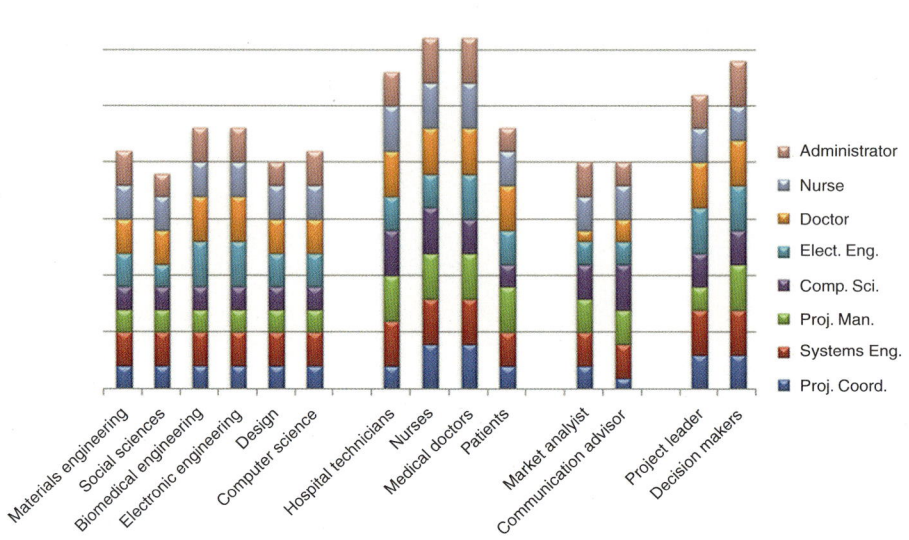

Fig. 6 Assessment of who has to become convinced by the laboratory-stage developed solution (with obvious implications on subsequent development stages)

a programmer, an electronics engineer, a medical doctor, a nurse, and a hospital administrator. In addition to the individual plots, the average value for each group is also represented.

We can see in Fig. 5 considerable similarities between the opinions of the inquired professionals. In fact, all those inquired agree on the level of challenges facing the development team, and there is almost unanimity regarding challenges on the users' side and also the interface/management aspects. Even regarding marketing/communication, opinions vary only within a range of 25%. Clearly, among those who answered the survey, the latter is seen as the aspect less challenging at the laboratory stage development (as one could expect). Conversely, major challenges are associated with both the technical development team and the project coordinator and managers.

Subsequently, people were asked to rank between 1 and 4 who has to become convinced by the developed solution so that it is considered successful (at the laboratory development stage, obviously). Results are shown in Fig. 6 as cumulative columns, using different colors for each of the inquired profiles.

In Fig. 6 we can identify again a reasonable consensus between the different inquired individuals. In fact, the overall ranks for each profile follow the general trends of individual answers. One should notice how project coordinators and managers tend to highlight the importance of the opinion of medical professionals, whereas researchers have a more homogeneous view. Opinions vary regarding marketing people, which can be explained by the fact that this varies considerably on a case-by-case basis, depending on the specific medical device being developed. The same applies for different areas of expertise among the development team.

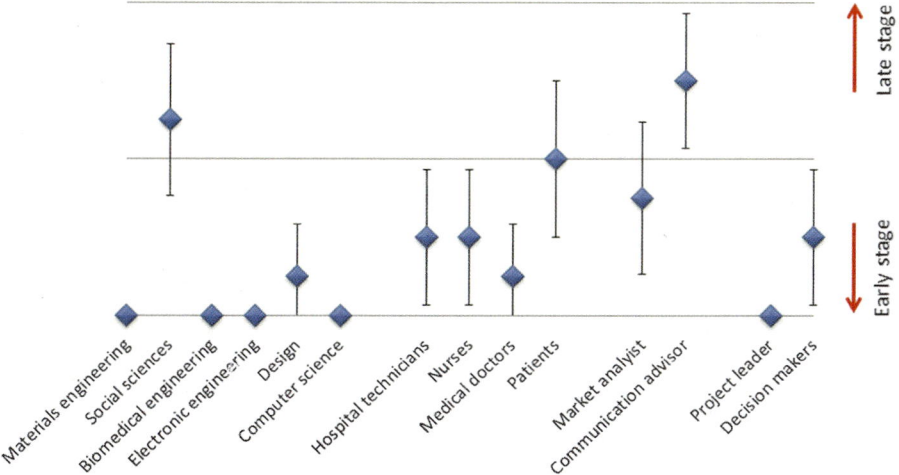

Fig. 7 Results regarding the suggested timing for involvement of the different profiles in the laboratory-stage product development process for medical devices

However, the results follow expectations, namely that doctors, nurses, and health-care facilities managers/administrators are those whose opinion will be critical when a decision is made regarding taking the project to the next level.

Finally, people were asked to indicate when along the development process (still considering only laboratory-stage development), each of the identified profiles should be involved in the project. The results are shown in Fig. 7.

Based on the individual input from all those inquired, the average timing and the respective standard deviation were calculated, for each of the profiles previously identified. Those values are represented in Fig. 7. In this figure, the bottom line of the plot corresponds to people being involved in the project from its very beginning. Conversely, the line at the top indicates a profile that should be involved in the project only after some preliminary development, typically after a first prototype is built or, at least, after a conceptual solution has been designed but not yet implemented. Thus, the higher we move on the vertical scale, the later should be the involvement.

It is important to emphasize again that these results have no statistical significance, nor do they attempt to be representative of all medical device development processes, which can vary tremendously in terms of complexity, technical level, scope, and goals.

The opinions of those inquired were relatively consensual in that highly technical researchers must become involved at the earliest possible time, and that doctors and nurses should become involved earlier than patients. However, it was suggested that some basic grinding be done before they are involved. Also, decision makers, such as hospital administrators, should be involved only after some preliminary work has been done.

5.3   *Analysis and Discussion*

The results shown in Figs. 5–7 illustrate the different opinions among the several individuals that are usually involved in the product design and development process of medical devices. This was expected from the fact that almost all those involved will only have immediately contact with a part of the entire process. Probably only the project coordinator is aware of the entire network of competences that contribute in some way to the process. However, despite the differences in opinions that were detected among the inquired profiles, the trends are similar, and there is clear consensus regarding the different roles that different groups have in the development process.

Understanding the expectations and the perspective of medical staff and decision makers is important to facilitate the development of projects in this field. Although this preliminary survey has enabled identifying some of those aspects, further work is clearly warranted.

6   Case-Study

Although the discussion above follows from personal experience through the involvement in several projects related to medical devices, with varying degrees of complexity (and ambition), as well as team size, a case-study project is useful to illustrate it.

From 2007 through 2010 a new concept for mobile health was explored in the scope of the Mobile Health Living Lab project in Guimarães, Portugal. It aimed at increasing mobility of patients in hospitals and their homes through continuous remote monitoring of vital signals, using wireless sensor networks (WSN). These networks are characterized by several features, such as self-organizing capabilities, short-range broadcast communication and multi-hop routing, frequently changing topology due to fading and node failures, and power limitations [12]. This solution has been selected due to similarities with scenarios tackled by other research groups, such as the SMART system [13] and a monitoring system developed at University of Texas [14]. These approaches are in contrast to solutions based on body area networks (BAN), which primarily collect data from wearable sensors and relay them to another network, such as the CodeBlue [15], BlueBio [16] and AID-N [17] systems.

The need was initially identified through discussions between decision makers and doctors at a healthcare provider and researchers from a university research center. It initially conceived the use of several support technologies and multiple support devices. It evolved along the first few months to a specific conceptual system design, including the need to develop hardware and software applications, narrowing the aims and goals, and defining project boundaries. During these 3 years,

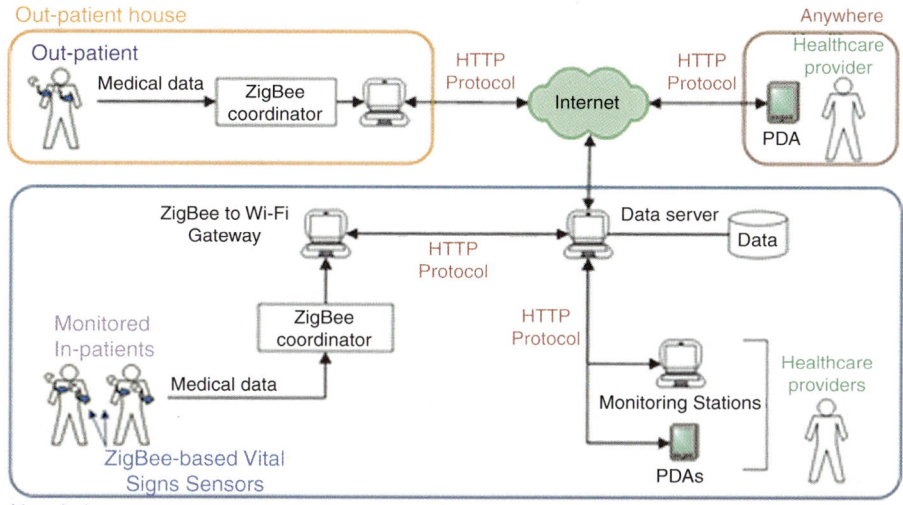

Fig. 8 Simplified view of the system architecture developed and implemented in the case-study project

it involved researchers from all areas described in §3.2 (and others), and the different healthcare professionals and end-users in the roles described in §3.1. The system architecture is represented in Fig. 8.

It is important to mention that the proposed architecture was designed for this specific type of use scenario. For example, in the case of intensive care units, where the use specifications and requirements are very different, but also where patients only move within a very restricted area, other solutions have been identified [18]. Only to illustrate the variety of applications within this field, one can mention also remote rescue and care [19], or disaster scenarios [15–17]. A plethora of other cases can be found in the literature [20].

The developed sensors, network gateways, applications, user interfaces, etc., are being field tested at the Guimarães Private Hospital (Grupo AMI – Assistência Médica Integral) and have been recently showcased in many media sources, including national television. This project paves the way for future innovation in the area, highlighting the advantages of user-centered development and synergic cooperation between universities and companies, and will have practical effect on the quality of healthcare for many patients.

7   Concluding Remarks

This chapter presents some considerations about the coordination of multidisciplinary teams for the development of medical devices. The different people that usually become involved in the process, even at a laboratory development stage, have been identified and their role discussed. The results from a small survey on this topic were presented and discussed, in order to provide a very preliminary assessment of the different perspectives held by different professionals who have participated in several medical device development projects.

Clearly, there are major challenges in today's development of medical devices that are related to the interface between all the different individuals involved in the process. The high complexity of products requires larger and more multidisciplinary teams. Effectively coordinating these efforts and managing the overall development project is not trivial, and can be a vital aspect in achieving a successful project. But this becomes increasingly problematic in the user-centered development framework that characterizes modern product development. In addition to researchers and technicians, end users (doctors, nurses, and even patients) are involved in early development stages, creating new challenges.

Vital aspects which could not be discussed here include medical device certification, and the different paradigms of developing medical devices within companies or in a university setting. These issues, and some aspects which could not be tackled in great depth, should be further explored in future work. An obvious example is expanding considerably the number of surveyed individuals for the discussion of Sect. 14.5.

Acknowledgments Colleagues involved in the case-study, namely José A. Afonso, Higino Correia, Adriano Moreira, Joaquim Mendes, and students Helena Fernandez-López, Ana Carolina Matos, Duarte Pereira, and Bruno Fernandes. Clinical and financial support for the case-study has been provided by Grupo AMI - Assistência Médica Integral (Casa de Saúde de Guimarães, SA), Portugal, under the partnership established between this healthcare company and the University of Minho. Financial support was also provided by the MIT-Portugal program. The author also acknowledges the Foundation for Science and Technology, Lisbon, through the 3° Quadro Comunitário de Apoio, the POCTI and FEDER programs, and Project PEst-C/CTM/LA0025/2011.

References

1. Zenios S et al (2009) Biodesign: the process of innovating new medical technologies. Cambridge University Press, Cambridge
2. Alexander K, Clarkson J, Bishop D, Fox S (2002) Good design practice for medical devices and equipment: requirements capture. Engineering Design Centre. Cambridge University, Cambridge
3. Simoes R, Sampaio AM (2009) Exceeding problem solving expectations in industrial design under severely restricted specifications, IRF - integrity, reliability and failure: challenges and opportunities, INEGI Editions, Porto, p 445, ISBN 978-972-8826-22-2
4. Fernandez-Lopez H, Afonso JA, Correia JH, Simões R (2010) HM4All: a vital signs monitoring system based in spatially distributed zigBee networks. In: Proceedings of pervasive health 2010 – 4th international conference on pervasive computing technologies for healthcare, Munich, 22–25 Mar 2010
5. Fernandez-Lopez H, Macedo P, Afonso JA, Correia JA, Simoes R (2009) Extended health visibility in the hospital environment. In: Biodevices 2009 – Second International Conference on Biomedical Electronics and Devices, Porto, Portugal, 14–17 Jan 2009, pp 422

6. Pereira D, Moreira A, Simoes R (2010) Challenges on real-time monitoring of patients through the Internet. In: Proceedings of CISTI 2010, Santiago de Compostela – Spain, 16–19 June 2010
7. Sampaio M, Pontes AJ, Simoes R (2009) Analysis of product design and development methodologies towards a specific implementation for embedded microelectronics. In: Proceedings of IDEMI09, Porto, 14–15 Sept 2009
8. Fernandez LH, Macedo P, Afonso JA, Correia JH, Simões R (2009) Evaluation of the impact of the topology and hidden nodes in the performance of a ZigBee network. In: Lecture notes of the institute for computer sciences, social-informatics and telecommunications engineering vol 24 (S-Cube 2009), Pisa, pp 256–271
9. Pugh S (1991) Total design - integrated methods for successful product engineering. Addison-Wesley Pub Co, Wokingham
10. Simoes R, Sampaio AM (2008) Effect of technology-driven products in the future of product design and development. In: Proceedings of RPD 2008 – rapid product development, Oliveira de Azeméis, 29–30 Oct 2008
11. Cruz-Cunha MM, Tavares AJ, Simões R (eds) (2010) Handbook of research on developments in e-health and telemedicine: technological and social perspectives. Information Science Reference, Hershey
12. Holger K, Willig A (2005) Protocols and architectures for wireless sensor. Willey, Networks
13. Dorothy C et al (2008) Physiological signal monitoring in the waiting areas of an emergency room. In: Proceedings of the ICST 3rd international conference on body area networks, ICST, Tempe
14. Hande A et al (2006) Self-powered wireless sensor networks for remote patient monitoring in hospitals. Sensors 6(9):1102–1117
15. Lorincz K et al (2004) Sensor networks for emergency response: challenges and opportunities. IEEE Pervasive Comput 3(4):16–23
16. Kramp G, Kristensen M, Pedersen JF (2006) Physical and digital design of the blueBio biomonitoring system prototype to be used in emergency medical response. In: Pervasive Health Conference and Workshops, 2006, Institute of Electrical and Electronics Engineers (IEEE), Innsbruck, Austria
17. Gao T et al (2008) Wireless medical sensor networks in emergency response: implementation and pilot results. In: 2008 IEEE International Conference on Technologies for Homeland Security, Waltham, MA, May 12–13 2008, pp 187
18. O'Donoughue N, Kulkarni S, Marzella D (2006) Design and implementation of a framework for monitoring patients in hospitals using wireless sensors in Ad Hoc configuration. In: 28th annual international conference of the IEEE EMBS, New York, pp 6449–6452
19. Kyriacou E et al (2007) m-Health e-Emergency systems: current status and future directions [wireless corner]. IEEE Antennas Propag 49(1):216–231
20. Dishongh TJ, McGrath M (2009) Wireless sensor networks for healthcare applications. Artech House, Norwood

A Process-Algebra Model of the Cell Mechanics of Autoreactive Lymphocytes Recruitment

Paola Lecca

Abstract Lymphocytes roll along the walls of vessels to survey the endothelial surface for chemotactic inflammatory signals, which stimulate the lymphocytes to stop rolling and migrate through the endothelium and its supporting basement membrane. Recent studies about the inflammatory process of the brain leading to the multiple sclerosis, have revealed that lymphocytes extravasation is a sequence of dynamical states (contact with endothelium, rolling and firm adhesion), mediated by partially overlapped interactions of different adhesion molecules and activation factors. These interactions are both concurrent and parallel, and consequently their modelling need to be specified in a language able to represent concurrency and parallelism.

Process calculi (or process algebras) are a diverse family of related languages developed by in computer science for formally modelling concurrent systems. Here, we propose the use of the biochemical stochastic π-calculus. This calculus is an efficient tool for describing the concurrency of the different interactions driving the phases of lymphocytes recruitment. It models a biochemical systems as a set of concurrent processes selected according to a suitable probability distribution to quantitatively describe the rates and the times at which the reactions occur. We use here this tool to model and simulate the molecular mechanisms involved in encephalitogenic lymphocytes recruitment. In particular, we show that the model predicts the percentage of lymphocytes involved in the rolling process on the endothelium of vessels of different diameters and the adhesion probability of the cell as function of interaction time. The results of the model reproduce, within the estimated experimental errors, the functional behavior of the data obtained from laboratory measurements.

P. Lecca (✉)
The Microsoft Research, University of Trento, CoSBi, Trento, Italy
e-mail: lecca@cosbi.eu

R.M.N. Jorge et al. (eds.), *Technologies for Medical Sciences*, Lecture Notes
in Computational Vision and Biomechanics 1, DOI 10.1007/978-94-007-4068-6_15,
© Springer Science+Business Media B.V. 2012

1   Introduction

The biophysics of cell adhesion is the most intensively investigated area of cell mechanics. These studies have been driven by the strong interest in many biological processes of which cell adhesion is an important element, leading to the development of a number of mathematical models. Cell attachment to and detachment from a surface, such as, for example, endothelial surface that lines the blood vessel wall is a central aspect in the inflammatory processes.

The lymphocytes are the cells whose adhesion mechanical properties are most deeply studied, because of their central role in the tissues response to inflammation. Lymphocyte adhesion under blood flow in microvasculature is mediated by binding between cell surface receptor and complementary ligands expressed on the endothelium, the surface lining the blood vessel wall. Lymphocyte adhere to the endothelium in a 4-phases mechanism: tethering and rolling (primarily mediated by selectins and in part also by integrins), firm adhesion (primarily mediated by integrins) and finally the cell migration through the endothelium toward the inflammation site. The rolling along the walls of vessels enables the lymphocytes to survey the endothelial surface for chemotactic signals, that stimulate their arrest and migration through the endothelium and its supporting basement membrane. This kind of mechanism is a critical event in the origin and evolution of the autoimmune diseases. In the ambit of this kind of pathologies, we mention the multiple sclerosis, an inflammatory disease of the central nervous system. A novel intravital microscopy model to directly visualize and analyze through the skull the interactions between lymphocytes and endothelium in celebral venules of mice has been created [24]. This technique allows to characterize each step and each species of adhesion molecules implicated in the lymphocytes recruitment in brain vessels. A realistic quantitative model and simulation *in silico* of the process leading to the extravasation of the lymphocyte from the blood vessels into the brain tissue may permit quantitative predications and subsequently a better control of the autoimmune attacks.

The most common approaches to the simulation of cell rolling process can be classified into three categories: mechanical, thermodynamic and kinetic. Mechanical models describe the lymphocyte rolling as peeling of a flexible and inextensible tape. The dynamics is formalized resorting the concept of adhesion energy. Analysis based on the energy conservation allows adhesion energy to be related to the work done by external forces and the energy stored in and dissipated by the deformed cell [10, 18, 30]. Thermodynamic models were developed concurrently to mechanical ones, in order to relate the adhesion energy to physicochemical properties of adhesive receptors and their interactions [3, 31].

The major result of the thermodynamical treatment is the expression of the adhesion energy in term of the number of bonds in the contact area. The adhesion energy density was found to be directly proportional to the number of molecular bonds between receptors and ligands and inversely proportional to the $K_B T$, where K_B is the Boltzmann constant and T the absolute temperature.

These mechanical and thermodynamic models are highly complex and with many parameters, yet they are still idealized and rely on a number of nontrivial assumptions, that often can not be supported by sufficient quantitative experimental observations. Furthermore, discrepancies appear when one tries to equalize the adhesion energy expression of the thermodynamic models with the one of the mechanical models. The disagreement is due to the inadequacy of the two-dimensional approximation of the thermodynamic analyses in treating the contribution of all the degree of freedom of a flexible tape in a three-dimensional space [32].

Recently a reaction kinetics approach has been reconsidered and it has been developed along with the experimental technologies. Kinetic models describe adhesive interaction using chemical reaction kinetics and relating the kinetic rates to the force applied to the rolling cell. They were conceptualized by Bell [2] and then refined by several authors [3, 8, 16] (See Appendix A for more details). Reaction kinetics is used in biology for describing the binding of ligands to cell surface receptors. The rationale for applying this framework to adhesive interactions comes from the physical characteristics of these non-covalent specific interactions: the receptor-ligand binding can be modeled as a key-to-lock type of interaction dynamically governed by reaction rates. The nature of the key-to-lock molecular interactions presents three inter-dependent features: (a) concurrency of different kinds of interactions that contribute to the expression of the same phenomenon, (b) inherently random competition between the various species of ligands in forming bonds with the same species of receptors, (c) discrete character of the quantity of components and low number of bond-mediated adhesion (single-bond condition). The inclusion of the kinetic equations into the mechanical and thermodynamical model enables the solution of the bond density, which, when combined with the force on a bond, provides the adhesive stress.

The three categories of models, mechanic, thermodynamic and kinetics, are usually deterministic and based on ordinary differential equations and algebraic equations. However, an ordinary differential equation model of the kinetics of the lymphocyte recruitment does not capture the concurrency and the parallelism that are inherent to the network of interactions. Moreover, usually deterministic differential equations are used to simulate a dynamics that is intrinsically stochastic, as the amount of the adhesion molecules responsible for the processes of tethering and rolling of the lymphocyte on the endothelium is low.

An alternative to the common approaches to model the kinetics of the molecular interactions governing the lymphocyte recruitment is a process calculus approach. Process calculi can represent interactions between independent concurrent and parallel processes as communication (message-passing), rather than as the modification of shared variables. They can describe processes and systems using a small collection of primitives, and operators for combining those primitives. Finally, process calculi define algebraic laws for the process operators, which allow process expressions to be manipulated using equational reasoning.

We focused on a stochastic extension [25, 26] of the π-calculus [21]. The biochemical stochastic π-calculus is an efficient alternative to the ordinary differential equations since it provides a stochastic modelling framework and it allows to describe concurrent and parallel interactions. The basic idea of this calculus is to model a system as a set of concurrent processes that interact according to a suitable probability distribution to quantitatively accommodate the rates and the times at which the reactions occur.

We adopted the framework of the stochastic π-calculus to model and simulate the molecular mechanism involved in encephalitogenic lymphocyte recruitment in inflamed brain microvessels. Here we review the data we obtained from simulations concerning the prediction of the rolling lymphocytes percentage versus vessels diameters and of the adhesion probability versus contact time [7, 17]. Our study, started in 2004 in collaboration with the Department of Pathology of University of Verona (Italy) [17], can also be interpreted as a comparison between the mechanical and kinetic methods to point out the ability of this new tool to perform a stochastic simulation of chemical interactions in a highly expressive and predictive way.

2   The Biochemical Stochastic π-Calculus Approach

In this section we first recall the basic syntax and intuitive semantics of the biochemical stochastic π-calculus, hereafter called *BioSpi*. We then discuss how the language is used to model generic biological phenomena and how its compositionality can be exploited to represent complex systems.

2.1   The Formalism

At the microscopic scale, biological processes are carried out by networks of interacting molecules. The interaction between molecules causes their biochemical modification. These modifications affect the potential of the modified molecules to interact with other molecules. The π-calculus represents the molecules as computational processes and the network of interacting molecules as a mobile concurrent systems. This kind of systems are composed of a community of co-existing computational process that communicate each other and that change their interconnection structure when they execute. Each computational process is defined by its potential communication activity. The communication between process, that is the abstraction of chemical interaction, occur via channels, denoted by their names. In order for two concurrent processes to communicate, they must share a common channel name on which the sender outputs a message with the receiver receives. The only content of messages transmitted in communication is channel names or tuples of channel names, which may be used for further communication. The π-calculus formally consists of a *syntax* for writing formal descriptions of the concurrent system state (specification), a set of *congruence laws*, that determine when two syntactic expressions are equivalent and an *operational semantics* consisting of *reduction rules* to define the potential changes in the state of the system induced

Table 1 The π-calculus

Process and channels	
$P, Q, \ldots$	Process names
$x, y, \ldots$	Channel names
$\overline{x}, \overline{y}, \ldots$	Channel co-names

Events	
$\pi ::= x(y)$	Receive y along x
$\pi ::= \overline{x}\rangle y\langle$	Send y along x

Process syntax	
$P ::= P_1 \mid P_2$	Parallel processes
$\pi . P_1$	Sequential prefixing by communication
$\pi_1 . P_1 + \pi_2 . P_2$	Mutually exclusive communication
$(v\,x)P$	Restricted communication scope
0	Inert process

Structural congruence	
$P \mid Q \equiv Q \mid P$	Commutativity of PAR
$(P \mid Q) \mid R \equiv P \mid (Q \mid R)$	Associativity of PAR
$P + Q \equiv Q + P$	Commutativity of summation
$(P + Q) + R \equiv P + (Q + R)$	Associativity of summation
$(v\,x)0 = 0$	Scope of inert process
$(\mu\,x)(\mu\,y)P \equiv (\mu\,y)(\mu\,x)P$	Multiple communication scopes
$((\mu\,x)P \mid Q)) \equiv (\mu\,x)(P \mid Q)$ if $x \notin fn(Q)$	Scope extrusion
$A(\vec{y}) \equiv \{\vec{y}/\vec{x}\}Q_A$	Recursive parametric definition
$x(y).P = x(z).(\{z/y\}P)$ if $z \notin fn(P)$	Renaming of input channel y
$(v\,y)P = (\mu\,z).(\{z/y\}P)$ if $z \notin fn(P)$	Renaming of restricted channel y

Reaction rules	
$(\cdots + \overline{x}\rangle x\langle.Q) \mid (\cdots + x(y).P) \rightarrow Q \mid P\{x/y\}$	Communication (COMM)
if $P \rightarrow P'$ then $P \mid Q \rightarrow P' \mid Q$	Reaction under parallel composition
if $P \rightarrow P'$ then $(\mu\,x)P \rightarrow (\mu\,x)P'$	Reaction within restricted scope
if $Q \equiv P, P \rightarrow P'$ and $P' \equiv Q'$ then $Q \rightarrow Q'$	Reaction up to structural congruence

by communication. The processes are constructed using channel names according to the syntax, show in Table 1, in which the channel are indicated with their names $x, y, \ldots$ and the process with the capital letters $P, Q, \ldots$. The simplest process is the empty process 0. The communication between to process consists of two types of atomic actions, denoted as π and called *prefix*: the *input* $x(y)$ to receive a name for y along the channel x and the *output* $\overline{x}\langle z\rangle$ to send the name z along the channel x.

A process P may be prefixed with an input or output action π: P will occur only after the action π is performed. Processes may also be combined to create more complex ones. The *mutual exclusive choice operator* $+$ allows summation of processes and denotes a complex process able to perform exactly one of several alternative actions. The choice between the actions is non-deterministic and depends on the actual communication that will occur. In fact, since several alternative communication may be possible, that actual communication that will be realized is unknown in advance and the behavior is non-deterministic. Two processes P and Q can also be composed in *parallel* by the PAR operator $|$. In this case, both are concurrently active and can act either independently or with each other.

Finally, the use of a certain channel name may be restricted to a particular process P by the *new* operator often indicates also as ν. The concept of scope of a process prefix abstracts the physical structure of two intersecting molecular domains and/or of a molecular complex: global channel names and co-names represent complementary molecular domains and newly declared private channels define complexes.

Thus, in the syntax of the calculus a process P is written as follows

$$P ::= \mathbf{0} \mid X \mid (\pi, r).P \mid (\nu x)P \mid [x = y]P \mid P|P \mid P + P \mid A(y_1, \ldots, y_n)$$

where $A(y_1, \ldots, y_n)$ is the definition of constants (hereafter, $\tilde{y}$ denotes $y_1, \ldots, y_n$). Each agent identifier A has a unique defining equation of the form $A(y_1, \ldots, y_n) = P$, where the y_i are distinct and $fn(P) \subseteq \{y_1, \ldots, y_n\}$ (see below for the definition of free names fn).

The parameter r is the single parameter of an exponential distribution that characterize the stochastic behavior of the activity corresponding to the prefix π. The replacement of the prefix πP of the original semantics of π-calculus with the stochastic variant $(\pi, r).P$ is the main modification needed to make π-calculus suitable to a realistic simulation of a chemical reaction. The other modifications concern an extension of the definition *structural congruence* $\equiv$ and the definition of the *race conditions*, governing the dynamic behavior of the system.

The *structural congruence* $\equiv$ on processes is defined as the least congruence satisfying the following clauses:

- P and Q α-equivalent (they only differ in the choice of bound names) implies $P \equiv Q$,
- $(\mathcal{P}/_{\equiv}, +, \mathbf{0})$ is a commutative monoid,
- $(\mathcal{P}/_{\equiv}, |, \mathbf{0})$ is a commutative monoid,
- $(\nu x)(\nu y)P \equiv (\nu y)(\nu x)P, (\nu x)(R \mid S) \equiv (\nu x)R \mid S$ if $x \notin fn(S)$, $(\nu x)(R \mid S) \equiv R \mid (\nu x)S$ if $x \notin fn(R)$, and $(\nu x)P \equiv P$ if $x \notin fn(P)$.
- $A(\tilde{y}) \equiv P\{\tilde{y}/\tilde{x}\}$, if $A(\tilde{x}) ::= P$ is the unique defining equation of constant A.

We recall the notion of free names $fn(\mu)$, bound names $bn(\mu)$, and names $n(\mu) = fn(\mu) \cup bn(\mu)$ of a label μ.

μ	Kind	$fn(\mu)$	$bn(\mu)$
τ	Silent	$\emptyset$	$\emptyset$
$\overline{x}y$	Output	$\{x, y\}$	$\emptyset$
$x(y)$	Input	$\{x\}$	$\{y\}$

The dynamic behavior of a process is driven by a race condition. All activities enabled attempt tp proceed, but only the fastest one succeeds. The fastest activity is different on successive attempts because durations are random variables. The continuity of the probabilistic distribution ensures that the probability two activities ending simultaneously is zero. Furthermore, the exponential distributions enjoy the *memoryless* property: the time at which a transition of state occurs is independent of the time at which the last transition occurred. Therefore there is no need to record the time elapsed to reach the current state. The race condition is implemented by the Gillespie stochastic algorithm [12, 13], that computes the time evolution of probability densities for chemical species concentrations. This algorithm models the kinetics of a set of coupled chemical reactions, taking into account stochastic effects from low copy numbers of the chemical species. In Gillespie's approach, chemical reaction kinetics are modeled as a markov process in which reactions occur at specific instants of time defining intervals that are Poisson-distributed, with a mean reaction time interval that is recomputed after each chemical reaction occurs. For each chemical reaction interval, a specific chemical reaction occurs, randomly selected from the set of all possible reactions with a weight given by the individual reaction rates.

The reduction semantics of BioSpi is the following

$$(\ldots + (\overline{x}\langle z\rangle, r).Q)|((x(y), r).P + \ldots) \xrightarrow{x, r_b \cdot 1 \cdot 1} Q|P\left\{z/y\right\}$$

$$\frac{P \xrightarrow{x, r_b \cdot r_0 \cdot r_1} P'}{P|Q \xrightarrow{x, r_b \cdot r_0' \cdot r_1'} P'|Q}, \quad \begin{cases} r_0' = r_0 + In_x(Q) \\ r_1' = r_1 + Out_x(Q) \end{cases}$$

$$\frac{P \xrightarrow{x, r_b \cdot r_0 \cdot r_1} P'}{(\nu x)P \xrightarrow{x, r_b \cdot r_0 \cdot r_1} (\nu x)P'} \qquad \frac{Q \equiv P, P \xrightarrow{x, r_b \cdot r_0 \cdot r_1} P', P' \equiv Q'}{Q \xrightarrow{x, r_b \cdot r_0 \cdot r_1} Q'}$$

A reaction is implemented by the three parameters r_b, r_0 and r_1, where r_b represents the basal rate, and r_0 and r_1 denote the quantities of interacting molecules, and are computed compositionally by the two functions In_x and Out_x. These two functions inductively count the number of receive and send operations on a channel x enable in a process. They are defined as follows

$$In_x(0) = 0$$

$$In_x\left(\sum_{i \in I}(\pi_i, r_i).P_i\right) = |\{(\pi_i, r_i)|i \in I \wedge sbj(\pi_i) = x\}|$$

$$In_x(P_1|P_2) = In_x(P_1) + In_x(P_2)$$

$$In_x((\nu z)P) = \begin{cases} In_x(P) & \text{if } z \neq x \\ 0 & \text{otherwise} \end{cases}$$

Out_x is similarly defined, by replacing any occurrence of In with Out and the condition $sbj(\pi_i) = x$ with $sbj(\pi_i) = \overline{x}$.

Table 2 Biochemical stochastic π-calculus specification for a heterodimer complex formation and breakage

$SYSTEM ::= Molecule1 \vert Moelcule2$
$Molecule1 ::= (\nu\ backbone) . (\overline{bind}\langle backbone \rangle, RA).Molecule1\_bound(backbone)$ $Molecule1\_bound(bb) ::= (\overline{bb}, RD) . Molecule1$
$Molecule2 ::= (bind(cross\_backbone), RA) . Molecule2\_bound(cross\_backbone)$ $Molecule2\_bound(cbb) ::= (cbb, RD) . Molecule2$

RA and RD are the channel communication rates between processes

The first axiom of the BioSpi reduction semantics corresponds to usual reactions involving two different molecules, the second one corresponds to homodimerization reactions, involving the same molecular species.

2.2 The Approach

The kinetic approach, treating the cell adhesion as a reactive rate process of the receptor and ligand molecules, is fit for a modeling and a simulation with BioSpi. This framework [1] is a stochastic extension of the π-calculus, a formal language originally developed for specifying concurrent computational systems [20]. In such systems, multiple processes interact with each other by synchronized pair-wise communication on complementary communication channels, and modify each other by transmitting channels names from one process to another. This feature, named *mobility*, allows the network structure to change with the interaction between processes.

The basic idea of the stochastic variant of the π-calculus is to model a system as a set of concurrent processes selected according to a suitable probability distribution to quantitatively accommodate the rates and the times at which the reactions occur. The stochastic π-calculus is particularly suitable to model biochemical networks as mobile communication systems. This language represents molecules and their domains as computational processes, where their complementary determinants correspond to communication channels. Chemical interaction and subsequent modification of the state of reagents coincide with communication and channel names transmission. In a stochastic π-calculus model of a system of interacting molecules, the time evolution of molecular populations levels is governed by the initial number of processes and by the communication rates between them. The communication rate associated to a channel is the parameter of an exponential probability distribution that characterizes the stochastic behavior of the activity corresponding to that channel. Precisely in this context activities denote actions with an associated duration. Therefore, the communication rate is the abstraction of the basal rate of a biochemical reaction, concerning the time that a molecular species takes to undergo a reaction.

The central molecular event in the cell adhesion mechanics is the complex binding and unbinding occurring between the receptors on the cell and the ligands expressed on the endothelium during the rolling of the cell along the vessel surface. The stochastic π-calculus representation of formation and breakage of a heterodimer complex between two molecules, Molecule1 and Molecule2, uses both private and public channels (see Table 2). The two molecules, represented by two processes, share a public *bind* channel, on which one process (Molecule1) is offering to send a message, and the other (Molecule2) is offering to receive. This complementary communication abstracts the structural molecular complementarity of the two molecules and the communication event represents the binding between them. The private *backbone* channel, indicated with the scope operator v, is sent from Molecule1 to Molecule2; it represents the formed complex. After the communication event the two Molecules change to a "bound" state (Molecule1_bound and Molecule2_bound). A communication between the two "bound" processes on the shared private channel *backbone* represents the complex breakage. As a result, the two processes return to the initial "free" state (Molecule1 and Molecule2), completing a full cycle. RA and RD are real numbers indicating the rates of communication between the processes.

In these last years the stochastic π-calculus has been used for modeling various molecular systems, including transcriptional circuits, metabolic pathways and signal transduction networks [26–29]. It has revealed its efficiency overall providing a unifying view of both the molecular data and the dynamic behaviour it underlies. Moreover, the stochastic π-calculus simulated evolution of the various considered biological system has been found to be in agreement either with the recent experimental results or with the most consolidated theoretical models.

The developments of the experimental technologies,[1] occured at the end of 1990s, have allowed to better understand the molecular mechanism driving the dynamics of lymphocyte interaction with vessels wall. The last studies based on the intravital microscopy [24] have revealed that the process leading to lymphocyte extravasation in inflammatory sites is a sequence of dynamical states (contact with endothelium, rolling and firm adhesion), mediated by partially overlapped interactions of different adhesion molecules and activation factors. On the basis of these studies, the lymphocyte recruitment, can be efficiently modelled as a set of concurrent processes. Furthermore, the BioSpi simulation of the time-evolution of the molecular bonds density occurring during the dynamical interactions of the rolling lymphocytes with the endothelium, can lead to predictive results about the number of cells that undergo an efficient rolling and recruitment in inflamed vessels. The stochastic π-calculus may, thus, open new perspectives for the simulation of this key phenomenon in the pathogenesis of autoimmune diseases, implicating not only better knowledge, but also better future control of the autoimmune attack.

---

[1] Major developments in the 1990s included experiments that provided direct measurements of kinetic rates, lifetimes and detachment force of adhesive interactions.

3 BioSpi Model of Autoreactive Lymphocyte Recruitment in Inflamed Brain Venules

In this section we briefly describe the physiology of the lymphocytes interactions with endothelial surface, then we shows our specification of the 4-phases of lymphocyte recruitment, and finally, we discusses the results of the stochastic simulation.

3.1 Molecular Mechanisms of the 4-Phases Model of Lymphocyte Recruitment

A critical event in the pathogenesis of multiple sclerosis, an autoimmune disease of the central nervous system, is the migration of the lymphocytes from the brain vessels into the brain parenchyma. The extravasation of lymphocytes is mediated by highly specialized groups of cell adhesion molecules and activation factors. The process leading to lymphocytes migration, illustrated in Fig. 1, is divided into four main kinetic phases: (1) initial contact with the endothelial membrane (tethering) and rolling along the vessel wall; (2) activation of a G-protein, induced

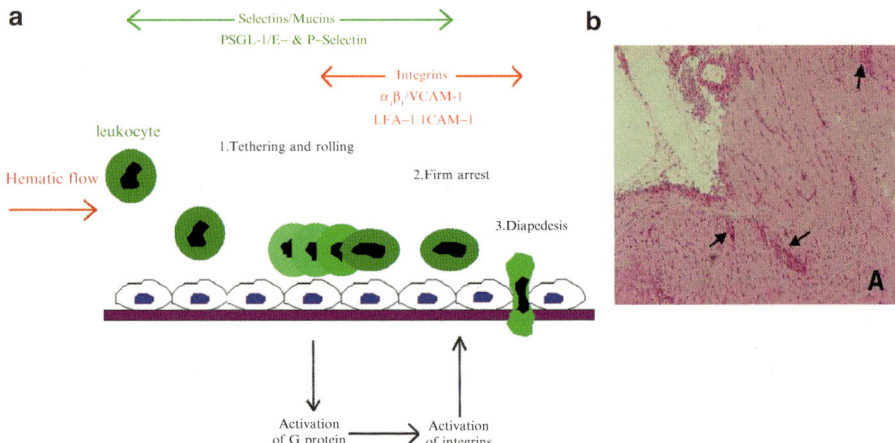

Fig. 1 (**a**) The process leading to lymphocyte extravasation is a finely regulated sequence of steps controlled by both adhesion molecules and activating factors. It involves: *1.* initial contact (tethering) and rolling along the vessel wall mediated by selectins (PSGL-1/E- and P-selectin) and integrins($\alpha_4\beta_1$/VCAM-1) and (LFA-1/ICAM-1); *2.* chemoattractant-induced heterotrimeric G protein-dependent intracellular biochemical changes leading to integrins activation; *3.* integrin-dependent firm arrest, due principally to LFA-1/ICAM-1 interaction: and *4.* diapedesis, i.e. the passage of the lymphocytes through the wall of a blood vessel into the surrounding tissues. (**b**) Transversal section of inflamed brain. The *black arrows* indicate the sites of inflammation at which the lymphocytes extravasation occur

by a chemokine exposed by the inflamed endothelium and subsequent activation of integrins (3) firm arrest and (4) crossing of the endothelium (diapedesis). For this study, we have used a model of early inflammation in which brain venules express E- and P-selectin, ICAM-1 and VCAM-1 [24]. The leukocyte is represented by encephalitogenic $CD4^+$ T lymphocytes specific for PLP139-151, cells that are able to induce experimental autoimmune encephalomyelitis, the animal model of multiple sclerosis.

Tethering and rolling steps are mediated by binding between cell surface receptors and complementary ligands expressed on the surface of the endothelium. The principal adhesion molecules involved in these phases are the selectins: the P-selecton glyco-protein ligand-1 (PSGL-1) on the autoreactive lymphocytes and the E- and P-selecton on the endothelial cells. The action of integrins is partially overlaped to the action of selectins/mucins: α_4 integrins and LFA-1 are also involved in the rolling phase, but they have a less relevant role.

Chemokines have been shown to trigger rapid integrin-dependent lymphocyte adhesion in vivo through a receptor coupled with G_i proteins. Integrin-dependent firm arrest in brain microcirculation is blocked by pertussis toxin (PTX), a molecule able to ADP ribosylate G_i proteins and block their function. Thus, as previously shown in studies on naïve lymphocytes homing to Peyer's patches and lymph nodes, encephalitogenic lymphocytes also require an in situ activation by an adhesion-triggering agonist which exerts its effect via Gi-coupled surface receptor.

The firm adhesion/arrest is mediated by lymphocyte integrins and their ligands from the immunoglobulin superfamily expressed by the endothelium. The main adhesion molecules involved in cell arrest is integrin LFA-1 on lymphocyte and its counterligand ICAM-1 on the endothelium. The action of α_4 integrins is partially overlaped to the action of LFA-1: α_4 integrins are involved in the arrest but they have a less relevant role [24].

3.2 BioSpi Implementation

The system of interacting adhesion molecules that regulate the lymphocytes recruitment on endothelial surface has been implemented in the biochemical stochastic π-calculus as a system composed by eight concurrent processes, corresponding to the eight species of adhesion molecules, that regulate the cell rolling and arrest: PSGL-1, P-Selectin, chemokines, α_4, VCAM-1, LFA-1 and ICAM-1. The implementation of 4-phases model of lymphocyte recruitment has been divided into three steps corresponding to the three principal involved molecular interactions:

1. **Selectin-lingand interaction**. The interaction between PSGL-1 on lymphocyte and P-Selectin expressed by the endothelium is responsible for the rolling motion of cell.
2. **Integrinic activation by chemokines**. The binding between the chemokines receptors on the lymphocyte and their ligands on the endothelium triggers the integrin-dependent adhesion of the cell on the vessel wall.

3. **Integrin-ligand interaction**. The interaction between the active form of integrins (α_4 on lymphocyte, the correspondent receptor VCAM-1 on endothelium; LFA-1 on lymphocyte and its receptor ICAM-1 on endothelium) causes the firm adhesion of the cell. It has also a less relevant role in rolling process.

We describe the implementative choices effected to model each of these molecular reactions and the subsequent kinetic state of the cell adhesion.

Selectin-lingand interaction Rolling is a state of dynamic equilibrium in which there is rapid breaking of bonds at the trailing edges of the lymphocyte-endothelium contact zone, matched by rapid formation of new bonds at the leading edge. To represent the formation and the breakage of a complex between the two molecules PSGL-1 and P-Selectin we use both public and private channels. Each of the molecules is represented by a process (PSGL1 and PSELECTIN in Table 3). The two processes share a public *bind* channel, on which one process, PSGL1) is offering to send a message, and the other, P-SELECTIN is offering to receive. These complementary communication represent the complementarity of the two molecular domanins involved in the bond formation. The communication event represents the binding. The private channel *backbone* offerend by the binding site of PSGL1 molecule (BINDING_PSITE process) is sent from PSGL1 to PSELECTIN and represent the formed complex. After the communication event the two molecule change to a "bound" state PSGL1_BOUND and PSELECTIN_BOUND. A communication between the two bound processes on the shared private *backbone* channel represents complex breakage. As a result, the two processes return to the "free" state (PSGL1 and PSELECTIN).

Integrinic activation by chemokines Integrins undergo dynamic functional changes, generically referred as "activation", which increase the ability of cells to interact with entracellular ligands. Their activation is a consequence of the binding of different kinds of chemokines with their receptors that generates both pro- and anti-adhesive intracellular signaling events, that are relevant to the kinetic adhesion and de-adhesion and to cell movement during diapedesis. However, because our implementation focus on the simulation of the kinetics of the lymphocyte, we model the integrinic activation by chemokines as a change of state of the integrinic molecules subsequtn to the binding of a generic chemokines species with its receptors. A process CHEMOKINE, representing the chemokine molecule offers a private channel *chemobb* on its binding domain BINDING_CSITE. The chemokine receptor, represented by the process CHEMOKINE_REC shares with the process CHEMOKINE the public channel *lig*, on which CHEMOKINE sends a message (the name *chemobb*) and CHEMOKINE_REC receives it. After communication CHEMOKIN change to a bound state CHEMIKINE_BOUND, that consists of the parallel composition of three processes ACT1, ACT2 and ACT3. The first two processes represent the activation of ALPHA4 and LFA1 integrins molecules and the third represent the breakage of the complex CHEMOKIN_BOUND. ACT1 and ACT2 processes send, with a communication rate A, the names *sign1* and *sign2* on the global channels *alpha_act* and *lfa_act* respectively.. After the communication the processes ACT1 and ACT2 don't change state. The process

Table 3 Biochemical stochastic π-calculus specification of 4-phase lymphocyte recruitment process

---

$SYSTEM ::= PSGL1|PSELECTIN|CHEMOKIN|CHEMOREC|ALPHA4$
$|VCAM1|LFA1|ICAM1$

$PSGL1 ::= (\nu\ backbone)BINDING\_PSITE1$
$BINDING\_PSITE ::= (\overline{bind}\langle backbone\rangle, RA).PSGL1\_BOUND(backbone)$
$PSGL1\_BOUND(bb) ::= (\overline{bb}, RD_0).PSGL1$
$PSELECTIN ::=$
$\quad (bind(cross\_backbone), RA).PSELECTIN\_BOUND(cross\_backbone)$
$PSELECTIN\_BOUND(cbb) ::= (\overline{cbb}, RD_0).PSELECTIN$

$CHEMOKIN ::= (\nu\ chemobb)BINDING\_CSITE$
$BINDING\_CSITE ::= (\overline{lig}\langle chemobb\rangle, RA\_C).CHEMOKIN\_BOUND(chemobb)$
$CHEMOKIN\_BOUND(chemobb) ::= ACT1|ACT2|ACT3(cbb)$
$ACT1 ::= (\overline{alpha\_act}\langle sign1\rangle, A).ACT1$
$ACT2 ::= (\overline{lfa\_act}\langle sign2\rangle, A).ACT2$
$ACT3(chb) ::= (\overline{chb}, RD\_C).CHEMOKIN$
$CHEMOREC ::=$
$\quad (lig(cross\_chemobb), RA\_C).CHEMOREC\_BOUND(cross\_chemobb)$
$CHEMOREC\_BOUND(ccr) ::= (ccr, A).CHEMOREC$
$ALPHA4 ::= (alpha\_act(act\_a), A).ALPHA4\_ACTIVE$
$LFA1 ::= (lfa\_act(act\_l), A).LFA1\_ACTIVE$

$ALPHA4\_ACTIVE ::= (\nu\ backbone2)BINDING\_ASITE$
$BINDING\_ASITE ::= (\overline{bind2}\langle backbone2\rangle, RA).ALPHA4\_BOUND(backbone2)$
$ALPHA4\_BOUND(bb2) ::= (\overline{bb2}, RD_1).ALPHA4$
$VCAM1 ::= (bind2(cross\_backbone2), RA).VCAM1\_BOUND(cross\_backbone2)$
$VCAM1\_BOUND(cbb2) ::= (\overline{cbb2}, RD_1).VCAM1$

$LFA1\_ACTIVE ::= (\nu\ backbone3)BINDING\_SITE3$
$BINDING\_SITE3 ::= (\overline{bind3}\langle backbone3\rangle, RA).LFA1\_BOUND(backbone3)$
$LFA1\_BOUND(bb3) ::= (\overline{bb3}, RD_2).LFA1\_BOUND$
$ICAM1 ::= (bind3(cross\_backbone3), RA).ICAM1\_BOUND(cross\_backbone3)$
$ICAM1\_BOUND(cbb3) ::= (\overline{cbb3}, RD_2).ICAM1\_BOUND$

$RA = 6.500 \quad RA\_C = RD_0 = 0.051 \quad RD_1 = 5.100$
$RD_2 = 1.000 \quad RD\_C = 3.800 \quad A = \infty$

Radius of vessel $= 25\ \mu m$ Length of vessel $= 100\ \mu m$
Volume of vessel $= 1.96 \times 10^5\ \mu m^3$ Radius of lymphocyte $= 5\ \mu m$

ACT3 can receive a message on channel *chb* with a communication rate RD_C and return a CHEMOKIN in a free state.

The processes ALPHA4 and LFA1, representing the integrins molecules, communicate with ACT1 and ACT2 on the channel co-names *alpha_act* and *lfa_act*. After the communication event, occurred at rate A, the processes ALPHA4 and LFA1 change into their "active" forms ALPHA4_ACTIVE and LFA1_ACTIVE, that are involved in the stable arrest of the lymphocyte on the endothelium.

Integrin-ligand interaction The active form of the integrins ALPHA4 and LFA1, abstracted by the processes ALPHA4_ACTIVE and LFA1_ACTIVE, are partially

Table 4 Deterministic rates
for the 4-phases of
lymphocyte recruitment

Process	k_{on} (sec^{-1})	k_{off} (sec^{-1})
Tethering	84	1
Rolling	84	100
Chemokines activation	0.5	75
Firm adesion	84	20

involved in rolling of the cell, so that they undergo an alternate binding/unbindig with their ligands represented by the processes VCAM1 and ICAM1. For the inter-action between the ALPHA4_ACTIVE and VCAM1 the implementation follows the same track of the previous cases of complex formation and breakage. The reaction between LFA1_ACTIVE and ICAM1 processes leads to the formation of a stable complex, represented by the "bound" states LFA1_BOUND and ICAM1_BOUND, implementing the firm adhesion of the lymphocyte.

We simulated the role and the contribution of the different interactions as bi-molecular binding processes occurring at different rates (Table 4). The selectins interaction PSGL1/PSELECTIN plays a crucial role in guaranting an efficient rolling, therefore the channels rates for the communication in the binding process between PSGL1 and PSLECTIN have been calculated from the deterministic rates of the kinetic model, that reproduce the tethering and rolling motion. Analogously, for the ALPHA4_ACTIVE/VCAM1 interaction, that contributes to rolling and, in part, also to cell arrest, the channels rate have been calculated from the deterministic rates that recreate the rolling motion. The interaction LFA1_ACTIVE/ICAM1 is the main responsible of firm arrest of the cell on the endothelium and thus the rates of communication between LFA1_ACTIVE and ICAM1_ACTIVE have been calculated from those reproducing the firm adhesion in mechanic simulations.

The whole process of lymphocyte recruitment occur in a space of $V = 1.96 \times 10^5$ μm^3, corresponding to a volume of a vessel of 25 μm of radius and 100 μm of length, and in a simulated time of 15 s. In the considered volume V, the number of molecules is of the order of 10^6. In our simulations the values of the volume and of the molecules number have been proportionally re-scaled by this factor, to make the code computationally faster.

The stochastic reaction rates for bimolecular binding/unbinding reaction are inversely propartial to the volume of space in that the reactions occur [13], in particular for the stochastic association rate we have that $RA = k_{on}/V$ and for the stochastic dissociation rate we have $RD = 2k_{off}/V$, where the k_i's are the deterministic rates.

4   Results

The output of simulation is the time-evolution of number of bonds (shown in Fig. 2) assuming the following densities expressed in μm^{-2}: PSGL-1 [23] and P-SELECTIN 5600, ALPHA4 [5] and VCAM-1 85, CHEMOREC and CHEMOKI-NES 15000, LFA-1 [14] and ICAM-1 5500.

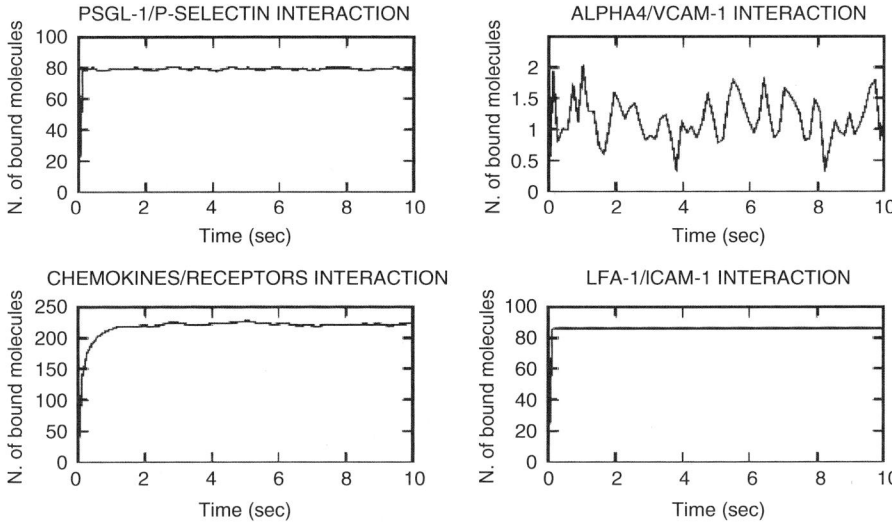

Fig. 2 BioSpi simulation of 4-phases model of lymphocyte recruitment

The BioSpi simulations reproduce the hyperbolic behavior predicted by the Dembo model. However unlike Dembo model, the BioSpi model is more sensitive to the variations of the dissociation constant rate k_{off}^0.

In Fig. 2 the curve describing the time-evolution of the bonds number of LFA-1/ICAM-1 interaction presents an approximately linear steep increasing followed by a clearly constant behavior: this curve represents the firm adhesion of lymphocyte and it is comparable with the state diagram of the mechanical model shown in Fig. 7. In fact, the firm arrest is reached when the number of bonds become stably constant in the time or, analogously, when the position of cell centroid does not change anymore. On the contrary, the plots representing PSGL-1/P-SELECTIN and ALPHA4/VCAM-1 interactions present, after a steep increasing with about the same slope of that of LFA-1/ICAM-1 binding, an oscillating behavior respect to the equilibrium positions given by the $y = 80$ and $y = 1$, respectively. This behavior represents the sequential bonds breaking and formation in the selectins and integrins binding during the rolling (see Fig. 7 for comparison).

4.1 BioSpi Prediction of Rolling Cells Percentage as a Function of Vessel Diameter

We have repeated the BioSpi simulation of lymphocyte recruitment for three groups of different values of the vessel diameter D_v (i. e., for different volumes V of the space in which the chemical interactions occur) given in Table 5. The result is the set of three groups of curves shown in Fig. 3.

Table 5 Three set of experimental values of rolling cell percentage (*RCP*) for different values of the vessel diameter D_v

D_v	RCP	D_v	RCP	D_v	RCP
16.6	18	40	9.8	74.6	1.13
16.6	15.5	43.2	5.4	68	6.2
20	14	43	6.7	65	3.7
21	13	42	5.8	65	3.5
20	9.3	45	4.2	68	6.2
25	17.3	43.6	4.7	66.6	2.4
23.8	10.1	44.6	6.5	66.6	3.4
16.6	15.5	40	5.4	66.6	4.7
23.3	9	40	4.9	73.3	1.5
23.3	14	40	7	75	4.8

Estimated experimental error on rolling cells percentage ±3

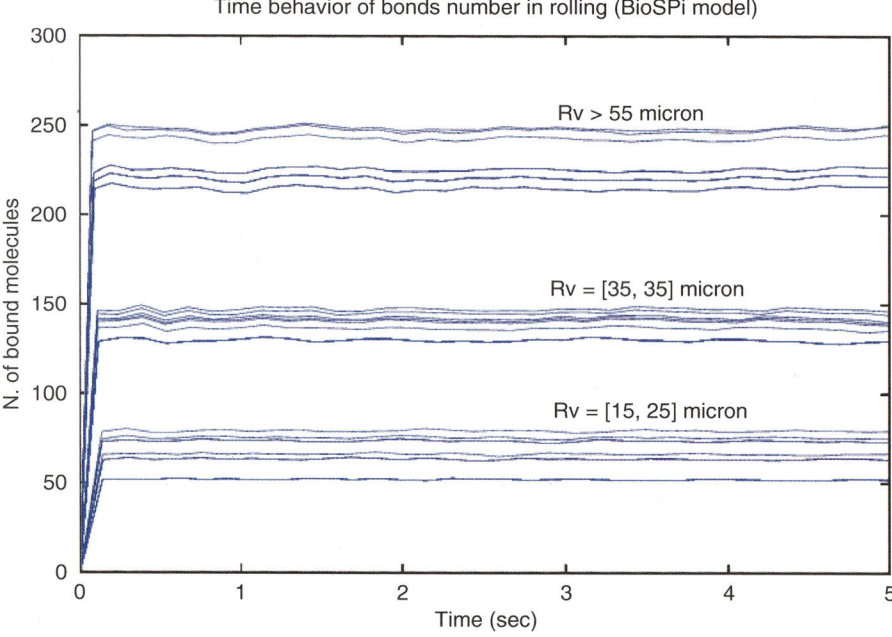

Fig. 3 Time evolution of number of bound molecules for three different sets of vessel diameters values

Dividing the number of bound molecules by the number of lymphocytes present in the blood flux in contact with the endothelium, we obtain the number of bound molecules per lymphocyte. This quantity is a measure of the propensity of the cell to interact with endothelium and to roll. In a simplified model and at the first order of approximation, the probability that a lymphocyte rolls on endothelium is directly proportional to this propensity. Writing the number of lymphocyte of the blood

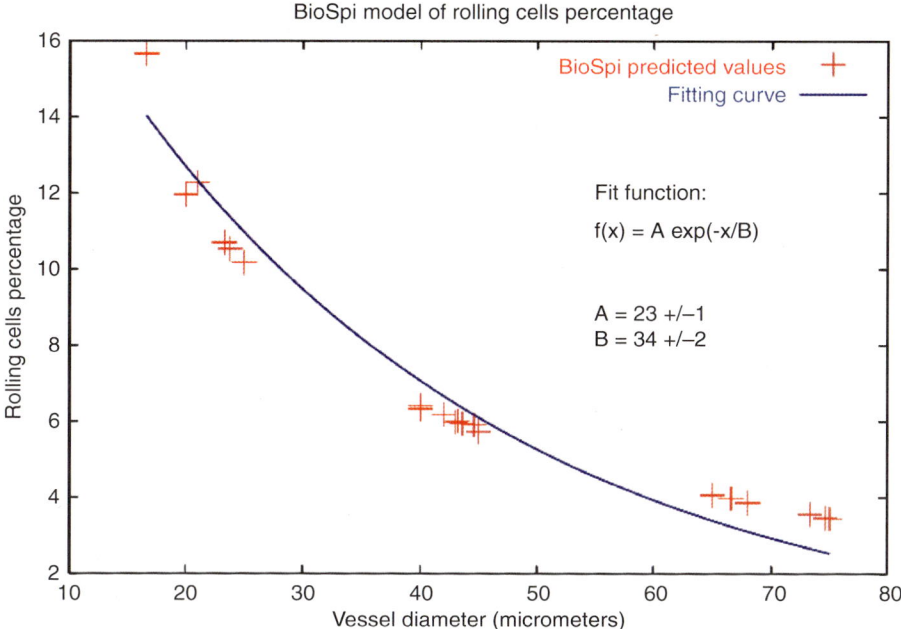

Fig. 4 Rolling cells percentage versus vessel diameter in BioSpi model

laminar flux on the endothelium as the ratio between the endothelial surface and the cell contact area ($\sim$200 μm^2 for a cell of about 10 μm of diameter), we express the rolling cells percentage (RCP) as in (1).

$$RCP \propto Pr(rolling) \approx C_1 N \frac{S_{contact}}{S_{endothelium}} + C_2 \tag{1}$$

where $Pr(rolling)$ is the rolling propensity, N is the number of bound molecules and the C's are proportionality constants depending on physical-chemical properties of the cell interaction with endothelium (overall intensity of the bond force and the rate of kinetic energy loss because of the intra- and extra-cellular frictions) and from the duration of the contact time with the endothelium [9,11,15,18,22,32]. In our model $C_1 = 1$ and $C_2 = 0$.

The value of RCP shown in the plot of Fig. 4 is obtained by getting from each simulation the value of N at the fixed time $t = 15$ s and substituting it in (1). Figure 5 shows the experimental value of the RCP versus cells diameters. Either in the simulated case or in the experimental one, the best fit has the same functional form of (2) and the fit parameters have values in overlapped error ranges.

$$RCP = a \exp\left(-\frac{D_v}{b}\right) \tag{2}$$

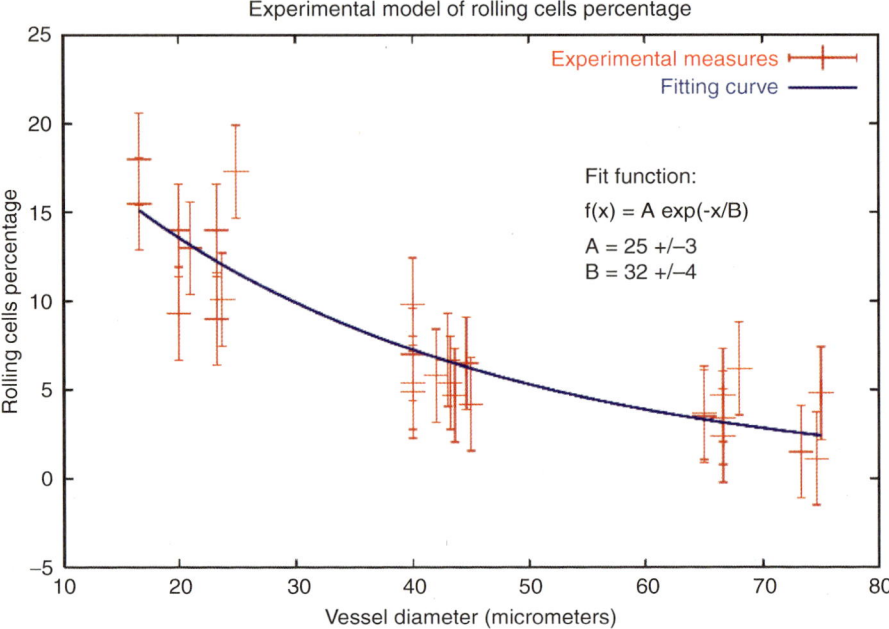

Fig. 5 Experimental measurements of the variation of rolling cells percentage at varying vessel diametxer

For the experimental observations $a = 25 \pm 3$ and $b = 32 \pm 4$, while for the BioSpi modeled data $a = 23 \pm 1$ and $b = 34 \pm 2$. The reduced chi-square for the fit of experimental observation is 0.69 and its probability is of 0.89.

For the fit of BioSpi simulated data the reduced chi-square is 0.75 and its probability is 0.83.

4.2 BioSpi Prediction of Cell Adhesion Probability

Only lymphocytes that express high levels of PSGL-1, high levels of LFA-1 and or α_4 integrins and the corresponding receptors for the activating factors presented by the endothelium will be able to efficiently be recruited in inflamed venules. Starting from this experimental evidence [24], the mathematical model of the cell adhesion probability is given by the following

$$Pr(adhesion) = \frac{1}{N_l} \sum_i w_i N_i \tag{3}$$

where $N_l = S_{endothelium}/S_{contact}$ is the total number of lymphocytes on the laminar flux in contact with endothelium given by the ratio between endothelial surface

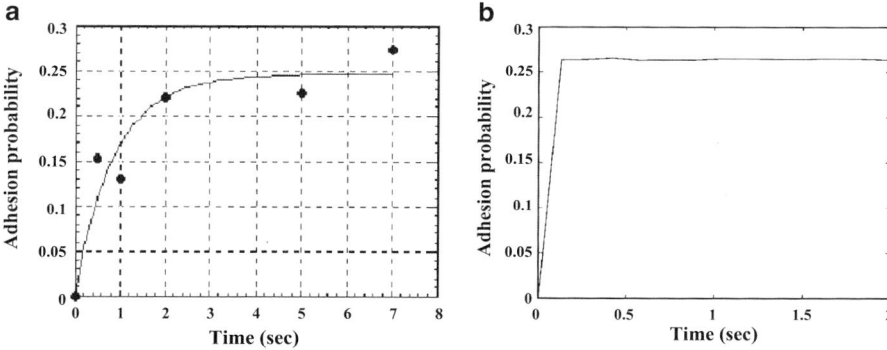

Fig. 6 (**a**) Experimental adhesion probability curve; (**b**) BioSpi model of cell adhesion probability versus contact time

($\sim$15,700 μm^2) and cell contact area ($\sim$200 μm^2), N_i indicate the number of bound molecules for the i-th molecular interaction, and the w's are the weights of the linear model, that quantify the statistical influence of the different molecular interactions in the cell adhesion mechanism. In our model the weights can take values in the range between 0 and 1. Because of the lack of experimental quantifications for the statistical influence of the different molecular interactions, we assume that $w_i = 1/8 = 0.125$ for all the considered interactions of all the eighth molecular species.

The model given in (3) is plotted in Fig. 6. It is in agreement, within the errors ranges, with the theoretical [22, 32] and experimental results [19].

5   Conclusion

The results obtained in this work assert that the formal description provided by BioSpi model represents in a concise and expressive way the basic physics governing the process of lymphocyte recruitment.

More generally, physics describes either microscopic or macroscopic interactions between bodies by means of the concept of *force*, that expresses the action of the field generated by a particle (or a set of particle) on the other bodies. BioSpi representation hits this remarks, that is just the central paradigma of the physical description of the nature and summarizes it in the new concepts of *communications exchange* or (*names passing*). Moreover, the rates of communication in stochastic π-calculus include all the dynamic of the system, because they contain the quantitative information about the intensity of the forces transmitted between the particles. Finally, the main advantage of the BioSpi model is that the π-calculus permits to better investigate dynamics, molecular and biochemical details. It has a solid theoretical basis and linguistical structure, unlike other approaches [6].

The usage of new languages such as stochastic π-calculus to describe and simulate the migration of autoreactive lymphocytes in the target organ will help us better understand the complex dynamics of lymphocyte recruitment during autoimmune inflammation in live animal. Furthermore, our approach may represent an important step toward future predictive studies on lymphocyte behavior in inflamed brain venules. In fact, the biochemical stochastic π-calculus simulation of experimental data offers the possibility to model and predict data of biological observations on a computer (*in silico* experiments). This new opportunity provided by the computer science may allow the biologists and medical researchers to save time by reducing the number of needed experiments in the case in which the computer simulation can exclude inadequate hypothesis.

A Dembo Adhesion Model

The kinetic reaction model proposed by Dembo et al. [8] simulates the rolling lymphocyte as a viscous newtonian fluid enclosed in a pre-stressed elastic membrane and the adhesion bonds formed between the rolling cell and its substrate are simulated as elastic springs perpendicular to the substrate. The adhesion bond force is assumed to be $f_b = N_b k (y - \lambda)$, where N_b is the associated bond density, k is the bond elastic constant, λ and y are the lengths of an unstretched bond and a stretched bond, respectively.

The bond density N_b, as function of time t, is computed using the following equations

$$\frac{\partial N_b}{\partial t} = k_{on}(N_l - N_{b0})(N_r - N_b) - k_{off} N_b \tag{4}$$

$$k_{off} = k_{off}^0 \exp\left(\frac{(k - \sigma_{ts})(y - \lambda)^2}{2 K_B T}\right) \tag{5}$$

$$k_{on} = k_{on}^0 \exp\left(\frac{(k - \sigma_{ts})(y - \lambda)^2}{2 K_B T}\right) \tag{6}$$

where k_{on} and k_{off} are the forward and the reverse reaction rates respectively, N_l and N_b are the ligands and receptors densities respectively and k_{on}^0 and k_{off}^0 are the equilibrium forward and the reverse reaction rates respectively. The parameters considered by this model are: $N_l = N_r = 400\,\mu m^2$, $k_{on}^0 = 84\,s^{-1}$, $k_{off}^0 = 1\,s^{-1}$, $k = 5\,dyne/cm$, $\sigma_{ts} = 4.5\,dyne/cm$, $K_B T = 3.8 \times 10^{-7}$ ergs and $\lambda = 20\,nm$. With these parameters values the solution $N_b(t)$ is given by the following

$$N_b(t) = -\frac{1}{84t} + 400 \tag{7}$$

and it is plotted in Fig. 7a.

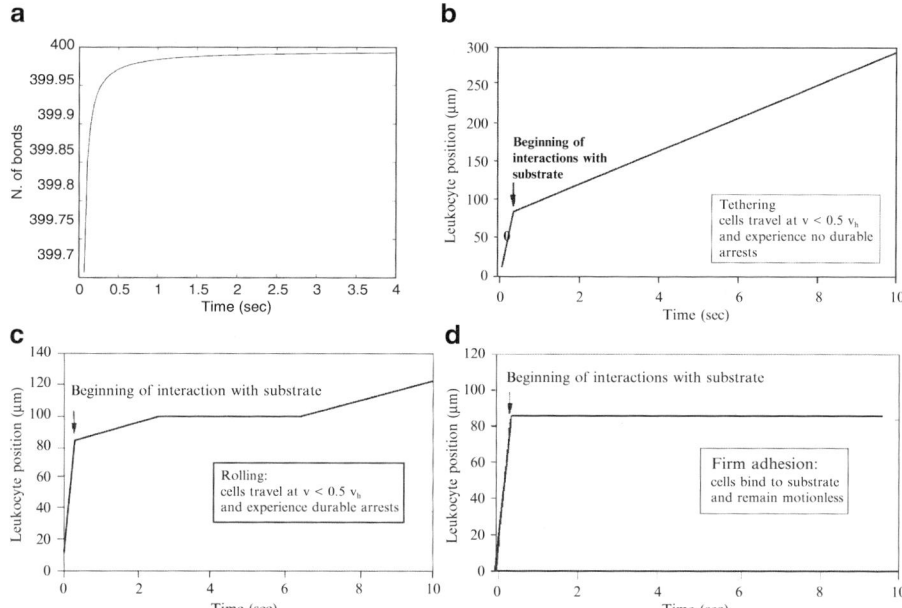

Fig. 7 (**a**) Time evolution of bond density in Dembo adhesion model. (**b**), (**c**) and (**d**) show representative trajectory of lymphocyte tethering at a mean velocity v equal to one half of the hydrodinamic velocity v_h. The parameters are the following: $\gamma = 0.001$ nm, $k_{on} = 84\,\mathrm{s}^{-1}$, $k_{off}^{0} = 1\,\mathrm{s}^{-1}$ (**b**). Representative trajectory of rolling motion of lymphocyte, with a mean velocity $v < 0.5v_h$, that experience durable arrests (**c**). Representative trajectory of lymphocyte for firm adhesion. The parameters are the following: $\gamma = 0.001$ nm, $k_{on} = 84\,\mathrm{s}^{-1}$, $k_{off}^{0} = 20\,\mathrm{s}^{-1}$ (**d**)

The physicochemical properties that give rise to the various dynamic states of cell adhesion are mainly the rates of reaction. From different values of rates constants, in particular of the dissociation rates [4] (see caption of Fig. 7), different motion state diagrams emerge [18]: *tethering*, in which lymphocytes move at a translational velocity $v < 0.5v_h$ (where v_h is the hydrodinamical velocity of the blood flow) but exhibit no durable arrest is shown in Fig. 7b; *rolling* for which cells travel at $v < 0.5v_h$, but experience durable arrests, is shown in Fig. 7c. Finally in *firm adhesion*, shown in Fig. 7d, cells bind to the endothelium and remain motionless.

References

1. BioSpi Project home page: http://www.wisdom.weizmann.ac.il/~biopsi/, 2002
2. Bell GI (1978) Models for the specific adhesion of cells to cells. Science 200:618–627
3. Bell GI, Dembo M, Bongrand P (1984) Cell adhesion. Competition between non-specific repulsion and specific bonding. Biophys J 45:1051–1064

4. Chang K, Tees DFJ, Hammer DA (2000) The state diagram for cell adhesion under flow: leukocyte adhesion and rolling. Proc Natl Acad Sci USA. doi:10.1073/pnas200240897

5. Chigaev A, Blenc AM, Braaten JV, Kumaraswamy N, Kepley CL, Andrews RP, Oliver JM, Edwards BS, Prossnitz ER, Larson RS, Sklar LA (2003) Alpha4beta1 integrin affinity changes govern cell adhesion, J Biol Chem 278(40):38174–38182

6. Curti M, Degano P, Baldari CT (2003) Casual π-calculus for biochemical modelling. In: Computational methods in system biology, CMSB, Rovereto, Springer, Berlin/New York

7. D'Ambrosio D, Lecca P, Priami C, Laudanna C (2004) Concurrency in leukocyte vascular recognition: developing the tools for a predictive computer model. Trends Immunol 25: 411–416

8. Dembo M, Torney DC, Saxaman K, Hammer D (1978) The reaction-limited kinetics of membrane-to-surface adhesion and detachment. Proc R Soc Lond B 234:55–83

9. Dong C, Cao J, Struble EJ, Lipowsky H (1999) Mechanics of leukocyte deformation and adhesion to endothelium in shear flow. Annu Biomed Eng 27:298–312

10. Evans EA (1995) Physical actions in biological adhesion. In: Lipowski R, Sackmann E (eds) Handbook of biophysics, vol I. Elsevier, Amsterdam

11. Fritz J, Katopodis AG, Kolbinger F, Anselmetti D (1998) Force-mediated kinetics of single P-selectin/ligand complexes by atomic force microscopy. Proc Natl Acad Sci USA 95: 12283–12288

12. Gillespie DT (1976) A general method for numerically simulating the stochastic time evolution of coupled chemical species. J Comput Phys 22:403–434

13. Gillespie DT (1977) Exact stochastic simulation of coupled chemical reactions. J Phys Chem 81(25):2340–2361

14. Goebel MU, Mills PJ (2000) Acute psychological stress and exercise and changes in peripheral leukocyte adhesion molecule expression and density. Psychosom Med 62(5):664–670

15. Goldman AJ, Cox RG, Brenner H (1967) Slow viscous motion of a sphere parallel to a plane wall: couette flow. Chem Eng Sci 22:653–660

16. Hammer DA, Lauffenburgher DA (1987) A dynamical model for receptor-mediated cell adhesion to surfaces. Biophys J 52:475–487

17. Lecca P, Priami C, Quaglia P, Rossi B, Laudanna C, Constantin G (2004) A stochastic process algebra approach to simulation of autoreactive lymphocyte recruitment. Simulation 80: 273–288

18. Lei X, Dong C (1999) Cell deformation and adhesion kinetics in leukocyte rolling. In: BED-Vol. 50, bioengineering conference, ASME

19. Marshall B, McEver RP, Zhu C (2001) Kinetics rates and their force dependence of the P-SELECTIN/PSGL-1 interaction measured by atomic force microscopy. In: BED-Vol. 50, bioengineering conference, ASME

20. Milner R (1989) Communication and concurrency. Internationa series in computer science. New Yourk, Prentice Hall

21. Milner R (1999) Communicating and mobile systems: the π-calculus. Cambridge University Press, Cambridge

22. N'dri N, Shyy W, Udaykumar HS, Tran-Son-tay R (2001) Computational modeling of cell adhesion and movement using continuum-kinetics approach. In: BED-Vol. 50, bioengineering conference, ASME

23. Norman KE, Katopodis AG, Thoma G, Kolbinger F, Hicks AE, Cotter MJ, Pockley AG, Hellewell PG (2000) P-selectin glycoprotein ligand-1 supports rolling on E- and P-selectin in vivo. Blood 96(10):3585–3591

24. Piccio L, Rossi B, Scarpini E, Laudanna C, Giagulli C, Issekutz AC, Vestweber D, Butcher EC, Costantin G (2002) Molecular mechanism involved in lymphocyte recruitment in inflamed brain microvessel: critical roles for P-selectin Glycoprotein Ligand-1 and Heterotrimeric G_i-linked receptors. J Immunol 168:1940–1949

25. Priami C (1995) Stochastic π-calculus. Comput J 38:6578–6589

26. Priami C, Regev A, Silverman W, Shapiro E (2001) Application of a stochastic name passing calculus to representation and simulation of molecular processes. Inf Process Lett 80:25–31

27. Regev A (2001) Representation and simulation of molecular pathways in the stochastic π-calculus. In: Proceedings of the 2nd workshop on computation of biochemical pathways and genetic networks, Villa Bosch

28. Regev A, Silverman W, Shapiro E (2000) Representing biomolecular processes with computer process algebra: π-calculus programs of signal transduction pathways. American Society of Artificial Intelligence Press

29. Regev A, Silverman W, Shapiro E (2001) Representation and simulation of biochemical processes using the pi-calculus process algebra. Proc Pac Symp Biocomput (PSB2001) 6: 459–470

30. Skalak R, Zarda PR, Jan KM, Chien S (1981) Mechanics of rouleau fromation. Biophys J 35:771–781

31. Vogler EA (1989) A thermodynamic model of short-term cell adhesion in vitro. Colloid Surf 42:233

32. Zhu C (2000) Kinetic and mechanics of cell adhesion. J Biomech 33:23–33

Printed by Printforce, the Netherlands